DIANE F~
S

D0425036

"This is the first book I have seen that marries culinary, hospitality, and nutrition management into one concise text. These three disciplines complement each other in so many ways."

Chef Kyle Shadix, MS, RD
Nutrition and Culinary Consultants, NYC
www.culinarynutritionists.com
American Culinary Federation
American Dietetic Association
American Institute of Wine and Food
Food & Culinary Professionals Dietetic Practice Group
Institute of Food Technologists
International Association of Culinary Professionals
James Beard Foundation
National Society for Healthcare Foodservice Management
Nutrition Entrepreneurs Dietetic Practice Group
Research Chef Association
Society for Foodservice Management
National Organization of Men in Nutrition (NOMIN)

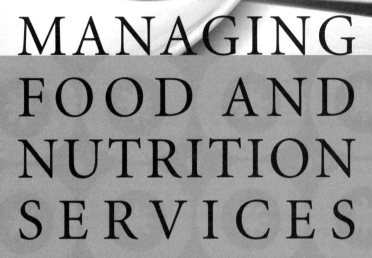

MANAGING FOOD AND NUTRITION SERVICES

FOR THE CULINARY, HOSPITALITY, AND NUTRITION PROFESSIONS

Edited by
Sari F. Edelstein, PhD, RD
Nutrition and Dietetic's Department
Simmons College
Boston, MA

Featuring
Foodservice Math in Easy Step-by-Step Instructions
and Foodservice Review for the Registered Dietitian Examination

JONES AND BARTLETT PUBLISHERS
Sudbury, Massachusetts
BOSTON   TORONTO   LONDON   SINGAPORE

World Headquarters

Jones and Bartlett Publishers	Jones and Bartlett Publishers	Jones and Bartlett Publishers
40 Tall Pine Drive	Canada	International
Sudbury, MA 01776	6339 Ormindale Way	Barb House, Barb Mews
978-443-5000	Mississauga, Ontario L5V 1J2	London W6 7PA
info@jbpub.com	Canada	United Kingdom
www.jbpub.com		

Jones and Bartlett's books and products are available through most bookstores and online book-sellers. To contact Jones and Bartlett Publishers directly, call 800-832-0034, fax 978-443-8000, or visit our website www.jbpub.com.

Substantial discounts on bulk quantities of Jones and Bartlett's publications are available to corporations, professional associations, and other qualified organizations. For details and specific discount information, contact the special sales department at Jones and Bartlett via the above contact information or send an email to specialsales@jbpub.com.

This publication is designed to provide accurate and authoritative information in regard to the Subject Matter covered. It is sold with the understanding that the publisher is not engaged in rendering legal, accounting, or other professional service. If legal advice or other expert assistance is required, the service of a competent professional person should be sought.

Production Credits
Publisher: Michael Brown
Production Director: Amy Rose
Associate Editor: Katey Birtcher
Production Editor: Dan Stone
Marketing Manager: Wendy Thayer
Manufacturing Buyer: Therese Connell
Cover Design: Kristin E. Ohlin
Composition: Maggie Dana/Pageworks
Printing and Binding: Malloy, Inc.
Cover Printing: Malloy, Inc.

Cover Credits
Fork and Plate © Karla Caspari/ShutterStock, Inc.; Background Pattern © Gina Goforth/ShutterStock, Inc.

Library of Congress Cataloging-in-Publication Data
Edelstein, Sari.
　Managing food and nutrition services : for the culinary, hospitality, and nutrition professions / Sari Edelstein. — 1st ed.
　　p. cm.
　Includes bibliographical references and index.
　ISBN-13: 978-0-7637-4064-1
　ISBN-10: 0-7637-4064-0
　1. Food service—Management. 2. Nutrition. I. Title.
　TX911.3.M27E33 2007
　647.95068—dc22
　　　　　　　　　　　　　　　　　　　2007005819

6 048

Printed in the United States of America
11 10 09 08 07　10 9 8 7 6 5 4 3 2 1

DEDICATION

To my wonderful husband and children

CONTENTS

Chapter 15   Disaster Planning for Foodservice Operations   385

Candace A Stewart, MS, RD, LD/N

Chapte 16   Food Safety and Bioterrorism   403

Sam Beattie, PhD and
Beverly McCabe-Sellers, PhD, RD

ABOUT THE AUTHOR

Sari Edelstein, PhD, RD
Nutrition and Dietetic's Department
Simmons College

BS, Florida State University
MS, Florida International University
PhD, University of Florida

Dr. Edelstein's present position is in the Nutrition and Dietetics Department at Simmons College. She presently teaches both food science and foodservice classes. Before coming to Simmons College, Dr. Edelstein had been in private practice and had served as a Hospital Food Service Director and Chief Dietitian. Additionally, Dr. Edelstein is a past president of the Miami Dietetic Association and has served in several other leadership positions in Florida. She is the author of many research articles and books.

CONTRIBUTING AUTHORS

Paul B. Baker, PhD
University of Arizona

Sam Beattie, PhD
Iowa State University

Bradley Beran, MBA, PhD
Johnson and Wales University
Syracuse University

Sheryl Boston, MEd, LD
Western Illinois University

Michelle Easterly, BS, MS
Syracuse University

Sari Edelstein, PhD, RD
Simmons College

Bonnie Gerald, PhD, DTR
Louisiana Tech University

Karlyn Grimes, MS, RD
Simmons College

Jacqueline S. Gutierrez, MS, RD, CDN
Red Apple Concepts

Robert W. Hartley
Truly Nolen of America, Inc.

Nancie H. Herbold, EdD, RD, LD
Simmons College

Julie Jones, MS, RD, LD
Ohio State University Medical Center

Cheryl Koch, MS, RD, LD, FADA, CNSD
Johns Hopkins Bayview Medical Center

Beverly McCabe-Sellers, PhD, RD
USDA, ARS Lower Mississippi Delta NIRI

Mary Angela Miller, MS, RD, LD, FADA
Ohio State University Medical Center

Darlene Moppert, MS, RD, LD/N
School Board of Broward County, FL

Julie M. Moreschi, MS, RD, LDN
Benedictine University

Esther C. Okeiyi, PhD, RD, LDN, CHA
North Carolina Central University

Raymond Papa, EdD, RD, LD/N
School Board of Broward County, FL

Carmen Roberts, MS, RD, CDE
Johns Hopkins Bayview Medical Center

Neeta Singh, PhD
University of the Incarnate Word

Dee Sanquist, MS, RD
Southwest Washington Medical
Center

Candace A. Stewart, MS, RD, LD/N
Private Practice

Chef Kyle Shadix, MS, RD
Nutrition and Culinary Consultants

Patrice L. Spath, BA, RHIT
Brown-Spath & Associates

Paul N. Taylor, PhD
Simmons College

PREFACE

Finally, the time has come! Culinary, hospitality, and dietetics food-service professions are now embraced in the common thread that holds us together in one foodservice textbook. These three disciplines complement each other in so many ways, and instead of being educated by three different texts, *Managing Food and Nutrition Services for the Culinary, Hospitality, and Nutrition Professions* focuses on the major concepts which bring together these three fields.

Before I became a registered dietitian (RD), I was a chef. No one thought cooks knew anything or cared at all about health and nutrition; after all the idea that *food must be bad for you if it tastes good* has been a widely accepted belief among Americans. On the flip side, people have often assumed that nutritionists or registered dietitians don't know anything about culinary arts. They are wrong! Dietitians all across the United States have a wide breadth of food knowledge and culinary skills that extend beyond the cafeteria. Oversimplified standardized ideas are nothing more than stereotypes. From hospitality foodservice to the classroom, nutrition and the art of cooking are beginning to share the spotlight in concert together.

As a chef and instructor at culinary schools in New York City, I have taught foodservice and menu management, supervision, and nutrition from a fundamental level which allows future chefs to translate what they've learned into real life experiences. I have taught and used several textbooks in various nutrition departments, and this is the first book to marry culinary, hospitality, and dietetics management into one concise text. This book is organized into 17 chapters, reflecting the major topics covered in a management book for dietitians, chefs, and hotel/restaurant/foodservice departments. Most textbooks are penned by one or two authors, but this book's chapters were written by respected experts within their specialized field of study, representing all three professions. The combined authority from culinary, hospitality, and nutrition professions shows a thorough proficiency that is often missing in generalized management texts.

As new restaurants open, and new food products hit the shelves, the need for qualified culinary nutritionists and hospitality specialists with a thorough understanding of the three disciplines arises. When I started my career, there were very few chef/RDs, but as the industry responds to the theory that nutrition is an important part of the foodservice industry, companies across the industry spectrum are eagerly seeking knowledgeable professionals with an appreciation of food, nutrition, and hospitality.

Chef Kyle Shadix, MS, RD
Nutrition and Culinary Consultants, NYC
www.culinarynutritionists.com
American Culinary Federation
American Dietetic Association
American Institute of Wine and Food
Food & Culinary Professionals Dietetic Practice Group
Institute of Food Technologists
International Association of Culinary Professionals
James Beard Foundation
National Society for Healthcare Foodservice Management
Nutrition Entrepreneurs Dietetic Practice Group
Research Chef Association
Society for Foodservice Management
National Organization of Men in Nutrition (NOMIN)

ACKNOWLEDGMENTS

Thanks to my teaching assistant, Christina Byrnes, and to Jones &
Bartlett, especially Mike Brown, Dan Stone, and Katey Birtcher.

PART I

ORGANIZATIONAL MANAGEMENT

Chapter 1   New Foodservice Trends for Culinary, Hospitality, Management Certificate, and Nutrition Professionals

Sari Edelstein, PhD, RD

Chapter 2   Management and Leadership Theory with Practical Applications

Sheryl Boston, MEd, LD and
Sari Edelstein, PhD, RD

Chapter 3   Corporate Culture and Communication

Dee Sanquist, MS, RD

Chapter 4   New Marketing Trends in Food and Nutrition Services

Nancie H. Herbold, EdD, RD, LD and
Paul N. Taylor, PhD

NEW FOODSERVICE TRENDS FOR CULINARY, HOSPITALITY, MANAGEMENT CERTIFICATE, AND NUTRITION PROFESSIONALS

Sari Edelstein, PhD, RD

Reader Objectives

After reading this chapter and reflecting on the contents, the reader will be able to:

1. Articulate how the three major foodservice professions overlap and how each contributes strengths to management and leadership.
2. Explain the routes to management for all food-related professions.
3. Map out the knowledge components that foodservice managers need to be successful.
4. Discuss how today's diverse customer will affect the business of foodservice.
5. Explain the major trends in all areas of foodservice management.
6. Discuss how HIPAA has changed medical areas of foodservice.
7. Articulate the meaning of business and clinical ethics.

Key Terms

Diversity: the differences between people; for example, ethnicity, gender, and age.

Hazard Analysis and Critical Control Point (HACCP): a quality or safety process for food during procurement, processing, and delivery of the finished food products; provides standards for each.

Health Insurance Portability and Accountability Act (HIPAA): this act necessitates privacy standards for consumer information, inclusive of health information.

Joint Commission on Accreditation of Healthcare Organizations (JCAHO): one of the major health care facility quality accrediting organizations in the United States.

Medical nutrition therapy (MNT): disease management, specific to nutritional intervention that may be reimbursable through sanctioned insurance billing.

Menu engineering: plan that brings together all aspects of foodservice to produce a financially successful and healthful, pleasing menu.

Quality management: the process of ensuring that all necessary activities are in place to design, develop, implement, and evaluate products and services.

Scope of practice: those elements of caring for patients for which one was appropriately trained.

Single line authority: a very linear chart where one supervisor dominates another down to the staff level employees.

Social marketer: the foodservice manager who advocates food that is healthy.

Team authority: a very flat chart where more supervisors collaborate for a team approach to management.

Merging the Three Foodservice Professions— Culinary, Hospitality, and Nutrition—in a Competitive Marketplace

The trends in foodservice management have always been a mixed bag—until now. Until recently, one could walk into a foodservice establishment and find that the manager had myriad backgrounds, both in work experience and/or education. Franchises, cafeterias, and catering companies, to name only a few, hired foodservice managers from the business world, an experienced chef, or a registered dietitian. Each professional brought a set of credentials to the table, but none had the full package for what it takes today to run a successful foodservice establishment. Foodservice establishments range from free-standing restaurants to hospital cafeterias—each needing a manager with a full range of expertise. The expertise that foodservice managers need for today's competitive marketplace include, but are not limited to, financial savvy, cooking expertise, management and leadership skills, marketing entrepreneurship, and food knowledge.

The three major education-based training grounds for foodservice managers lie in culinary, hospitality, and nutrition college programs. While each of these programs has a different emphasis, they still must turn out industry leaders and managers who are chock-full of expertise. This is the unique feature of management. When management skills alone are not enough anymore, managers must bring additional expertise to the table to fully understand all aspects of a foodservice business. In addition to college programs, several foodservice management certification programs are available. These include *ServSafe®, Certified Food Protection Professional® (CFPP), National Certified Professional Food Manager® (NCPFM), Certified Food Safety Manager®,* and *Certified Dietary Manager® (CDM).* These programs are designed to produce individuals with foodservice expertise in different areas. A brief description of each is available in Table 1.1. Figure 1.1 shows the shared expertise that must come from each of the foodservice professions, coming from our three major educative programs.

How Can We Best Serve Our Customers?

Diversity

The customers of today are quite different than customers of yesterday. The population has grown, leaving the foodservice industry with more customers than ever before.[1]

This population has a growing interest in food because of many factors. First, there is an emphasis on eating out in U.S. culture, and today's population continues to purchase more meals away from home than ever before. Second, the U.S. population is also more diverse than ever before. **Diversity** can be represented by age, such as baby boomers who will become the majority of the U.S. population by 2011 and will total 77 million people by 2029.[2] The baby boomers are more interested in consuming healthful foods and being engaged in cooking and nutritional factors than generations previously.[2] The customer demands of baby boomers related to food

Table 1.1   Foodservice Certification Programs*

ServSafe®

A comprehensive food safety education and training program developed by the Educational Foundation of the National Restaurant Association that is widely recognized by many federal, state, and local jurisdictions. (www.edfound. org)

Certified Food Protection Professional® (CFPP)

The Dietary Managers Association's CFPP credential is geared toward the foodservice professional. Options for the food protection course are a 16-hour classroom food safety training course, independent study via print materials, or independent on-line study. (www.dmaonline.org)

National Certified Professional Food Manager® (NCPFM)

The NCPFM exam tests knowledge, skills, and abilities related to food protection, and the ability to organize and supervise employees within the work environment. The NCPFM exam is appropriate for site supervisors, managers, or first-line supervisors in establishments that prepare and serve food. (www.experioronline.com)

Certified Food Safety Manager®

The Food Safety Manager Certification Examination is designed to be used with any food safety training program available on the market. (www.nrfsp.com)

Foodservice Management Professional® (FMP)

The Foodservice Management Professional credential distinguishes restaurant and foodservice managers who achieve the high level of knowledge, experience, leadership, and professionalism. (www.nraef.org)

Certified Dietary Manager® (CDM)

A Certified Dietary Manager has the education, training, and experience to competently perform the responsibilities of a dietary manager and has proven this by passing a nationally recognized credentialing exam and fulfilling the requirements needed to maintain certified status. CDMs work together with registered dietitians to provide quality nutritional care for clients in a variety of noncommercial settings, including health care, public schools, corrections, and others. (www.cdmonline.org)

*Not all existing programs may be listed.
Compiled by the author from the Web sites listed under each certification type.

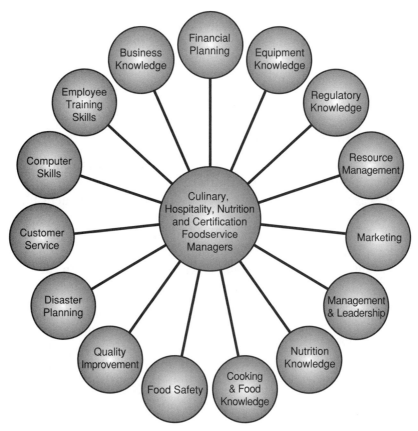

FIGURE 1.1   Proposed Shared Expertise of All Foodservice Managers

will spill over into restaurants, hospitals, assisted living centers, and nursing homes.

Diversity also can be represented by ethnicity, with present minority groups becoming the U.S. majority in the twenty-first century. Foodservice managers must become knowledgeable about the eating habits and food consumption, nutritional concerns, marketing techniques, and pricing to meet the needs of the rising U.S. population.[1] This knowledge will be necessary for providing services to the population as well as for business financial success.

New Trends in Management and Leadership

New trends in management and leadership demand that the manager-leader must be multi-skilled in many areas, as discussed previously. The one-dimensional manager is now a dinosaur and will not be successful in today's foodservice industry. Managers must realize that their arsenal of problem-solving skills must have many methods and theories. Managers must have the ability to:[3]

1. Assess the organization's goals and needs in long-term, short-term, and day-to-day operations.
2. Assess the individual employee for proper job placement for success.
3. Encourage employees to become members of a team, empowering them with a feeling of ownership.
4. Provide motivation for employees by linking goals in the workplace to personal values.

Organizational charts reflect this change from a single manager-leader to a more team approach. Single manager-leaders had ultimate authority and passed down their orders through the ranks of the organizational chart, with little input from anyone else. Team management approaches combine the skills of many to produce ideas that have been considered from many vantage points and different areas of expertise. The result is usually a more feasible answer to a problem than the single-minded problem solving from the past. Figure 1.2 illustrates the **single line authority** (linear looking) as opposed to older organizational charts, and the newer **team authority** approach (compact or flat looking) organizational chart is illustrated in Figure 1.3. Figure 1.4 gives another view of an organizational chart where the clinical staff of dietitians is separate from the foodservice department.

New Trends in Corporate Culture and Communication

Just as the organizational chart has evolved into a team approach to management, so have the foodservice corporate culture and methods of communication. The *team approach* dictates that there

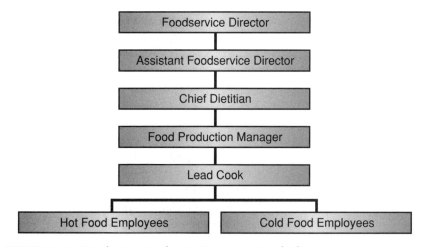

FIGURE 1.2 Single Line Authority Organizational Chart

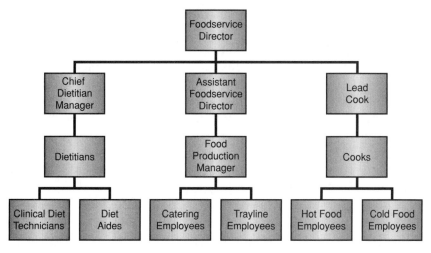

FIGURE 1.3 Team Authority Organizational Chart

is a play of interchange and feedback among team members that allows for abundant communication.[4] A respect for each member's expertise and what they can add to serve the customer is both needed and welcomed. Businesses that have continued the top-heavy one manager literally ruling the roost will fail because employees lack the empowerment necessary to feel a part of the

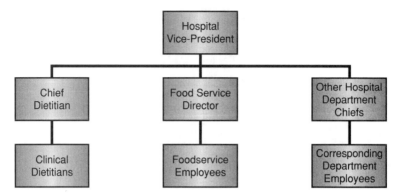

FIGURE 1.4   Separating the Clinical Nutrition Component from
Foodservice in an Organizational Chart

entity. Qualified, creative, and interested managers will not tolerate
a one-dimensional foodservice operation and will seek employment
elsewhere.

The leader of today's new management team must support individual ideas and embrace the instincts of staff. The importance will
be on what the team brings to the business, no matter who first
brought a good idea to the table. When ideas can be freely brought
to the table through nonthreatening, even welcoming communication, a trust is built. The corporate culture becomes one of trust and
freedom. The savvy leader knows that when a management team
reaches this level of communication, the business works and the
customer is better served.

New Trends in Customer Privacy: Health Insurance Portability and Accountability Act (HIPAA) Issues

The Health Insurance Portability and Accountability Act (HIPAA)
necessitates privacy standards for consumer information, inclusive
of health information. The act was passed in Congress in 1996.
Healthcare facilities and professionals had a compliance date of
October 16, 2002, with smaller entities complying by 2003. This privacy standards issue arose because of the electronic transactions
that occur in standard operations, such as billing and scheduling
patients, where personal information is transmitted. The impact on

healthcare foodservice and clinical nutrition was substantial. Most facilities and practitioners had to change their standard operation in the following ways:[5]

1. Establish policies and procedures for maintaining patient information privacy.
2. Areas of patient information privacy should at least include:
   a. The patient's written authorization and consent to disclose private information in a permissible manner (can pertain to treatment, billing, and research).
   b. Establish ways the personal information can be secured.
   c. Develop a notice to patients on how their personal information will be used and to whom their information will be accessible.
3. Ongoing education and training for staff in order to ensure compliance.
4. Performance of ongoing monitors, shown by written tracking of information privacy.

In foodservice, the patient's information should be kept private, limiting those personnel who need to work with the information. Many operations have gone to using coded menu titles for patient's names and/or modified diets to limit access to this information on the hospital floors. Private practice dietitians will have to develop their own consent forms, as well as secure transmission of any and all patient data.

New Marketing Trends in Food and Nutrition Services

Incredibly, marketing in the United States has changed. One might not have noticed the slow evolution that has brought us to today's standards, but we are certainly here....in the new era of social marketing![6] While we watched the cigarette ads from the 1950s slowly disappear from the media as a link was found between smoking and health, so are we seeing more ads than ever before in the twenty-first century for healthful eating. While this is not the standard yet in marketing, it is a growing trend.

As more educated individuals take positions in the food industry, it is hoped that the thrust toward marketing those foods and products that are most healthy will take over the advertising of that which is injurious to health. By including nutrition as a subject in culinary and hospitality programs, this understanding of social conscience and food should result. Graduates of nutrition and dietetics programs, when management skills are recognized, will also serve as **social marketers**.

New Trends in Sanitation and Food Safety: Hazard Analysis and Critical Control Point (HACCP)

HACCP made its way into the foodservice arena and has continued as the standard for keeping food safe to consume. HACCP's main thrust is identifying *critical control points* that could affect quality or safety of the food during procurement, processing, and delivery of the finished food products and providing standards for each. These points can be determined anywhere in the production process or recipe of a food item where controlling the food or action could prevent, eliminate, or reduce the potential hazard to levels that are acceptable. These include points in time from when the item is raw and still is with its producer or grower to the time it is consumed by the customers. At each step during the workflow of food production, there is a risk that contamination can occur.[7] A well-educated manager should be able to implement HACCP and train employees on their roles in any size foodservice operation.

New Trends in Fiscal Management

The new trend in foodservice fiscal management is that the manager must have expertise beyond those who held the position in the past. In the past, the foodservice manager, in some cases, could defer to the comptroller or the facility accountant to help with labor, food, supplies, and capital equipment evaluation and cost. But, as previously noted, today's foodservice manager must be as adept at fiscal management as he or she is in food knowledge and human resource management.

New terms, such as **menu engineering** and contribution margin, are as important today as the old terms of "as purchased" and "edible portion." The new fiscal manager must be able to input food cost formulas such as variable cost and variable rate ratios into software, such that appropriate food purchasing specifications can be sent to a purveyor.[8]

New Trends in Reimbursement of Nutrition Services

With the advent of disease management or **medical nutrition therapy (MNT)**, the need for nutrition counseling services has expanded to the private practice. With private practice, dietitians must be knowledgeable of the MNT reimbursement process to be legally compliant with reimbursement regulations, help their client maximize the benefit of their healthcare plan, and be paid for the services they provide.[9] Thus, nutrition knowledge alone will not be enough. The dietitian will have to expand his or her knowledge base to fiscal and business management and all it entails.

New Trends in Information Technology

Information technology (IT) has revolutionized business and communication. Any foodservice business that did not integrate IT into its operation in the last 5 years will be in the minority.[10] It is almost impossible to operate a business in today's world without the use of IT. IT has brought a long list of information systems that affect food and nutrition services. For one, the new requirements by regulatory agencies such as the **Joint Commission on Accreditation of Healthcare Organizations (JCAHO)** will necessitate the application of information systems for the purposes of data collection, data management, and data reporting. It will not be feasible to collect, evaluate, and report data by hand in a world where quality improvement systems are mandatory.

In addition, information systems have created management control systems, such as software packages that are designed to manage information for clinical management and meal service; menu planning; forecasting and purchasing; production; catering; inventory management; food safety; payroll; financial management; and material data sheets. Foodservice vendor orders can now be synchronized to cut down on calls and paperwork. And, computerized technology has brought about the electronic medical record, where intellectual property regarding clinical information systems has evolved.[10]

New Trends in Quality Improvement and Benchmarking

Customer and regulatory quality demands have driven healthcare facilities to build strong **quality management** systems that include benchmarking indicators of quality. Quality management is the process of ensuring that all necessary activities are in place to design, develop, implement, and evaluate products and services. The quality management process is one of ongoing evaluation and constant readiness. All businesses and organizations are renewing their focus on the customer. The quality and effectiveness of services provided to customers must be systematically evaluated and revised to produce the best overall outcome and to remain competitive within the marketplace.[11]

New Trends in Disaster Planning for Foodservice Operations

With the onslaught of natural disasters like Hurricane Katrina, the United States found out how little prepared it was to feed and house people in need. The "how to" plan for a disaster of this magnitude will be new for every foodservice manager in the United States. Developing an effective disaster plan requires that foodservice managers do the research regarding the regulations specific to their institution. Who will they serve? What services will be needed? And, how best can these services be rendered? This research can be called a hazard analysis, where disaster scenarios are planned for with policy and procedure development and task identification. The writing of the disaster plan should be in simple terms, feasible and complete with staff training and drills.[12] The management team members and foodservice staff should all participate in disaster plan critique and revision for the best possible preparation.

New Issues in Food Procurement and Bioterrorism

The threat of bioterrorism targeted at the food supply is a new area that all food managers will have to address.[13] Prior to 2001, food-service managers planned only for natural disasters but will now have to be concerned with intentional contamination and have a plan in place to serve the public if this occurs. Safe food sources and distribution under untenable circumstances will take masterful planning and execution. We need to be ready for this potential problem.

New Trends in Entrepreneurship

Many culinary, hospitality, and nutrition students of today hope to own and manage their own restaurant or private practice during their career. When this stage of one's career is reached, a few questions need to be answered by researching the total market, market niche, competition, and finances. Questions such as "Who is the market and what are their demographics?" need to be asked. One can begin by breaking down a market into manageable segments, analyzing a potential segment, and gleaning relevant demographic data to support a proposed business. This research will help determine if the business can be supported by the chosen market niche, what check averages could be supported, further define the client or customer base, and help assess what services may be required or desired. Depending on the type of restaurant or private practice, different income levels, professions, ethnic backgrounds, commute times, and job locations will all influence how a niche is filled.[14]

Once a business idea is fully researched, many more questions pertaining to business type and finances will have to be explored. Inclusive in the research is the business plan, which can help the entrepreneur explore capital equipment and personnel requirements. A poorly written business plan is one that has not fully explored all of the details and factors that can affect a business. The time commitment to produce a useable business plan as a blueprint for success is considerable. The level of knowledge, detail, and work is great, but the rewards are many.

New Trends in Business and Clinical Ethics

While ethics has always been a concern in both business and health care, it has been recently placed in the spotlight. This fact is confirmed by a higher incidence of white-collar crime in the business arena and is a result of the advancement of medical treatment in the healthcare arena.

Business ethics in foodservice encompasses many of the same ethics that any business has to concern itself with. For example:[15]

1. Discrimination in any shape of form should not be a business practice. Examples include discrimination in hiring, supervising, or serving any persons.
2. Having unsafe working conditions is unethical. Conditions must be made safe by the standards determined by regulatory agencies for both employees and customers.
3. Hiring illegal immigrants displaces jobs and is against the law.
4. Overserving alcohol causes unsafe conditions for patrons.
5. Serving unsafe food puts persons at a health risk. The foodservice establishment must show its loyalty to the customer by serving wholesome, safe food at all times. This also pertains to the Truth in Menu law that stipulates a food item on the menu must be a true representation of what is served to the customer.
6. Sexual or any other type of employee harassment should not take place.
7. Stealing is probably the most common legal and ethical wrong in foodservice. Stealing can come in many forms, such as purchasing food and supplies from friends and accepting kickbacks and gifts from purveyors.

Many may have to be convinced that dietitians face ethical dilemmas in their everyday positions, but actually medical ethics affects dietitians in several ways. The violation of the dietitian's **scope of practice** is the major ethical dilemma most dietitians must confront.[16] Because medical technology has advanced so much in this era, dietitians may be asked to participate in medical care for which they have not been properly trained. For example, dietitians have been asked to write parenteral nutrition orders in scenarios where it may be unsafe for the patient. In other scenarios, the dietitian may have had training and certification to write orders. A hospital policy should state the qualifications of those writing these types of medical orders. Individual dietitians can check with the American Dietetic Association for assistance on scope of practice and certifications. Dietitian managers should be aware of the qualifications of dietitians in the different medical specialty areas.

The American Dietetic Association has issued a code of ethics for dietitians and diet technicians.[17] In brief, the code asks that dietetic professionals conduct themselves with honesty and integrity, basing all their practices on proven scientific knowledge. In addition, the nutrition professional should exercise good judgment, collaborate with other healthcare professionals, and provide respectful information to their clients that allows full disclosure, while allowing informed decision making in a confidential environment. Other code points include many of those presented in the previous business ethics section. The complete code of ethics is available at www.eatright.org.

Summary

Foodservice management will require myriad skills with a requirement for a larger knowledge base than in the past. This knowledge base will include concepts such as leadership, finances, culinary expertise, and food knowledge. Within each of these areas are subgroupings that this text will address to serve today's customer. The chapters that follow explain these concepts to all foodservice professionals in training.

Student Activities

1. Call three healthcare facilities to find out the academic background of the foodservice director. Discuss why the background of each foodservice director is appropriate or inappropriate for the facility.
2. Interview a foodservice director by telephone or in person and ask how important background was in choosing him or her for the position.
3. Interview a restaurant manager by telephone or in person and ask how he or she serves the diversity of customers he sees today.
4. Call a hospital and ask where dietitians are placed in the organizational chart and the reasoning for that decision.
5. Call or visit a healthcare facility of any medical office and ask how HIPAA has impacted the facility.

6. Call or visit a foodservice department of a healthcare facility and ask how HIPAA has impacted the department.
7. Discuss examples where restaurants have been social marketers.
8. Call or interview a foodservice manager about the existence of a disaster or bioterrorism departmental policy plan and procedure.
9. Discuss the terms *illegal* and *unethical.* How are these terms alike and/or different?
10. Interview a dietitian by telephone or in person and ask about any scope of practice issues that have affected him or her.

Web Sites

American Culinary Federation, Inc.
www.acfchefs.org

American Dietetic Association (ADA)
www.eatright.org

American Institute of Baking (AIB)
www.aibonline.org

Dietary Managers Association (DMA)
www.dmaonline.org

Food Marketing Institute (FMI)
www.fmi.org

HIPAA
www.healthprivacy.org

National Restaurant Association Educational Foundation
www.edfound.org

References

1. Jarratt, J. & Mahaffie, J.B. (2002). Key trends affecting the dietetics profession and American Dietetic Association. *Journal of The American Dietetic Association, 102*(12), 1821–1839.
2. Chappa, S., Chao, S. & Edelstein, S. (2004). Boomer ready initiative: Identification of wellness needs. *Journal of The American Dietetic Association,104*(6), 878–882.

3. Boston, S. & Edelstein, S. (2007). Management and leadership theory with practical applications. In S. Edelstein (Ed.), *Managing food and nutrition services for hospitality, culinary, and dietetic professionals.* Sudbury, MA: Jones and Bartlett Publishers.
4. Sanquist, D. (2007). Corporate culture and communication. In S. Edelstein (Ed.), *Managing food and nutrition services for hospitality, culinary, and dietetic professionals.* Sudbury, MA: Jones and Bartlett Publishers.
5. Michael, P. & Pritchett, E. (May 2001). The impact of HIPAA electronic transmissions and health information standards. *Journal of The American Dietetic Association, 101*(5), 524–529.
6. Herbold, N. & Taylor, P.N. (2007). New marketing trends in food and nutrition services. In S. Edelstein (Ed.), *Managing food and nutrition services for hospitality, culinary, and dietetic professionals.* Sudbury, MA: Jones and Bartlett Publishers.
7. Gutierrez, J.S. (2007*).* In-service education and meeting regulations: Sanitation, Safety, and HACCP. In S. Edelstein (Ed.), *Managing food and nutrition services for hospitality, culinary, and dietetic professionals.* Sudbury, MA: Jones and Bartlett Publishers.
8. Okeiyi, E. (2007). Fiscal management in foodservice. In S. Edelstein (Ed.), *Managing food and nutrition services for hospitality, culinary, and dietetic professionals.* Sudbury, MA: Jones and Bartlett Publishers.
9. Beran, B., Easterly, M. & Miller, M.A. (2007). Entrepreneurship: Writing a business plan for establishing your own restaurant or private practice and reimbursement for RD services. In S. Edelstein (Ed.), *Managing food and nutrition services for hospitality, culinary, and dietetic professionals.* Sudbury, MA: Jones and Bartlett Publishers.
10. Singh, N. (2007). Computerized information systems for managing food and nutrition services. In S. Edelstein (Ed.), *Managing food and nutrition services for hospitality, culinary, and dietetic professionals.* Sudbury, MA: Jones and Bartlett Publishers.
11. Koch, C. & Roberts, C. (2007). Managing quality in food and nutrition services. In S. Edelstein (Ed.), *Managing food and nutrition services for hospitality, culinary, and dietetic professionals.* Sudbury, MA: Jones and Bartlett Publishers.
12. Stewart, C. (2007). Disaster planning for foodservice operations. In S. Edelstein (Ed.), *Managing food and nutrition services for hospitality, culinary, and dietetic professionals.* Sudbury, MA: Jones and Bartlett Publishers.
13. McCabe, B. & Beattle, S. (2007). In S. Edelstein (Ed.), *Managing food and nutrition services for hospitality, culinary, and dietetic professionals.* Sudbury, MA: Jones and Bartlett Publishers.
14. Beran, B., Easterly, M. & Miller, M.A. (2007). Entrepreneurship: Writing a business plan for establishing your own restaurant or private practice and reimbursement for RD services. In S. Edelstein (Ed.), *Managing food and nutrition services for hospitality, culinary, and dietetic professionals.* Sudbury, MA: Jones and Bartlett Publishers.
15. The seven cardinal sins of foodservice. (2004). *Nation's Restaurant News, 38*(21), 53.

16. Visocan, B. & Switt, M. (2006). Understanding and using the scope of dietetics practice framework: A step-wise approach. *Journal of The American Dietetic Association, 106*(3), 459–463.
17. American Dietetic Association. (1999). Code of ethics. *Journal of The American Dietetic Association, 99,* 109–113.

## CHAPTER 2

MANAGEMENT AND LEADERSHIP THEORY WITH PRACTICAL APPLICATIONS

Sheryl Boston, MEd, LD and Sari Edelstein, PhD, RD

> *"Human relationships, like life itself, can never remain static."*
>
> Eleanor Roosevelt

Reader Objectives

Upon completion of the readings and practical solutions, the reader will be able to:

1. Identify the historical background of management theory and identify the founders of management theory.
2. Identify contemporary management and leadership theories.
3. Examine questions about management and leadership theories as they apply to employee problems in foodservice management.
4. Assess the potential of future employees by application of theories and practices in management and leadership theory.

Key Terms

Authoritative: having authority, ascendancy, or influence.
Benevolent: intending or showing kindness.
Consultative: advisory, giving advice.
Hierarchy: a system of ranking and organizing things or people where each element of the system (except for the top element) is subordinate to a single other element.

Hygiene: factors affecting health, such as cleanliness.

Leadership: a process by which a person influences others to accomplish an objective and directs the organization and its vision in a way that empowers others to make the organization more cohesive and coherent. Leaders carry out this process by applying their leadership attributes, such as beliefs, values, ethics, character, knowledge, and skills.

Management: characterizes the process of leading and directing all or part of an organization often through the deployment and manipulation of resources (human, financial, material, intellectual, or intangible).

Motivation: the initiation, direction, intensity, and persistence of behavior.

Participative: models of change that recommend managers consult widely and deeply with those affected to secure their willing consent to the changes proposed.

Introduction

The economic indicators for the United States and other parts of the world predict that more jobs and more careers will fall into the service-related fields over the next few years. Foodservice management has been an important part of the service industry for many years and will also continue to grow in the need for skilled and motivated employees and supervisors. In the most challenging of economic situations, people still eat, whether it is in casual dining experiences, in hospital rooms, or on a military base. One recurring problem in the foodservice industry is effective managers who stay in the business for their whole career and the practice of **leadership** that inspires others to seek a career in foodservice management.

To enable managers and future managers to see a career in foodservice **management**, one approach includes examining historical theories and gleaning from that history a strong base for management theory. There is a new collection of research in management and leadership theory that assists foodservice managers in assessing their staff, developing a plan for action, and measuring the progress in leadership and motivation. New theories have been developed that assist managers in understanding human behavior as it applies to the work force.

Historical Approaches to Management

Considered by many as the father of motivational theory, *Abraham Maslow* developed the **Hierarchy** of Needs in 1943.[1] The basis of Maslow's theory included identifying five levels, which he called deficiency and growth needs, that continually shape human behavior. These needs include:

- Level 1: Physiological Needs—air, water, food, clothing, and shelter
- Level 2: Safety Needs—protection against danger, freedom from fear, and an overall feeing of security
- Level 3: Social Needs—love, belonging, affiliation, and acceptance
- Level 4: Esteem Needs—achievement, recognition, and status
- Level 5: Self-Actualization Needs—realizing one's potential, growth, using creative talents

According to the theory, a person will not be able to move ahead until the needs that are on the lower level (Level 1) of the hierarchy are partially or completely fulfilled, and once one of the needs is satisfied, it will not longer motivate the person. For the foodservice manager, the first step in using this managerial approach will include determining where on the hierarchy each employee may be. In our current society, this determination is very difficult. There are persons who have needs that fall all over the hierarchy. In the inner city areas, there are many more opportunities for jobs. Foodservice employees can come to the facility, even having attended a magnet school that included using their creative talents and achieving a great deal of status in their schoolwork. But, when they head home, the family may be struggling to meet their needs for food, shelter, and the environment in which they live. This may include crime in the streets and in the housing project in which they live.

The theories of *Elton Mayo* were developed after studies were completed at the *Western Electric Company in*

> **Learning Point:** In theory, some persons will not be able to reach the top of the hierarchy in life. Thus, some may conclude that the hierarchy theory, while a good basis to begin the study of **motivation,** may not be appropriate in the new work force that exists today.

Chicago between the years of 1927 and 1932.[2,3] This theory states that recognition in the workplace serves as a motivator. Employees who demonstrate special ability or high-level job skills in the workplace will continue to work at this high level if they receive recognition. Also, if the employee can transfer this feeling into his personal or educational life, he will be successful there as well. There are four factors that best sum up the results of the research at the Western Electric Company:

1. Intelligence is a poor indicator or predictor of how well an employee will produce in the job environment. Rather, the social environment of the workplace is a stronger predictor of job success.
2. The informal relationships within the workplace affect productivity. Research indicates that when a positive relationship exists between the supervisor and the employees, the employees are more willing to work toward organizational goals.
3. Work groups have the ability to set their own productivity levels or they reach a consensus about what constitutes a productive day's work. This phenomenon was always considered, but this set of research set up the first confirmation. As long as the supervisors agree with the productivity level, this group will continue to be successful.
4. The workplace has it own separate and important social system. The amount of time and commitment that is part of a full-time job leads the relationships at work to have an important social system.

Frederick Herzberg's theories are referred as **Hygiene** *Theories.*[4] The theory in this approach includes a belief that the activities associated with work, including being supervised, having job benefits, and job satisfaction, can be negative motivators and are therefore

Learning Point: If the Hygiene Theory is one of motivation, then employees in the foodservice industry should be very motivated. This industry remains one with the most opportunity for upward movement. The number of supervisors and managers that have come up through the ranks still outnumber the people who are educated in foodservice management.

viewed as hygiene factors. Employees will not be motivated by these factors because they are present in all types of work environments. Instead, job motivation takes more; it takes interesting work, added responsibility, the availability to advance in the job to a supervisory or managerial position, and the opportunity for personal growth. These *factors* lead to employee motivation.

Dr. Rensis Likert's Theory of Human Behavior in organizations entails defining the relationship between the manager/leader with the employees in four possible situations. These four scenarios are summarized below[5]:

1. Exploitive-**authoritative** system. In this system, decisions are imposed on subordinates, and the power to achieve goals comes from *threats* from upper management. The front line employees are given little if no responsibility and have no communication or joint teamwork efforts.
2. **Benevolent**-authoritative system. The relationship is often compared to the *master-servant* trust. The upper management is responsible for the work and the achievement of goals, and lower level employees have no responsibility. There is no communication or teamwork.
3. **Consultative** system. In this system, employees are not completely trusted, but supervisors do look to the staff for some *input*. The overall feeling is that front line employees can provide some input, but it is limited and there is not a significant amount of teamwork.
4. **Participative**-group system. Considered by Likert as the optimum solution in management, in this system supervisors have complete confidence in their subordinates, and those persons are given financial rewards based on completion of the goals of the organizations. In order to reach goals, there is a high level of communication and cooperative teamwork.

To convert a foodservice organization to a participative-group system, the management must provide an environment that fosters modern principles and techniques and does not use the old system of rewards and threats. The employees must be viewed as people who have needs, desires, and values. Also, the foodservice organization must be a tight-knit group that works together in a highly effective manner. The group must be committed to achieving the goals and objectives. Finally, supportive relationships must exist in

Learning Point: To convert a foodservice organization to a participative-group system, the management must provide an environment that fosters modern principles and techniques and does not use the old system of rewards and threats.

the work group; there must be a high level of mutual respect among the employees and their supervisors.

There are some particular situations that make the participative-group system of leadership work well. The members of the group are skilled in leadership and have an easy interaction with other employees and supervisors. The goals and values of the organizations are shared. These groups have been together long enough to share department goals and are loyal to each other and the organization. This is a challenge for many foodservice employers due to the high level of turnover and the lack of leadership that expresses goals and objectives.

David McClelland is another motivational theorist. He is most noted for the three types of motivational needs that were identified in his 1988 book, *Human Motivation,* that was published just 10 years before his death.[6] The three needs of motivation are described as:

1. The Need for Achievement Motivation. The *needs achievement* employee is a person who seeks achievement and wants to attain challenging goals that will lead to advancement in the workplace. For the employee to achieve his goals, he requires a high level of feedback as he strives for work accomplishment. This employee will then be motivated by the sense of accomplishment and will work on subsequent goals.
2. The Need for Authority and Power. This employee is motivated by *the need for authority and power* and strives to be influential and effective in the workplace. The employee measures worth by looking at whether he or she has made an impact in the workplace. In this situation, the employee has a need to lead and wants her ideas to prevail. Supervisors, in this situation, work hard so that they can increase their personal status and assure themselves a prestigious place in the workplace.
3. The Need for Affiliation. In this situation the employee is motivated by the need for *friendly relationships and affiliations* and enjoys interaction with other people. These people are team players and work best when the employees working with them like them.

David McClelland indicates that most people have characteristics of each of these needs in their personality, but that some people have a very strong bias to a particular motivational need. This influences strongly their manner in working and managing people.

Prior to David McClelland, *Douglas McGregor* proposed the *Theory X and Theory Y* of human motivation, with each being the opposite of each other.[7] In Theory X, the organization takes the attitude that workers are lazy and will avoid work if left unsupervised. In Theory Y, the organization assumes the worker is motivated and desires to do a good job.

Modern Theories of Motivation and Leadership

John Stacy Adams is a workplace and behavioral psychologist who developed a theory in 1965 related to job motivation called Equity Theory. The Equity Theory assumes that all employees in an organization expect to find justice, fair play, and equality in the manner that they are treated by their employers. The theory holds that there are two variables:

1. Inputs: Characteristics that the employee brings to the job, including experience, special knowledge and job-related skills, and personal characteristics.
2. Outputs: The rewards for contributions made by the employee to the facility. The outputs often include pay, promotions, recognition in the workplace, status for his or her work, and fringe benefits.

The balance of inputs and outputs makes this system work. If the employee feels that there is a just or equal balance of input and outputs, then the employee will be motivated to work. If the situation ever reverses where the worker is giving more inputs and is getting less adequate outputs, such as compensation, then a sense of *demotivation* occurs. The level of demotivation is proportional to the imbalance of inputs to outputs.

The foodservice employee who is willing to work extra shifts, be on-call, or train others for additional responsibility will continue to be motivated if he or she feels that he or she is getting additional pay and/or other benefits. But if this situation becomes expected or is not appreciated, then the employee will begin to sense that he or she is giving more to the job than he or she is receiving. An impor-

Learning Point: For some employees, a simple *thank you* and inclusion in the team are adequate outputs; others may wish for more outputs. In this situation it is sometimes impossible to achieve a balance.

tant consideration of this theory is to recognize that it is the employee's "perception" of balance.

Charles Handy is a twenty-first century researcher involved in *motivation* and *leadership theory*. In 1997, he authored a book called *Leader to Leader* and has a newsletter and workshop series to educate persons in his method of leadership.[8] Handy is from Europe, where there may be a different view of leadership than in the United States. The author feels that the U.S. system of capitalism is not going to be sustained well into the new millennium. Handy feels that the most valuable asset of a company is not the buildings or property, but instead it is the people who are employees of the company. The value of labor, expertise, and knowledge base can be termed as intellectual property, which can be up to 40 times as valuable as the actual value of the tangible, physical place of business. In recent economic conditions with the declining value in the market and/or fierce competition, companies are downsizing, leaving only the business core intact. In effect, these companies are getting rid of the most valuable commodity of the business—the employees.

Handy's theory includes the premise that company stock purchase is the purchase of the intellectual capital. For example, when one buys stock in Microsoft™, one is actually purchasing the belief that Bill Gates can continue to motivate employees to work for his company. Handy's theory about ownership of the company states that the way to reward employees is to reward by stock options and/or the voting rights to determine the direction the company will go. When businesses are owned by people who have careers riding on the decisions of the company, you see real motivation to work hard and a reward in the feeling of ownership, as opposed to being owned. Handy's theories about the meaning of work include:

1. Institutions and individuals all have something to contribute to the work. Individuals are all in search of meaning and feel the need to find out what can be contributed throughout their lifetime.
2. If you are not of use to anyone, why survive?

3. All people have a need to be strongly affiliated with an organization.
4. Everyone should find out at an early age what he or she can learn to do best; this does not mean by figuring an IQ score. People have different aptitudes, and we need to know each child's characteristics in order to prepare him or her in school and for a life's work.

> **Learning Point:** Leaders need to remind the employees that it is the characteristics of the individual that make him or her valued and that each person, not the superstructure, is important to the business.

To summarize, Handy states that it is the responsibility of good leaders to believe that the future of the organization is up to the people who work there. Leaders need to make sure that an individual knows that he or she is an integral part of the organization.

Bruce Tuckman's research interests include motivation and how that manifests itself into self-regulatory behavior.[9] The research work had led to a theory called *Forming, Storming, Norming, and Performing: A Developmental Sequence of Groups*. The following list defines each of these areas in Tuckman's work:

- Forming: Occurs when groups initially begin the orientation process. At this point there are boundaries set by the group for interpersonal and task behaviors, and relationships are developed. Group members find out what their level of dependency will be on the leader and other members of the group. Each member has his or her own "testing" method for the group dynamics.
- Storming: Occurs when a conflict emerges in the group. All of the personal issues from each of the group members will surface and the group will have conflict about its task. The group finds out what the strengths and weakness of the members are and in what areas each can be approached.
- Norming: Occurs in the group dynamics when each member of the group has accepted the other members and has over-come some of the differences. The group begins to form a feeling of cohesiveness, and a set of unstated stands begin to evolve. Roles for each member of the groups evolve from

established communication. Each member of the group can express personal opinions.

- Performing: Occurs when the group has reached the final point of being ready to take on a task. The established interpersonal structure can be used as a tool for accomplishing the group task. Each member's role has become more relaxed and accepted. Each person's strength is used for the purpose of doing the work.

Tuckman's research on these types of group dynamics has gone on for 20 years and indicates that this method exists in a variety of groups. For the foodservice leader, group dynamics can be very important. Managers soon learn that if groups have been formed and undergone the development of structure, placing a new employee in the mix can create problems. The group will have to go through the whole reforming again, and the role may create conflict for a new member. The employee's ability to fit into a group will have a large impact on his or her ability to feel accepted and to stay. When employees are asked what single reason they left a position, they say that they were never accepted by the group and felt that they would never fit in.

The one factor that makes this situation easier for the employee is that these groups appear to be cyclical, meaning that they have a tendency to automatically recycle when new tasks or groups members are added. So, if employees are able to withstand the "storming" cycle of the group's dynamics, then they will find their fit in the group.

Another modern theorist of leadership is *William Ouchi*, who developed the *Theory Z* of management, which states that organizations should work on increasing employees' loyalty and that both employer and employee will benefit from this reciprocal relationship.[10] The organization gains the employee's loyalty by allowing individual responsibility, promoting for loyalty, including the employee in corporate decision making, and showing a genuine concern for the worker and his family.

Learning Point: It is the leader's role to assess the new employee's ability to fit into groups and determine whether he or she has the ability to withstand the tests or conflict that will plague the group in the first few weeks of employment.

In addition, Stephen Covey wrote *Principled Centered Leadership*, *The 7 Habits of Highly Effective People*, and *The 8th Habit*, which contend that good leadership is the product of the leader's personal character and discusses the criteria that lend themselves to building character.[11-13] Good character from a position of leadership in a company allows for others to become empowered and self-actualized. The company can build on a work force that is creative and loyal from an example of good character, leadership, and communication. Helping others find their voice within an organization is an inspiration to both parties.

Pop Psychology Theories

In the arena of motivational and leadership theory, a particular series has evolved that has come to be known as *pop* psychology. Each of these has been rooted in historic theories or is a new spin on behavioral theories. The next section will feature a few of these pop psychology theories.

Fritz Heider's Attribution Theory[14]

Attribution Theory examines the difference between *High Achiever* thinking and others.

Characteristics of high achievers are:

1. High achievers think success and future success is due to the high ability and the high level of effort that is put into a project. They never think that they will fail and if they do, it is not due to anything that they could have controlled. Instead, failure is due to back luck. In this way, the high achiever's self-esteem is never attacked. Success, pride, and confidence are continually built up as high achievers find the successful solution to a problem.

2. High achievers believe that they have to persist when work gets hard and that if there is a failure, it is because they have not given enough effort.

3. High achievers build their skills by selecting work-related problems that are not terribly challenging at the first; this enables them to take challenges that increase in difficulty as

time goes by. In this way, high achievers build their ability to solve problems.

4. High achievers believe that they will be successful if they work with a lot of energy. They assume that they will not be evaluated totally by results but instead with how hard they work or how hard they try.

Other Pop Theories

Harvey Mandel and *Sander Marcus* developed a theory about *how to motivate persons who are considered to be unmotivated.*[15] This researcher pair state that a lack of motivation is best described as a fear of achievement and a desire to avoid responsibility. Those employees who fall into this category have developed a set of excuses as to why they cannot be successful. This situation makes it very difficult for such employees to move ahead because they so firmly believe their own excuses. Through professional counseling, these persons can begin to deal with the self-perception and fear, and only then can they begin to look honestly at themselves.

The *Law of Least Effort* was devised by *Eisenbuerger* in 1992, and the main thesis deals with how the value of goals differs with each person.[16] These value differences are accounted for in employees who simply know that they need to work harder and longer in certain situations. This is called the *Law of More Effort*. Those employees realize that hard work pays off and is the springboard for promotion and success. These persons take into consideration all of the work conditions, which include the attitudes and personality traits of the employees with whom they are working. They understand that positive relationships must be developed in work settings. Employees who operate under the *Law of Least Effort* are the opposite. They do not put forth much effort and do not have the work ethic required to be successful.

> **Learning Point:** Efforts must be made by the supervisor to assess persons who are seeking employment and determine their level of effort related to the job that needs to be filled.

The last theory to be examined is by *Victor Vroom*.[17] In 1973, Vroom began to develop the Vroom-Yetton *model for leadership and motivation.* The basis for this new model was rooted in the historical work of Hersey and Blanchard's *Theory of Situational Leadership.*[18] In Hersey and Blanchard's model, leadership styles were identified as:

- Telling: The leader provides clear instructions and specific direction and is best matched with an employee who is not very mature and does not have a high readiness to learn.
- Selling: The leader encourages two-way communications among the supervisors and employees or learners. This leadership style encourages employees to build confidence in their abilities, and, while still depending heavily on the skills of the leader, this is a step closer to building employees into leaders.
- Participating: The leader and the employees share the decision making, and there is no longer a need for the leader to be very directive. The employee is at a moderate level of readiness to take over leadership.
- Delegating: The leader and the employee have come to a point where both are ready to accomplish a task and both are motivated to take full responsibility for the outcome.

It is from this basis that Vroom developed his model. The main difference between Vroom's model and Hersey and Blanchard's model is that leadership styles lie in the focus and on the amount and form of employee decision-making participation. Hersey and Blanchard's model of leadership is very explicit that the decision-making powers can be shared by leaders and employees. A second difference is the manner in which a situation is evaluated. For Vroom, any situation is a problem or decision that is faced exclusively by the leader. In the Vroom model, the problem is believed to present a distinctive combination of characteristics that will influence the leader's choice of leadership style. In order to determine the most effective decision style, the leader uses a set of seven attributes or factors that affect or help clarify the decision. Those attributes are listed below:

1. Attribute A: The Importance of Decision Quality. This decision is defined as high quality and consistent with the organizational goals to be attained.
2. Attribute B: Leader's Information Relevant to the Problem. This decision has been determined to have a quality level, then is analyzed as to whether the leader has all of the information

required to permit an intelligent decision. This can be technical data and does not take into consideration whether this decision will please anyone.

3. Attribute C: Extent to which the Problem is Structured. The leader has knowledge about the current state of the organization, the desired state of the organization, and the ability to transform the organization from its current state into its desired state.

4. Attribute D: Importance of Acceptance of Decision by Subordinates to Effective Implementation. In this attribute, subordinates will execute the decision and will be evaluated on their decision making. Also in that role, subordinates will be evaluated on whether their decision was based on a set of routines and preplanned steps or whether they actively participated. The higher the level of participation, the more likely the subordinate will accept and take ownership in the solution.

5. Attribute E: Probability that the Leader's Decision Will Be Accepted by Subordinates. The bases of power come in three descriptors. First, *legitimate* power is best described as the person who has the power to enforce organizational rules because of his or her position in the company. Next is *expert* power or power that is based on a knowledge level related to the problem. A person who is an expert can be utilized in making a decision because he or she holds expert authority related to a problem. The last is called *attraction* power, the positive feelings that are shown toward a leader. These feeling include trust, respect, and admiration. If a leader makes a decision using all three power sources, the probability of acceptance by subordinates increases.

6. Attribute F: Congruence of Organizational and Subordinate Goals. Common purposes pave the way for a joint decision. Others involved see the value in the decision and have greater interest in it. There also needs to be power-sharing.

7. Attribute G: Conflict or Disagreement among Subordinates. For many in management and leadership roles, conflict is not viewed as positive. You can understand that there are employees who have congruent goals that are locked in conflict or disagreement about how to achieve those goals. Vroom looks at conflict in a different way and feels that conflict will lead to four implications:

- Conflict among people increases the time that it takes to implement a decision.
- Conflict among people stops progress and causes a division in the relationships of the subordinates and supervisors.
- Conflict can lead to clearer thinking and better overall decisions.
- Conflict among people is a sign that they should interact more in their attempt to arrive at a decision.

In this model, one can see that in the third and fourth implications, conflict may lead to better results from collaborative decision making that was initially based in conflict.

Practical Applications

In the material that was presented above, there is no one model or leadership style that is guaranteed to be the method that needs to be adopted by all leaders or managers in all situations. Instead, managers must realize that their arsenal of problem-solving skills must have many methods and theories. What works for one person in one particular situation might not work in a problem that presents itself in another situation.

Labor sources are changing every moment as well. The needs of employees are constantly changing, and work conditions need to be considered. The list below summarizes the different considerations a manager must make in the workplace.

Managers must have the ability to:

- Assess the organization's needs. Managers must determine a set of skills that are to be used to demonstrate effective job performance. Managers must be able to determine through interview the basic behaviors that are expected by staff of the foodservice industry.
- Assess the individual. The manager must be able to assess the key behaviors that are required by a person for a particular job. This assessment must be completed in an analytical manner, or rather a collection of data about the person applying for the job and the list of job skills.
- Deliver the assessment with care. In an attempt to get useful information about job applicants that will make their train-

ing and actual job performance easier and more successful, individuals must feel that they are not being picked at or torn apart. After the assessment, the applicant requires feedback that shows how the employer is trying to match the job needs to the employee in a manner that will make him or her the most successful.

- Maximize learner choice in the job place. Research indicates that employees are more motivated to change when they choose to do so. To the greatest extent possible, employees need to be permitted to make the choice to participate in a program that promotes change as well as set the goals for the program.
- Encourage persons to participate. When employees determine that programs that promote change are valuable and worthwhile to them, the supervisor will not have a problem getting persons to participate. This process involves building trust and creditability among the staff.
- Link learning goals in the workplace to personal values. People are motivated to change when it affects them personally; the buy-in will be greater.
- Adjust expectations. When the supervisor is able to build positive expectations for potential learners and show them that improvement will affect the outcome of their lives, employees will be able to look at the program and have realistic expectations of the effect it will have on their lives and their jobs.
- Gauge readiness. The supervisor is responsible for assessing whether the employee is ready for training. If that person is truly not ready for change, then it will not happen and the employee will experience another disappointment.

Summary

This chapter's summary can most effectively be represented by a list of *Best Practices*. Best Practices are a list of guidelines managers may apply to their supervision of employees and serve as a summary for this chapter:

1. Foster positive relationships between employees and supervisors.

2. Make change self-directed.
3. Set clear goals.
4. Break goals into manageable steps.
5. Provide opportunities to practice.
6. Give performance feedback.
7. Rely on experiential methods.
8. Build in support.
9. Use models.
10. Enhance insight.
11. Prevent relapse.
12. Encourage use of skills on the job.
13. Develop an organizational culture that supports learning.
14. Evaluate.

Student Activities

1. E-mail or telephone a foodservice manager in your city and ask for an example of a problem he or she was confronted with and which leadership methods were used to problem solve.
2. Interview a foodservice employee and ask his or her perception of the group or team dynamics where he or she is employed.
3. Research the phrase "group dynamics" and report findings that were not covered in this chapter and are applicable to foodservice situations.
4. Research the phrase "leadership style" and report findings that were not covered in this chapter and are applicable to foodservice situations.
5. Research a "management theory" and report findings that are applicable to foodservice situations.

CASE STUDY #1: THE LEADERSHIP EXPECTATIONS OF BAILEY FOODSERVICE INCORPORATED

Bailey Foodservice Incorporated is a small independent foodservice company that provides meal service to long-term care facilities. At the end of the last quarter, the owner, George Bailey, had determined that the leadership needed to

---

continues

be replaced. He currently has contracts with five long-term care facilities, and he would like to acquire more. The change in the manner in which the government funded long-term care for meals, and the private pay clients, has led to a financial crunch and created more competition in the business arena. George Bailey called upon a college friend, who was a foodservice consultant, to assist in assembling a report on the issues and financial conditions of the Bailey company. George realized that he needed an independent view of his business. Below is the report that the consultant provided to George Bailey.

Human Resources

The facilities that are owned by Bailey Foodservice Incorporated are all managed in a similar fashion. The dietary managers have been promoted according to seniority, do not possess supervisory skills, and have had not formal training. Many of the supervisors have been placed in positions of authority and have taken advantage of this position when it comes to hiring friends and family and in the decisions regarding staffing and scheduling.

Cafeteria Dining Room Staff

The staff in the cafeteria have done a good job in satisfying the needs of the client's family and the employees who use the dining room. It was then observed that one of the staff, Delores, was unkind to assorted customers and she gave free food to those whom she liked and small portions to those whom she disliked. It appeared that similar problems occurred in each of the facilities. The dietary manager had her favorites and gave preferences in work shifts. Any overtime was offered to those whom she felt were the most deserving.

Kitchen Operations

The kitchen staff is competent, although they are not formally skilled. The leadership in the kitchen is lacking, and the staff are often in conflict. The supervisors are highly stressed and often do not cope well with the job-related responsibilities. They often bring problems from their personal lives to work. All of the stress and conflict have a negative effect on the attitudes in the kitchen department.

When new staff were added to the kitchen department, they were often not trained for an adequate length of time and not in a formal manner. A person was trained for only a few days. If the person responsible for training had bad habits, the new staff picked up those same bad habits.

The items included in inventory and budgeting were in the hands of Sally, the Dietary Manager in one of the locations. She did not let anyone know her routine for doing inventory. When George Bailey questioned the manner in which she kept records, Sally was unsure if the books were indeed correct. Since Sally was the staff member with the longest tenure, she had trained managers in the other facilities, and they used her same system.

The consultant made the following summary related to the facilities that were owned by George Bailey:

- The dietary manager is perceived as unapproachable. She gives the appearance that she is right in every situation, thus making it difficult for employees to have a fair employment opportunity.
- The morale of the employees is greatly dependent on the mood of the supervisory staff. If they are in a good mood, then the day goes well for the staff of the kitchen.
- The general manager in several of the facilities intimidates some of the employees, especially the cafeteria staff person, who shows favoritism to some staff. They run off both the staff outside the dietary department and within the department.
- The dietary manager tries to impress the owner when he is on site. She goes the extra mile with the staff when he is present. This confuses the staff and adds to the poor morale.

continues

Questions for Discussion

After reading the case study above, have students break down into small groups and answer each of the following questions:

1. According to the research on leadership, employees have to feel that they can see a better future before they will get on board for participating in a radical change. With this in mind, what steps will George Bailey have to make immediately to resolve the leadership problems with each of his facilities? How can George make his vision for change real to the employees of the foodservice management company?
2. Could George Bailey have made this report himself or was it valuable for him to have a "neutral" set of eyes look at his business?
3. Identify and explain the supervisory challenges in the kitchen, cafeteria, and dietary manager's areas.

CASE STUDY #2: MOTIVATION AT WORK

Objectives

At the completion of the case study, the student will be able to:

1. Describe the importance of motivation at work.
2. Explain the value of the relationships between the foodservice management department and human resource department.
3. Evaluate all the concepts, aside from job skills, that affect employees in the workplace.
4. Describe the effect that human resource laws have on the employee.

The Foodservice Management Story

A small Midwestern university has a foodservice company that provides foodservice in all four of the university's resident halls. The daily meal count across campus is about 5,000 meals per meal period. The foodservice company was faced with a decline in employee morale and motivation to work. The employees had been facing a freeze in their salaries and had received only small cost of living increases over the past 2 or 3 years. They were beginning to be very vocal in their complaints about this situation. The management company had used the excuse that, due to the cost of energy and transportation, the company is not making money at the same levels as in previous years. Because the company had not announced the financial situation to the employees, the employees were not aware of the deep financial problems facing the management company. Instead, they felt that the problems with the company were rooted in the leadership and management of the company. The employees also felt that the upper levels of management did not understand or appreciate the work ethic most of the employees contribute to the management company. The employees worked extra hours when asked and did additional tasks that were not part of their workload. This situation has led the employees to begin to look for other jobs with competing companies. In all areas of the hospitality industry, employee turnover is high and has been for a number of years.

The foodservice management company does not have a very clear understanding of the staff that they employ. The workers are not highly educated and do not possess highly developed skills, and the administration of this company feels that for every person working, there are plenty more waiting to come to work for their company. As with many corporately owned firms, the administration of this company and the local units are very well paid individuals. The

continues

administration/management is also perceived by the staff as overpaid and underworked. In many situations when the front line staff could use an additional set of hands, managers in their offices, rather than out with the staff.

The practice that has led to the greatest dissatisfaction is when staff are asked to come in early or stay late, off the clock. This is mandatory. This is a measure that has been explained as a cost-saving effort. This practice further divides the front-line staff from the management. These front-line employees feel underappreciated and taken advantage of. Management feels that the staff are so uneducated that they do not understand the labor laws and their rights under the law. Employees fear that they will lose their jobs if they pursue a complaint with management.

In the past, the foodservice management has had a good reputation of being fair to its employees. In fact, these managers were considered good employers. With the decline in profits, the benefits and other employee packages have been cancelled or cut back, thus increasing the cost to the employees.

These problems have resulted in employee morale and motivation falling. Employees feel that they just come to work and give the minimal effort and then move on to a better job when they get the opportunity.

Questions to Consider

After reading the narrative above, break into groups of three or four and discuss the situation. Please complete the questions below, and determine how to turn this situation around.

1. List all of the issues that management handled incorrectly.
2. List everything the staff of the foodservice company might have to complain about.
3. Identify what you think the management can do to improve the situation.
4. Identify all the laws and regulations that management has broken in the situation. How can employees protect their rights?

5. Explain how management views their employees and further explain how this view affects the employees' morale.
6. How can management's view be changed?
7. List what ideas you have about how to decrease employee turnover in the foodservice industry.

References

1. Maslow, A. (1952). *Motivation and personality.* New York: Harpers.
2. Wallis, D. (1986). The humanist temper: The life and work of Elton Mayo. D. Wallis. *Journal of Occupational Psychology, 59*(2),158.
3. Mahoney, K.T. & Baker, D.B. (2002). Elton Mayo and Carl Rogers: A tale of two techniques. *Journal of Vocational Behavior, 60*(3), 437–450.
4. Bockman, V.M. (1971). The Herzberg controversy. *Personnel Psychology, 24*(2), 155–189.
5. Likert, R. (1967). *The human organization: Its management and value.* McGraw-Hill.
6. McClelland, D. (1988). *Human motivation.* Cambridge, MA: Cambridge University Press.
7. McGregor, D. (1960). *Human side of enterprise.* New York: McGraw-Hill.
8. Handy, C.B. (2005). *Understanding organizations.* New York: Penguin Business Books.
9. Tuckman, B.W., Abry, D. & Smith, D.R. (2001). *Learning and motivation strategies: Your guide to success.* Upper Saddle River, NJ: Prentice-Hall.
10. Ouchi, W.G. (1982). *Theory z.* Mass Market Paperback.
11. Covey, S.R. (2004). *The 8th habit: From effectiveness to greatness.* New York: Free Press.
12. Covey, S.R. (1991). *Principled centered leadership.* New York: Simon & Schuster.
13. Covey, S.R. (1989). *The 7 habits of highly effective people.* New York: Simon & Schuster.
14. Martinko, M. (1995). *Attribution theory: An organizational perspective.* Delray Beach, FL: St. Lucie Press.
15. Mandel, H.P. & Marcus, S.I. (1988). Psychology of underachievement. New York: Wiley.
16. IIE solutions. (2000). *Punchline, 32*(9), 66.
17. Vroom, V.H. & Yetton, P.W. (1976). *Leadership and decision-making.* Pitt Paperback.
18. Hersey, P. (1985). The situational leader. New York: Warner Books.

## CHAPTER 3

CORPORATE CULTURE AND COMMUNICATION

Dee Sanquist, MS, RD

Reader Objectives

After studying this chapter and reflecting on the contents, you should be able to:

1. Review corporate culture and current trends.
2. Discuss how management style affects decision making and communication.
3. Learn communication strategies and negotiation.
4. Discuss meeting formats.

Key Terms

Accountability: the principle that individuals, organizations, and the community are responsible for their actions and may be required to explain them to others.

Alliance: close association of nations or other groups formed to advance common interests or causes.

Coaching: a process providing an individual with feedback, insight, and guidance on achieving their full potential in their business or personal life.

Collectivistic culture: a group of people with a tendency to understand someone better than that person understands himself.

Communication: the exchange of thoughts, messages, or information, as by speech, signals, body language, and writing.

Competency: having substantial knowledge in an area of expertise and the ability to recount the facts in a logical, coherent manner based on the truth.

Corporate culture: refers to a company's values, beliefs, business principles, traditions, ways of operating, and internal work environment.

Mentoring: assisting individuals in order to advise, counsel, and/or guide them.

Negotiation: discussion intended to produce an agreement.

Introduction

There are many approaches to **corporate culture** and even more definitions. No one culture is right for all organizations. Corporate culture is formed from a pattern of commonly held values, beliefs, and assumptions. Corporate culture sets a particular company apart from the rest; it's the company's unique personality or characteristics. Healthy cultures have positive energy and provide for recruitment and retention of employees and customers. People feel included and valued and work together toward a common goal. **Communication** and corporate culture are continually changing and developing. Both are a "work in progress" that require adapting to the changing environment, financial, and regulatory guidelines from which all companies must adhere.

Corporate culture and communication can be approached from a cumbersome process and in-depth analysis, or this process can be simplified to mean that corporate culture and communication are the result of every conversation, every day, by every employee. Some organizations need a great amount of structure and formality. Other organizations are more flexible and informal. Consider the fact that corporate culture is an evolution and must adapt and change based on the goals of the organization. The foodservice culture needs to be consistent with corporate culture and communication style within the organization to provide reinforcement and consistent messages for employees.

As hierarchical corporate structures break down, the leadership challenge is to embrace the mobile, adaptable, transparent organization. The challenge of foodservice leadership is keeping organizational culture in balance amidst change. High-performing departments work within the organizational culture to get results. It takes more than knowing what to do. Once the goals are set, focus on the "how to" implement and "how to" be flexible when circumstances change.

Trends

In the Industrial Age, corporate culture was dictated by management. Today's corporate culture differs from the past because it is created by employees rather than by dictating managers. Today's culture includes bottom-up decision making. Team members are empowered to make decisions within the boundaries of financial constraints.[1] As the culture is set for spreading the wings of each team member, the leader is able to have time to anticipate the needs of customers, grow the business, and develop new products or services to be on the cutting edge of the competition.[2] Tables 3.1 and 3.2 list the definitions and levels found in the corporate culture.

Learning Point: Corporate Culture Can Be Approached by Asking Four Questions:

1. Where do we need to go strategically?
2. Where are we now?
3. What are the gaps between where we are and where we need to go?
4. What is our plan of action to get to where we need to go?

It is a challenge for foodservice leaders to build, guide, influence, and maintain a strong culture that is consistent with the strategic plan, values, and goals of the organization. The foodservice leader can gain consistency by linking organizational goals to department goals.

Table 3.1 Definitions of Corporate Culture

Adaptive: Leaders care about customers and team members. People are strongly valued and a process is created for useful change. Leaders pay attention to customers (internal and external) and initiate change when necessary. These leaders are risk takers. They continually think outside the box and try new products and services. Team members are included in decision making and planning to support change.

Unadaptive: Managers care about themselves, the immediate work group, or product. They do not like risk taking and are less likely to take initiative. The workgroup is not empowered and must seek permission for even small changes. Communication tends to be on a "need to know" basis.

Table 3.2   Levels of Corporate Culture

1. Surface:

Culture is reinforced through visible appearances and behavior. Examples are physical facility layout, dress code, organizational structure, policies of the organization, procedures, and behaviors.

Are the uniforms for foodservice employees formal looking or casual?

Does the facility layout reflect a certain food preparation or service area (formal dining room, cook, chill, cook-serve, room service)?

2. Middle:

Culture is based on beliefs and values.

Are organizational values reflected in foodservice policies, procedures, structure, and behavior expectations?

Are meetings organized around the mission and values of the organization? Does performance appraisal include values as criteria?

3. Deepest:

Basic assumptions of culture are automatic responses and established opinions. Workers are consistent and genuine in daily actions that support organizational values and beliefs.

Some examples are when employees anticipate needs of lost visitors and take them to the correct location.

Are policies easily obtainable and understandable by staff or are they locked in an office?

Is there a mentoring program for new staff?

Unacceptable behaviors are dealt with in a prompt manner and negative behaviors are not tolerated.

Negative behaviors can quickly break down years of building a positive culture.

How does profit status affect corporate culture? Generally the difference is subtle. For for-profit businesses, the concern is to provide dividends to investors. Non-profit organizations tend to provide money or services according to a specific mission and use any net revenue to reinvest in the business rather than give dividends to investors. Corporate goals are generally defined by a board of directors who also determine the mission, vision, and values that provide a framework for operations and decision making.

The Nature of Culture

The hospitality industry is a business that consistently focuses on customer service and creating exceptional experiences for guests. Dealing with people can result in varying levels of stress for the people within a corporation. A healthy corporate culture can help individuals cope with a high stress business environment. Edgar Schein, MIT Professor of Management and author of *Organizational Culture and Leadership: A Dynamic View,* states that "Today, organizational leaders are confronted with many complex issues during their attempts to generate organizational achievement." A leader's success is dependent upon his or her understanding of corporate culture. For example, if a manager's new vision or plan is inconsistent with the company's corporate culture, it will fail because the organization will not support it.

Corporate culture affects the basic decisions and behaviors made within the organization. (For example, Walt Disney Productions™ has a corporate culture that dictates strict dress codes for hair, facial hair, and body jewelry.) There are many definitions of the concept of corporate culture. The corporate culture relates to organizational values. Values are important to the organization and guide the decisions and behavior of the organization. This influences the way people behave in a variety of areas that include how customers are treated, performance standards for team members, and innovation. Increasingly, successful organizations find part of their success is from effective culture management. For example, Starbucks™ has grown from two retail stores to more than 2,500 stores worldwide. The company believes that the way it treats its employees affects the way those employees treat customers, which affects the overall success of the company, including financial performance. Starbucks™ has adopted human resource practices that help team members feel valued.

How does corporate culture affect the bottom line? Eric Flamholtz, author of *Corporate Culture and the Bottom Line,* found a statistically significant relationship between corporate culture and financial performance.[3] In addition, corporate culture influences behavior and decision making. Flamholtz found that four areas influence behavior and decision making:

1. How customers are treated.
2. How team members are treated.

3. Standards and values of organizational performance.
4. Demonstration of accountability.

There are other areas of organization performance that contribute to culture and communication, however, the list above tends to be synergistic with respect to innovation, corporate citizenship, and change management. Other areas include support for innovation, openness to change, and the support of organization by the employee.

Strategies for Building a Growth Culture

New leadership styles encourage emphasis on the future, not the past, and the possibilities, not the constraints. Strategies that support a hospitality department culture, such as rewarding a team instead of an individual, help to reinforce the new corporate culture. However, it is important to maintain clear individual accountabilities within the team.

Learning Point: Generally Characteristics of Building a Successful Culture Include the Following:

- Emphasize the future, not the past.
- Focus on possibilities, not constraints.
- Reach customers through employees.
- Discourage politics and encourage risk taking.
- Reward team success, not individual success. Maintain clear individual accountabilities.
- High level of freedom and trust.
- Debate before consensus.
- The successful hospitality leader will have processes in place that support these strategies.

Communication

A key part of a successful corporate culture is communication. Setting and communicating goals are important for strong corporate cultures. Behavior is the outcome of communicating the corporate culture message. Words are meaningless unless they are transformed into behavior. Of utmost importance, is linking the communication strategy with organizational goals. Leaders must facilitate and communicate rather than command and control. People with responsibility need to define clear expectations to employees.

Key components for communicating include look, listen, and learn. Often management focuses on dispersing information. They need to find ways to listen to the employees. Concentrate on building a team of consensus and self-regeneration. Get procedures and policies to align with the behaviors that are expected.

The process of communication is a continuous loop. Feedback leads to feedback, which leads to action. We live in an age where we are constantly overwhelmed with information. It's important to provide enough pertinent information yet not overwhelm the employees with minor details. The challenge is finding how much information your team can handle and providing options for people who have a need for more information. Defining the strategy provides a concrete, not abstract, method for establishing criteria and process. It helps people make day-to-day decisions and provides a template for communication. Communication goals can be reinforced by setting department and individual performance goals that are consistent with those of the organization. For example, a foodservice manager could write a script or include in-depth orientation to foodservice staff regarding answering questions in the cafeteria about the preparation of a product. This may include having the ingredients available for the staff or customers. An individual staff member may have a goal focused around anticipating the needs of a customer.

Communication needs to constantly tie the corporate *mission, vision, and values* back to the people who perform the work. When performance standards and expectations use similar terminology as the corporation, employees can begin to identify with the larger picture. Open and timely communication includes both the good and the bad. Encourage a team atmosphere where members can easily ask for clarity. Use of a scripted vocabulary can support the organizational goals and provide consistency. Consider first the organization, then the department. Typically, a strong communication and culture will contribute to increased motivation by employees, which will help the bottom line.[3]

Holding product meetings will provide a powerful avenue for communication and allow employees to participate. *Plan ahead.* There are many frameworks for holding a successful meeting. The best one is the one that works for a particular team. An agenda with timelines can be helpful if a timekeeper is appointed to keep the meeting on track. A facilitator other than the manager can provide a neutral atmosphere. A recorder will write key points so that everyone can have a consistent message to take away from the meeting. Minutes need to be approved by management before they are distributed. One of the most important parts of any meeting is to assign next steps or action to be taken. Accountability for completing the action with a timeline must be assigned. If time permits, it may be helpful to have a part of the meeting where each team member can briefly update the team about current challenges or outcomes in their areas.

Making a decision can be difficult for teams. Dialogue is the best way to make a quality decision. Dialogue can lead to new ideas. This includes successful follow-through and feedback. The setting for dialogue affects corporate culture. Openness, candor, informality, and closure can enhance communication. Openness means that there is no predetermined outcome. Candor is a willingness to speak the unspeakable. People express their real opinions, not what they think the team wants to hear. Informality loosens the atmosphere. Closure means that at the end of the meeting, people know what is expected of them. Accountability and deadlines are assigned. Leaders get the behavior they expect. Table 3.3 gives the reader a list of dialogue killers.

Holding productive meetings will enhance decision making and communication within the organization. Usually there are three

---

Learning Point: Important Components of Any Communication Include:

Vision: Where the department is headed and how the employee can contribute.
Goals: Must be measurable and specific enough to be achievable.
Priorities: List the order of focus.
Corporate reputation and values: Describe the slogan for the department.
Stakeholder beliefs: What do you want each stakeholder group to believe about your business?
Communication objectives: Focus and define priorities. Pick three to six areas.

Table 3.3   Dialogue Killers

1. Dangling Dialogue: The meeting ends without a clear next step and confusion prevails. People create their own conclusion to the meeting.
2. Information clogs occur when there is a failure to get all the relevant information. perhaps an important fact or opinion is brought forth after the decision is made. To remedy this situation, make sure the appropriate people are in attendance in the first place.
3. Piecemeal perspective is where people have narrow views and demonstrate self-interests. There is a failure to acknowledge the interests of others. Solve this by drawing people out until you are sure all sides of the issue have been represented. Keep restating the common purpose to keep employees focused. Talk about alternatives.
4. Free-for-all occurs when there is a failure to direct the flow of the discussion and negative behaviors are demonstrated. Some people may try to hold the team up until others see it their way. Others may delve into unnecessary detail. Solve this by repeatedly reinforcing acceptable and unacceptable behaviors. Remove people who consistently demonstrate negative behavior.

Compiled by the author from Charan, R. (2006, January). Conquering a culture of indecision. *Harvard Business Review*, pp. 108–116.

types of communication strategies. First, the master strategic plan looks at the overall organization and attempts to build a high-level communication. Secondly, the operating plan addresses how it will be done and contains the behavioral outcomes and methods that are needed for each target audience. This plan identifies issues, specific strategies, and time frames in which the communication takes place. And, thirdly, individual "project plans" are detailed about specific desired behaviors, audience, and timing.

The communication plan needs to include objectives, target audience, desired outcome, the issue, implementation strategy and timing, and measurement of progress.

Include issues that can impact success, such as lack of systems, support, and training, and assign responsibility. Look for the same return on investment from communications as from other functions, such as human resources and marketing. The communication can guide decision making around advertising, internal communication, and resources, which should drive the budget and resource allocation.

A common trait among great leaders is that they demonstrate great communication skills—both one-on-one and in a group. The job of the leader is to mentor and give the team the strength and skills to grow and then let them spread their wings. If you, as a leader, hang on to the employees, you will hold them back. Leaders should give away power and gain as many avenues for communication for fellow team members.

A new team member generally is excited and motivated to learn a new job. A more directive approach is used at this beginning stage so that communication is clear, concise, and leaves no room for misinterpretation. For example, the leader sets the rules, " This is the expectation I have for the team...." The next stage involves the leader shifting from directing to coaching. Coaching is a softer approach where the leader will reiterate the rules and help the team member succeed if he or she is willing to put forth the effort.

It is important for coaches or mentors to understand the peaks and valleys of the process. Performance includes balance—the same as a person balances day and night.

The next step is to let the team member know he or she is competent and that you are always available when needed. It takes strength for a coach to sit back and allow the team to take the glory. This ability is critical to increasing communication within the corporate culture. The team members are the corporate culture, and it's important that they demonstrate the values of the organization throughout their work. The goal is performance. The coach must have the confidence that the team will demonstrate corporate values through their interaction with internal and external customers.

The savvy leader knows that rough times are part of leadership. "Rough diamonds don't fit into a mold. It's not about controlling; just don't hurt other people in the team."[4] Table 3.4 lists the steps to changing corporate culture and communication.

Group Communication and Problem Solving

There are several well-used methods for group communication, problem solving, and decision making. Among these are the Delphi Technique, the Nominal Group Technique, and brainstorming. The Delphi Technique does not require that the participants of the group

Table 3.4 Steps to Changing Corporate Culture and Communication

Many performance improvement models exist. Use the model for the organization and adapt it for the hospitality environment. Define the following:

1. What is the current culture?
2. Write a definition that demonstrates behaviors that would define the desired culture.
3. Develop a plan using a variety of members from all level of the foodservice department. Include people from other departments or customers on an ad hoc basis.
4. Implement the plan.
5. Measure the outcome and make adjustments.

Compiled by the author from Flamholtz, E. (2001). Corporate culture and the bottom line. *European Management Journal*, Vol. 19, No.3, pp. 268–275.

meet or discuss issues with one another. Instead, a trained facilitator may send out questionnaires to a group asking for individual ideas to solve a problem. When the questionnaires are returned, the facilitator compiles all the ideas and sends these out to the group again. Participants then respond to all the ideas and send them back to the facilitator. The process continues, pointing out the strengths and weaknesses of ideas, until a resolution is decided upon.

The Nominal Group Technique is similar to the Delphi Technique, except the group members usually meet. In the Nominal Group Technique, ideas are generated in written form and group members can ask questions of the individual who has created the idea. This questioning usually takes a few rounds, ending with a ranking or voting for the solutions to the problem or the idea.

In brainstorming, the members of the group list their solution to a problem out loud and produce an exhaustive list of possible ideas. These ideas are then organized and discussed for practicality to solve the problem at hand. At the end, a consensus for handling the problem is reached by the group.

How does the foodservice leader improve departmental culture and communication? Just as there is no one perfect corporate culture, there is no right or wrong way to improve communication. It's what works best for a particular business or department at a particular point in time. What will work may depend on:

1. Your current reporting relationships.
2. Your business model (central vs. decentralized).
3. A command and control approach vs. collaboration and consensus.
4. The needs of your audience (knowledge workers vs. task workers).
5. Individual learning and communication styles of employees (oral, written, touch, experience).
6. Seeking out knowledge about generational management and how to best reach workers from various age groups.

Start with defining the goal. Once this is done, all communications can reflect that goal. For example, use goals as a basis in making decisions, addressing staff concerns, and in operational challenges. Approach the phrase "best practices" with a touch of skepticism and with curiosity. Insights into best practices require the need to fit an organization's culture, legacy, personalities, physical plant, and strategies. It allows management to ask themselves important questions about the way they work, which provides rewarding insights into change. Table 3.5 lists several different types of communication methods.

Consider gender differences in communication strategies. The gender gap is the phenomenon that prevents women from advancing careers at the same rate as men. **Mentoring** can help bridge this gap. Mentoring is a behavior that will provide a developmental relationship between senior and junior colleagues, at any level in the organization. Mentors provide psychosocial and social connections. Organizational citizenship is discretionary and helps contribute to maintain a social system and indirectly contributes to the workgroup. **Collectivistic culture** emphasizes cooperation. Tables 3.6 and 3.7 list the characteristics of the masculine organizational culture and the collectivistic organizational culture.

After hiring, the organization takes care of overall personnel welfare.[5] Each gender has unique communication styles and strategies. Males tend to find pay, benefits, achievement, success, status, and authority important. Women rank friendships and other relationships, recognition and respect, and communication and collaboration as higher priorities.

Table 3.5   Communication Methods

Develop a model that will provide a consistent framework in which to share communication.

1. Keep it simple. Cut to the "bottom line" and focus on the core message(s) that are the priority. Limit this number to between three and five messages. Too many messages are hard to manage and they get misinterpreted.

2. Write simple core messages, Use a fifth to seventh grade reading level. Avoid acronyms, abbreviations, and jargon. Use active, not passive verbs.

3. Keep it short. The goal is to turn 20 words into a few focused sentences.

4. Justify your message. Give an example. What's the reason? Include the word "because."

5. Don't overwhelm them. Tell people what they need to know and provide a website, phone number, or other information for people who need more information.

6. Respect the time of other people and time your contact. Everyone is busy. Be concise. Give people time to think about the information. Make sure it's an appropriate time to communicate the information.

7. Use multi-touch and multi-timed communication. According to adult education experts, the average adult needs to hear, feel, and experience the message for up to six times before they remember the message. Use a variety of methods to communicate the message:
   - Individual
   - Small Group
   - Department
   - E-mail
   - Voicemail
   - Web
   - Newsletters
   - Posters, bulletin boards

8. Messages need to be redelivered. Reinforce major messages with periodic updates or reminders.

9. Use a question and answer format. Have one central location where staff know they can re-check information, or check for updates.

10. Treat employee concerns as valid and helpful. Everyone has a different perspective and that perspective must be grown and nurtured.

Compiled by the author from *SCM*, (2005, October/November).Vol. 9, No. 6.

Table 3.6   Masculine Organizational Culture

1. More males than females in leadership roles.
2. Men tend to choose other men for collaboration.
3. Men chair important meetings.
4. Top management believes it is more important for men to have a professional career than women.
5. Women are not visible in management.

Table 3.7   Collectivistic Organizational Culture

1. Management and supervisors are protective of their workers.
2. Employees take each other's views into consideration regardless of hierarchy.
3. Decision is made jointly by the supervisor and employees.
4. Employees are treated as members of the family.
5. Workers are informed about major decisions that affect the success of the organization.
6. Everyone shares responsibility for the organization's failures as well as successes.

There is no one correct culture or communication technique. Consideration should be given to the cultural, age, and gender diversity of the work force in the communication process. Eight mistakes can deter from otherwise effective communication strategies:

1. Silence. When silence is used, the employees will make up their own information.
2. Over analyzing before acting.
3. Managing by power creates a culture where staff are fearful and do not engage fully in a process.
4. Self-centeredness produces managers who spend their time on their personal quest for recognition.
5. Being too distant. E-mails are replacing human contact. Relationships are the heart of corporate culture and communication.

6. Unclear messages. Focus the message and the communication. This is best done face-to-face rather than via e-mail where messages are often misinterpreted.
7. Leading by taboos.
8. Leading by miracle strategies. There is no quick fix.

Lead by Insight and Innovation

A mistake many leaders make is to lead by *numbers* rather than by *people*. Numbers and reports can be used as information, but including a team of people to set goals will provide a positive, supportive, and innovative environment. The boundaries or framework must be articulated. When a team of people is used, this collaborative effort will enhance communication strategies.

Leaders must have consistency between words and actions. Using terminology such as "we" instead of "I" will recognize the value of each person as a contributing member of the team. Develop a cohesive culture and focus on systems instead of individual mistakes made by people. Place the customer at the forefront. Mutual support and consistency will provide an enlightened culture that will allow supportive communication opportunities.

Enhance communication through storytelling. Think about the people on your team and the emotions you experience when you're with each team member. What tools are available to help you work more productively with each member and with the team as a whole? The practice of storytelling is an effective tool leaders can use; however, the stories must be picked carefully to match the situation. Analysis can intrigue the minds, but storytelling can activate the emotions of the heart. Storytelling can turn a list of dry numbers into an inviting picture of the communication. It's important to make the story concise in a matter of *seconds*, not minutes.

There are a variety of storytelling techniques used to achieve goals. Storytelling can spark action and help to provide information for various learning styles. Communicate the complex nature of the change and inspire skeptical team members to carry them out. Tell a story based on an actual event. A recent event will be more realistic. This springboard story can provide a picture for the listener to accept the need for change and to act. Of course, there must be a happy ending. The story needs enough detail to be credible but not so much as to overwhelm or bore the listener. For example, if you want to use a new piece of equipment or technology, tell a story about successful implementation and outcomes using the equipment elsewhere.

People need to trust you. Tell them who you are, where you have come from, and why you hold the views that you do. Generally, this type of story gives some strength and vulnerability to who you are as a person. This type of story may entail more detail so make sure enough time is allowed for the narrative. The story may be used to communicate values, similar to a parable. The story is generally from the past. Facts may be hypothetical but need to be believable. For example, a story of how certain company (or jobs) went by the wayside when it couldn't provide new products for a new set of circumstances is a story most employees could relate to.

The grapevine is often an inaccurate version of storytelling. Consider harnessing the grapevine to defuse a rumor. The grapevine story highlights the disconnect between the rumor and reality. Work with, not against, the underground network.

Often knowledge is not written down but is stored in someone's head. Knowledge stories are about a problem, setting, and solution, and how and why it was resolved. Include a description of the problem, including how and why the problem got to where it is. This can be a challenge because people don't like to admit mistakes. Focus on the systems and how they can be improved.

The leader must prepare people for the future. A story can help take people from where they are now to where they need to be. The challenge is to tell a narrative that is credible and believable. Listeners should be able to remember the story, and it should portray the situation in a positive way. Show people where to aim instead of what to avoid. Hearing a story about what happened elsewhere can help workers prepare for the future.[6]

Word of mouth is powerful. Ideas, behaviors, and messages are transmitted just like an epidemic. There are no rules. Little changes can have big effects.

We need to match the tone to the message. For example, if we are communicating good news, the tone is far more vibrant and energetic than if we are communicating bad news.

Our voice is quieter and we carefully choose the right words. Word-of-mouth communication multiplies with inconsistencies every time the message is repeated.

Corporate culture and communication can spread through a team very much like an epidemic. The challenge is to provide a positive epidemic that is of interest to all.

The role of internal communication is at the heart of any change process. Communication and timelines are needed in all messages. It is important to support internal communications with simple key messages and role modeling. The person communicating the message must provide a supportive and positive environment and consistent messaging. Don't be afraid to overcommmunicate. Consistency is the key.

Truly changing corporate culture can take years. A consistent message that identifies short- and long-term goals, successes, and celebration can provide a supportive structure for corporate change and consistent communication. Table 3.8 lists the lessons one can learn regarding cultural change and communication.

Technology can support communication and change. Are there newsletters, bulletin boards, paycheck stuffers, or information question and answer opportunities to reinforce the key messages.[7]

Today's organizations are moving away from the "3 Rs"—*restructuring, rightsizing, and reengineering*—and moving to the "3Cs"—*culture, communication, and competencies.*[8] The key to making change is people, not structure. Structural changes can provide increased productivity, higher quality, and increased customer service.

Table 3.8 Lessons Learned on Cultural Change and Communication

1. The vision must be shared and supported by the top.
2. Develop a clear, simple message.
3. Establish the reason for change.
4. Establish the sense of urgency.
5. What is the long-term identity of the change?
6. Establish a strategy.
7. Be consistent.
8. Empower others.
9. Leaders must be change role models.
10. Create short-term wins and celebrate.

However, people create the culture and give and receive communication. Organizations don't create culture and communication; people do. As a result, organizations are starting to more strategically manage human capital more srategically. Engaged and committed employees result in increased productivity, quality, recruitment, and retention of employees.

Employers are creating new ways of working, such as job sharing, flexible work schedules, telecommuting, and team scheduling. This flexibility creates new opportunities to redefine corporate culture and communication methods. Communication is more open and honest and is both upward and downward. Clear and frequent communication from the top makes employees feel included in the process. By understanding the goals, employees realize reasons for change and how they can best contribute.

Competencies

Employers are finding that matching the skill sets and strengths of the employee supports a high-performing corporate culture. Each team member within the same job description has individual strengths. The savvy leader will hone those strengths and provide opportunities for developing the weaker areas of performance. By shifting the focus from the job to the person, employers rely upon **competencies** to ensure quality and consistency. Competencies include knowledge, applied skills, abilities, and behaviors of the employee that are essential to perform the work. These competencies can be used to help employees understand the corporate strategy and goals and to communicate how goals will be achieved. In today's flattened hierarchy in the workplace, competencies allow employees to complete additional competencies to advance in the organization. Competencies can be used in foodservice to increase an employee's skill set to provide a platform for qualifying for another position. Competencies create a sense of ownership and provide flexibility. Respect for the individual is demonstrated through appropriate training and mentoring. A survey of more than 1,000 North American organizations done by Watson Wyatt found that competency-based departments outperformed those without competencies. Those that used competencies had a 36% lower turnover rate and a higher productivity rate by 43%.[8] Table 3.9 delineates competent communication structure.

Table 3.9 Communication Structure

Find a method that works for you in your organization. There is no one approach.

- Know your industry, benchmark best practices.
- Understand the demographics of your work force. What is important to them?
- Tailor your communication specifically to each demographic group.
- Clearly communicate the reasons for change, expectations, and accountability.
- Seek input and make adjustments frequently. Consistency is important.
- Keep it simple.
- Cleary describe assumptions, never assume.
- Speak a common language.
- Discuss resources.
- Identify priorities.
- Monitor performance.

Compiled by the author from: The high performing organization. *Harvard Business Review*, July–August 2005, pp. 64–72.

At some point in time, every team struggles and encounters a rough patch due to employee changes, facility challenges, or a major project. What do you do when your back is against the corporate wall? The rule in communication is to assume that you have been misunderstood. Refrain from using words such as "fault," "blame," or "failure." Of utmost importance is to check with listeners and ask them to repeat key points from what they think you said. Develop **alliance**. Remind employees of the goal at hand and what's in it for them. Analyze the situation and ask: "What's possible? What's missing? What's next? What does the grapevine say?" Defuse your hot buttons. Everyone has them, and they're different for each individual. Keep your cool. A person who values autonomy and independence might have a difficult time working for a micromanager. Some individuals need to receive regular and frequent thanks and appreciation. If someone seems to be avoiding you, consider what behavior you may be displaying that is causing avoidance.

When things get tough, generate several options and potential solutions. Get help. Most organizations have a human resources or education department that can provide another person outside the department to facilitate the process or issues at hand. Watch your language. Be positive and build hope even in a bad situation. One thing you can control when circumstances are challenging is your conversation. Think before you speak. Questions can be intimidating. Why did this happen? Who was there? Neutral language such as using "what" and "how" instead of "who" and "why" can help provide background information. Turn misinterpretation into communication. People make speak figuratively, and the listener may interpret literally. Ask, "what did you hear me say?"[9]

Don't get so tangled up in the web of blame that nothing gets done. Employees respect that someone at the top is willing to tell the truth. Only by using the truth can deep-rooted problems be identified and resolved. Why are organizations afraid to admit problems? Several dynamics work together to create cultures of misinformation and unproductive speculation. Too much distance between the top and the people who are closest to the work invites a gap in communication, leading to half-truths and avoiding difficult topics.

Leaders assume that employees should be spared from "management issues." In addition, people don't like to admit mistakes, and many bosses feel that they are expected to know all the answers. In the face of uncertainty, most managers are too busy to explain the situation to every employee. They believe that employees trust that management knows what it is doing. This lack of information does not build trust, and a negative interpretation of the situation will arise. Because no one feels free to talk about the situation, the culture becomes poisoned with speculation, blame, or self-protecting and defensive behavior.

Graham is convinced this negative culture can be overturned, and a culture of honesty can be built.[10] The quickest way to get honesty is to reverse the top-down communication structure physically, visibly, and immediately. Conducting expensive by-the-book employee surveys is the worst thing a company can do in this situation. Instead, assign a coach who has been trained to ask questions and gather specific information from the workers about the leadership openness and honest communication. The coach is also trained to ask probing questions to find out specifics that help to sort out vague complaints from facts. "Did the managers keep their office door open?" "Did they talk to employees by name and in the hallways?" "Did they listen and respond genuinely to concerns?" "Was the manager hard to reach when an employee tried to contact him or her?" "Did they know why the manager was away?" Once a quarter, meet with the coach and receive the information. Here the manager will find out what matters to employees, not what management thinks is important to the employees. For example, it's easy for a manager to be out of the office for work-related issues. To the employee, that may be viewed as the manager losing connections with employees. Consider adding walk-around to the daily schedule. Eat in the cafeteria rather than the office. Hold a brown bag lunch with employees throughout the year so they can voice opinions directly.

In order to solve deep-rooted problems, two things are needed: to be open about the problem and to ask for participation in solving the problem. Managers feel responsible for responding to employee feedback; in addition, employees must feel responsible to help solve the problem. Talk about goals and why they were reached or not reached. Show the summary of the numbers. Talk about what was learned. Answer questions from employees.

One method is to have management ask employees directly for help in solving problems. Lay out the facts. Explain the situation. What are the barriers? Shared experiences can solidify the culture of honesty. Telling stories of challenging experiences can provide a framework for a challenging issue. Stories of difficulty remind employees that they have the ability to make a difference and that management can support them in unusual ways. New employees find that storytelling is a valuable way to learn the culture of the organization. Rituals can also help to reinforce the culture. Shared experiences can be serious or humorous. Being honest doesn't mean you need to talk about every issue. Honesty dictates that you mean what you say and do what you say you're going to do. Own up to any mistakes. This pays dividends, and employees will do the same.[10]

Communication messages can be organized based on under-standing three basic motivations that determine and guide human behavior:

1. Need for growth. Humans are motivated to learn. Learning gives joy and energy. When a worker is fully challenged, he or she experiences less stress.

2. Need for control. People like to work independently and control their work. The leader can communicate opportunities for control by being clear about goals and letting the worker determine the means to reach the goal. **Coaching** by the manager will help to fill in the gaps of the employee's skills.
3. Need for belonging. Humans are social and need to feel they belong. This gives them a security in their relationships where they both give and receive. The leader should help employees feel they are making a contribution and that they are valued and respected.

Working in teams increases an individual's sense of belonging and leads to better organizational performance, which includes creativity and innovation. Teams will work more effectively if both the team and each individual are clear about the goals. Goals must be negotiated within the team and should be challenged by all members. This produces a stronger end product. Team members need to know they can trust others. This trust allows problems to surface, and improvements can be made.

The skill of **negotiation** is important in any interpersonal communication. Successful negotiation is measured by three criteria:

1. Produce an agreement that meets legitimate interests of each side to the extent possible.
2. Be efficient.
3. Improve or at least not damage the relationship between the parties.

The method of negotiation is as follows:[11]

1. Separate the people from the problem. Think about how the other party perceives the problem, and put yourself in his or her shoes. Detach emotionally.
2. Focus on interests, not positions. The most powerful interests are human needs such as security, economic well-being, a sense of belonging, recognition, and control over one's life.
3. Invent options for mutual gain. Be creative and find new options for a solution. Brainstorm.
4. Insist on using objective criteria. If there is a credible resource that is a best practice or evidence-based, use it. Frame each issue as a search for objective criteria. Establish in advance the

worst-case scenario, and resist pressures to go beyond that pre-determined limit.

The community of culture is strengthened by communication links, both formal and informal, and between different levels of the organization. Good employee management increases productivity and makes a difference. Alienation of people results in negativity and damaged team performance. Trust within a department is complicated by the fact that people refer to the word "trust" in three different ways. Strategic trust is the trust employees have in people at the executive level to make the right decisions. Second is personal trust. Do the managers have vision and competence to pursue the right course and resource allocation? Are employees treated fairly? Do managers consider employees' need when making decisions, and do they put the company's needs ahead of their own desires? Third is organizational trust, which is the level of trust people have in the organization. Are processes well-designed, consistent, and fair? Does the company keep its promises? It is of critical importance to maintain trust within the organization. There is a link between trust and corporate performance. People who trust their management will be able to work through disagreements. They will work harder, longer, contribute better ideas, and dig deep to help the company. If they don't trust the organization and its leaders, they will disengage from the work, believe rumors, participate in office politics, and decrease performance.

Building trust includes consistency, clear communication, and a willingness to tackle difficult questions. In addition, it requires a defensive game. Protect trust from enemies. Because trust can take years to build, it can suffer serious damage in just a moment.

Enemies of trust can be a person, a punishing culture, or broken promises. It could be a person, a supervisor who voices contempt for management, a culture that buries dissent and conflict, layoffs, or inconsistent messages. Inconsistent messages are a fast destroyer of trust and communication. They can occur any time, any place, and in any conversation. For example, a manager tells employees she will meet with them weekly to discuss relevant issues, but then the meeting is cancelled most of the time. Inconsistent standards arise when employees believe that an individual manager or the company plays favorites. When employees do not have all the information, their perception prevails. Misplaced benevolence is demonstrated by the employee who regularly steals, cheats, or humiliates co-workers. It may be difficult to address this behavior because it's difficult to prove. Incompetence is encountered when a person is out of his or her league, leaving everyone amazed at why the person is in the position in the first place. Employees who directly report to that supervisor learn to work around the person and wonder why that person's supervisor doesn't intervene. In essence, incompetence destroys value and all trust.

There are employees who are volatile or just mean. These employees get away with horrible behavior because of their technical competence in some valued area of the company. Typically, they may steamroll colleagues, destroy teamwork, and put their own agendas ahead of the organization's interests. Sometimes this employee can be coached, but sometimes he must be terminated. Troubling behavior sidetracks everyone.

In the work environment, it is important to treat employees like adults. This can be accomplished by sharing data and reasons that make the action necessary. Be cautious about using terms such as "hidden agenda" and "layoffs," and don't tell an employee this is the "hardest thing" you've ever had to do. Many times damage occurs not because of an incident but because of how it's handled internally. People get distracted by external pressure, and they don't address the immediate crisis. Employees need trust and need to have a reason to trust their leaders. They are quick to find reasons why they don't trust management. In times of stress, competent managers feel fragile, overwhelmed, and unable to cope. These feelings makes it difficult to act like a leader. Employees feel this just as much as the manager does. Employees need a calm vision. Don't withdraw. Let employees know that you are aware of the situation and that you will update them as information becomes available. Set a schedule and stick to it even if the news is no news. If you ignore or downplay the situation, employees will be skeptical and suspicious. Choose your words carefully. You don't need to have all the answers. Let people know that you are aware of the issue and its impact on them. Let them know when they will hear more. Figure out what it will take to restore trust. List changes you will make. How will these changes affect employees? What's a reasonable time frame to expect the changes to take place?

Build and maintain trust; restore it when it's damaged. Trust is the crucial ingredient of organizational communication and culture in the hospitality industry. Simply listening and allowing others to speak shows compassion. Every person who works for an organization is an ambassador. People remember how you made them feel.[12]

Summary

The organization and ensuing departments reflect the overall values, belief, mission, vision, and goals through corporate culture and communication. Success can be defined through financial, customer, and employee satisfaction. Communication alone is not enough; all staff must reflect the overall values, beliefs, mission, vision, and goals in everyday conversations and interactions. Without a culture driven by these beliefs, an organization will most likely have unhappy middle managers who do not have a consistent framework for making decisions or consistent communication.

Communication includes using small steps and a vision to grow and adapt to an ever-changing world. It's not one change. It is the continual small changes that contribute to meeting the overall goals that support the vision. Communication can create an environment where change can flourish and build momentum. Communication can include "best practices," case studies, and moments of inspiration and can demonstrate how each individual can contribute. There is no one correct method of communication.

Student Activities

1. Email or telephone a foodservice manager in your city and ask for an example of how communication occurs between management and employees. Based on what you learned in this chapter, analyze the responses.
2. Interview a foodservice employee and ask their perception of departmental communication.
3. Research the phrase "communication style" and report findings that were not covered in this chapter and are applicable to foodservice situations.
4. Research the phrase "corporate culture" and report findings that were not covered in this chapter and are applicable to foodservice situations.

5. Research a "communication theory" and report findings that were not covered in this chapter and are applicable to foodservice situations.

References

1. Dann, M. (2000). *Corporate culture in the new economy.*
2. Charan, R. (2006). Conquering a culture of indecision. *Harvard Business Review,*108–116.
2. Seel, R. (2000). New insights on organizational change. *Organizations and People 7*(2).
3. Flamholtz, E. (2001). Corporate culture and the bottom line. *European Management Journal, 19*(3), 268–275.
4. Heller, R. (2006). *Communication skills: The art of coaching and motivation.* Retrieved March 2006 from http://www.thinkingmanager.com/.
5. Jandeska, K. & Kraimerk, M. (2005). Women's perceptions of organizational culture, work attitudes, and role-modeling behaviors. *Journal of Management Issues, XVII* (4), 461–467.
6. Denning, S. (2004). Telling tales. *Harvard Business Review.*
7. Galford, R. & Drapeau, A. (2003). The enemies of silence. *Harvard Business Review.*
7. (2003). *SCM, 7*(2).
8. O'Dannell, E. (1999). *Benefits Quarterly,*18–25.
9. Hood, S. (2004). Monkey business. *Canadian Business, 77*(16), 83–85.
10. Graham, G. (2002). If you want honesty, break some rules. *Harvard Business Review,* 42–47.
11. Fisher, R. & Ury, W. (1991). *Getting to yes: Negotiation agreement without giving in* (2nd ed.). New York: Penguin Books.
11. The high performing organization. (2005). *Harvard Business Review,* 64–72.
12. Bogoroch-Dikofsky, M. (2005). The bounds of silence. *Canadian Business,78*(10),189–193.

## CHAPTER 4

NEW MARKETING TRENDS IN FOOD AND NUTRITION SERVICES

Nancie H. Herbold, EdD, RD, LD and Paul N. Taylor, PhD

Reader Objectives

After reading this chapter and reflecting on the contents, the reader will be able to:

1. Compare and contrast simple marketing, business marketing, and social marketing.
2. List and define the four Ps of marketing and some additional Ps of social marketing.
3. Discuss types of market research and how these can be used in preparing a plan for food and nutrition services.
4. Compare and contrast the ethics of business marketing and social marketing.

Key Terms

Branding: a collection of images and ideas representing an economic producer; more specifically, it refers to the concrete symbols such as a name, logo, slogan, and design scheme.

Business marketing: the practice of organizations, including commercial businesses, governments and institutions, facilitating the sale of their products or services to other companies or organizations that in turn resell them, use them as components in products or services they offer, or use them to support their operations.

Caveat emptor: a Latin term meaning "let the buyer beware." A legal maxim stating that the buyer takes the risk regarding quality or condition of the property purchased, unless protected by warranty.

Consumer sovereignty: the principle that assumes that consumers dictate the types, quality, and quantity of the goods and services provided.

Continuous quality improvement: an approach to quality improvement in which past trials of change are used as the basis of future trials and something is always being tested for its effects on improvement.

External secondary data: data obtained from outside the firm.

Formative evaluation: method of judging the worth of a program while the program activities are forming or happening.

Internal data: data generated by an organization's operations, such as sales and purchase orders, inventory transactions, etc., instead of being provided from a third party study or database.

Qualitative: relating to quality or kind.

Quantitative: involving the measurement of quantity or amount.

Simple marketing: communication about a product or service for which the purpose is to encourage recipients of the communication to purchase or use the product or service.

Social marketing: the application of commercial marketing concepts and techniques to target populations to achieve the goal of positive social change.

Summative evaluation: a method of judging the worth of a program at the end of the program's activities.

Marketing Defined

The opening years of the twenty-first century clearly indicated that foodservice managers and dietitians must understand the nuances of marketing and how its concepts are used, not only to promote their businesses, but also to counter messages that may not be in the best interests of the public concerning health. The obesity crisis, as well as other concerns, should not be ignored by those who market food in the United States. For example, one would be hard pressed to find My Pyramid (www.mypyramid.gov) explained in a television or newspaper advertisement, but it is easy to find examples of marketing for weight loss supplements, meal replacements, and "low-carb" foods.

Relatively recently, health careprofessionals and organizations realized the value of marketing to reach desired objectives. The dietitian, as an important member of the health care team, must understand the power and value of marketing as a tool and use marketing concepts to inform and educate the public as part of effective food and nutrition services.

How, then, does one define marketing, keeping in mind the need for promoting good health? The National Public Health Leadership Institute provides this comprehensive definition:

> "Marketing" can denote a continuum of efforts and activities ranging from simple "marketing" to the more complex "media advocacy;" each form of marketing involves a relationship and two-way interaction between the marketer and those to whom the marketing is being directed. "**Simple marketing**" involves targeted communication of information based on audience research. "**Social marketing**" aims to create attitudinal and/or behavioral change in a target audience by emphasizing relevant benefits to that audience. "**Branding**" strives to define and establish a positive image or impression for a product via a linked association with a visual or auditory cue that will, when re-experienced, stimulate a quick, almost hard-wired short-cut reminder of the positive value of the product. "Media advocacy" is a strategy designed to bring about a political action and/or policy change through the reframing of issues in mass media.[1]

In this chapter we will focus on social marketing, although other forms of marketing will be mentioned. We should also distinguish between traditional, or **business marketing**, and social marketing.

Business Marketing versus Social Marketing

A practical definition of business marketing is given by Pride and Ferrell:

> The process of creating, distributing, promoting, and pricing goods, services, and ideas to facilitate satisfying exchange relationships with customers in a dynamic environment.[2]

In business marketing, therefore, an exchange of goods or services occurs between a buyer and a seller such that both buyer and seller are satisfied. The dynamic environment in which these exchanges occur consists of uncontrollable forces (consumers, competition, the economy, politics, government, the media, and technology) that affect the marketing mix. Because the marketing environment is dynamic, the most successful marketers continuously evaluate their marketing plans and change them as necessary to ensure that their product is available at the right time, in the right place, at an acceptable price.

Social marketing, when introduced in 1971, was defined as:

> the design, implementation, and control of programs calculated to influence the acceptability of social ideas and involving considerations of product planning, pricing, communication, distribution, and marketing research.[3]

More recently, Andreasen described social marketing as:

> the application of commercial marketing technologies to the analysis, planning, execution, and evaluation of programs designed to influence the voluntary behavior of target audiences in order to improve their personal welfare and that of their society.[4]

These definitions should describe the activities of food entrepreneurs and dietitians who desire to change food choices and eating behaviors among their constituents. Whereas, business marketing focuses on maximizing organizations' profits by fulfilling customers' needs and desires, social marketing focuses on benefiting the target audience and the general society by influencing social behaviors.[5]

Andreasen[6] proposes six benchmarks to identify approaches that could be legitimately called social marketing:

1. Interventions are designed and evaluated using behavior change as a benchmark.
2. For all projects, formative research is conducted to understand the target market, intervention elements are pretested before implementing, and interventions are monitored as they are introduced.
3. Resources are used to maximum efficiency and effectiveness by carefully segmenting target audiences.

4. Influence strategies are designed to create attractive, motivational exchanges with target audiences.
5. All four Ps of the traditional marketing mix are considered in developing strategy: create attractive benefit packages (products); minimize costs (price); make the exchange convenient and easy (place); and communicate powerful messages through media appropriate to the target audiences (promotion).
6. The competition likely to be faced by the desired behavior is anticipated and accounted for in the program strategy.

In the 30+ years since the advent of social marketing, there have emerged two separate lines of thought regarding its definition. Thus, a dietitian implementing a program to inform the public about the role of trans fatty acids in the prevention of heart disease is following the premise of Kotler and Roberto: social marketing programs are "aimed at increasing the acceptability of a social idea or practice in one or more groups of target adopters."[7] In contrast, the "5 A Day" campaign, a joint venture between the National Cancer Institute (NCI) and the Produce for a Better Health Foundation that encourages the public to eat five servings of fruits and vegetables per day, is following Andreasen's premise that the ultimate objective should be behavior change in the target population.[6,8,9] In the foodservice industry, a restaurant can elect to use monounsaturated oil in cooking, offer more healthy foods, and reduce portion sizes for a target population.

> **Learning Point:** The use of social marketing to develop a business plan requires commitment from top-level management, adequate funding and personnel, marketing skills, and vision.

As with any business or nutrition program, the foundation of marketing is thorough research, beginning with defining the goal or problem. Once data have been collected and analyzed, recommendations can be made to form the outline of the program and to delineate the marketing plan.

Marketing Research

Marketing research is necessary to plan, develop, and implement a successful marketing program for an organization. Market research begins with defining the goal or problem and gathering data to understand all aspects. Data will consist of both objective and subjective information. Marketing research provides information on the knowledge, beliefs, attitudes, wants, and practices of the targeted population necessary to develop strategies.[10] The better the problem is understood, the greater the likelihood of developing a successful plan.

Secondary Data

Secondary data include information collected by other groups and agencies. Health and sales indicators collected by the federal government, such as the National Health and Nutrition Examination Survey, is one example of secondary data. Private polling data collected by organizations such as AC Nielsen and the Roper Center may also be helpful. There are many helpful Web sites for data collection; some are listed in Table 4.1.

Secondary data collected within an organization is referred to as **internal data**. The number of patients who visit the nutrition cardiac program or customers who frequent a restaurant, costs of the services, and popular days and times for services are all considered internal secondary data. In contrast, the data collected by an outside entity are regarded as **external secondary data**. It is important to gather as much secondary data as possible to save time, effort, and money.

A review of the professional literature is an important part of collecting information. This review can provide clarity on the problem and uncover successful and unsuccessful approaches to the same or similar problems. A literature review can also lead to helpful Web sites. For example, Project LEAN (Leaders Encouraging Activity and Nutrition) and Team Nutrition both address the issue of healthy eating and physical activity in school children. The Web sites provide background information and examples of activities used in these programs.[11,12] The literature discusses details of the programs and provides authors' names and affiliations, making it easy to contact someone for additional information. The review of the literature can also uncover food, nutrition, and health trends, such as the increase in consumer use of fortified foods,[13] attention to body image prompting adherence to low-fat diets,[14] and increased fish consumption to aid heart disease prevention.[15]

Table 4.1 Helpful Web Sites

www.eatright.org	American Dietetic Association
www.apha.org	American Public Health Association
www.diabetes.org	American Diabetes Association
www.americanheart.org	American Heart Association
www.marketingpower.com/	American Marketing Association
www.social-marketing.org	Social Marketing Institute
www.restaurant.org	National Restaurant Association
www.fao.org	Food and Agriculture Organization
www.ift.org	Institute of Food Technologists
www.who.org	World Health Organization
www.cdc.gov	Centers for Disease Control and Prevention
socialmarketing-nutrition .ucdavis.edu/	Center for Advanced Studies in Nutrition and Social Marketing
www.cdc.gov/mmwr Report	Morbidity and Mortality Weekly
www.cdc.gov/nchs	National Center for Health Statistics
www.census.gov	National Census Bureau
www.phli.org	National Public Health Leadership Institute
www.fda.gov	Food and Drug Administration
www.fedstats	Fedstats
www.hhs.gov	Department of Health and Human Services
www.usda.gov	U.S. Department of Agriculture
www.healthstats.gov	Healthstats
www.ropercenter.uconn.edu	Roper Center

Data can also be gathered from trade association research. The National Restaurant Association (NRA) collects information on food eaten away from home and the latest trends on new foods, diners' preferences, and spending patterns. Forty-two percent of the household food dollar is spent on food away from home, and August is the most popular month to eat out, according to information retrieved from the NRA website.[16] *American Demographics* and *Brandweek* are other sources of information on consumer trends and buying practices.[17] *Brandweek,* for instance, reports women were targeted with an advertising campaign for a new cereal forti-fied with nutrients and vitamins (Harmony™) that described the product as a "support system for women."[18] After gathering the sec-ondary data, the foodservice manager/dietitian should assess what is lacking. Once gaps in the collected secondary data are identified, primary data collection should begin.

Primary Data

Primary data include information collected from focus groups, observations, mail or telephone surveys, interviews, etc. Primary data help to focus the problem and define targeted audiences. For example, after interviewing mothers with young children, it was discovered that fresh fruit was not being offered to children at home. The parents did not lack knowledge about the health benefits of fruits and vegetables, but the local supermarket had closed recently. Parents now shopped at a local convenience store where only a limited variety of fresh produce was available and was more expensive than what had been available at the supermarket.

Qualitative and Quantitative Data

Primary information includes **qualitative** and **quantitative** data. Qualitative data are usually small samples of the targeted group and frequently use open-ended questions in focus group formats, or in-depth interviews with key informants to obtain knowledge about the problem. Key informants are individuals who are knowledgeable

Learning Point: Collecting primary data can provide insight on the attitudes, beliefs, and consequent nutrition, health, and eating behaviors of a population. For example, if a cultural group believes in the humoral theory of health, where illnesses are classified as either "hot" or "cold" and remedies and food are classified into the same two categories, a "hot" illness needs to be treated with a "cold" remedy to bring the body into balance.[19] A person ill with a cold might not be willing to consume orange juice because orange juice is classified as a "cold" food by humoral theory health practi-tioners.[20]

about the targeted population and can provide insight and history on the specific problem. Because of the small sample size, the results cannot be generalized to the larger target population. Stakeholders (owners, board members, prominent community leaders) should also be interviewed. They are individuals who are interested in addressing the goal.

Formative evaluation uses qualitative data to help understand attitudes, beliefs, and perceptions. Formative evaluation is undertaken during the development of a marketing program. It includes pre-testing of ideas and materials, allowing for revisions prior to implementing the full business or program.[21]

Quantitative data are objective indices from a selected sample where results are expressed in numerical terms. As an example of quantitative data, Yussman reported that "17% of adolescents and children reported using herbal remedies."[22] Both qualitative and quantitative data are used in the planning of social marketing strategies.

Market Segmentation

Market segmenting is used to target a social marketing strategy to a particular group. Rather than apply the "average" approach where mean age, income, and education are used to produce an "average American,"[23] market segmenting more narrowly focuses on groups, such as Latina-American women, adolescents, urban dwellers, etc.

Market segmentation is based on:

- Demographics: age, race, gender, income, education, etc.
- Geographics: country, state, urban/rural, climate
- Psychographics: attitudes, values, beliefs, personality traits
- Behavioral: desired benefits, usage

It is important in marketing to consider the multicultural nature and beliefs of our society and the media habits of the various ethnic groups.[24] Even when a market is targeted to Asian-Americans, you may want to subdivide this market even further. For example, is the population you want to reach Chinese-American or Vietnamese-American? Both groups share many cultural values, but there are differences as well. Most Asian cultures are rooted in Confucianism, where deferring to the father/husband and holding elders in high esteem is part of the Confucian practice.[25, 26] However, the extent to which these behaviors and cultural norms are practiced may be influenced by how long the group has lived in the United States, income level, and education (Table 4.2).

Age can also be a factor when segmenting a market. Different generations have different identifying characteristics. For example, adults over the age of 45 have an increase in alcohol consumption at dinner because of their exposure to the message that alcohol may decrease heart disease.[28] Children are another segmented market, one with influence on purchasing decisions. For example, 40% of children were considered to have "a lot of influence" on the purchasing of cold cereal.[29] By market segmenting, a customized plan and strategy can be developed that increases the likelihood of yielding greater success.

The Social Marketing Mix

In traditional business marketing, the specific combination of marketing elements used to achieve objectives and satisfy the target

Table 4.2   Selected Socio-demographic Characteristics of the Population 18 Years and Older by Race

Race	Income 3-yr average 2000–2002	Not high school graduate	High school graduate or higher	Less Than Bachelor's some college	Bachelor's degree/ or higher
		Percent	Percent	Percent	Percent
Caucasian	$47,194	16.3	83.7	75.2	24.8
African-American	$29,982	22.4	77.6	85.1	14.9
Hispanic-American	$33,946	42.8	57.2	90.6	9.4
Asian/Pacific Islander-American	$54,999	12.6	87.4	57.4	42.6

Source: www.census.gov/hhes/income/income02/3yr_avg_race.html and www.census.gov/population/socdemo/education/ppl-169/tab01a.pdf.

market is known as the marketing mix. Those variables over which an organization has control include the four Ps of marketing: *product, place, price, and promotion.* [30] Social marketing plans also use the four Ps, and some authors espouse additional Ps for social marketing (*partnership, policy, politics, positioning, publics, and purse strings*).[31-33] These additional Ps, with the possible exception of *positioning,* usually pertain to the uncontrollable variables of the marketing environment. Alcalay and Bell[33] regard "positioning" as "a psychological construct that involves the location of the product relative to other products and activities with which it competes."

Product

In traditional business marketing, the product is a good (tangible), a service, or an idea (intangibles). Nutrition services are usually intangible, such as distributing weight control counseling or consulting on developing foodservice menus. Tangible products are restaurant food and services associated with eating out.

In stark contrast to business marketing, the social marketing product may be offered or provided to the customer without considering whether the customer wants or needs the product. For example, patients who are diagnosed with diabetes or cardiovascular disease may be automatically referred for nutrition counseling whether or not they want the service. To overcome reluctance or outright denial of service benefits, the product must be carefully designed, implemented, and followed-up on to maximize the probability of the patient's acceptance of a need for the service and eventual beneficial behavior change.

Product Design

Designing a restaurant or nutrition product or service that will have maximum potential for success requires careful planning. Some of the following factors should be considered:

- Product name, nutrition private practice, or foodservice establishment (establishing a brand)
- Product packaging
- Product differentiation (set product apart from its competitors)
- Product lifetime

- Product flexibility (continually revising to adapt to a changing market environment)

When developing a restaurant or nutrition product/service, include long-range planning to ascertain the probable lifetime of the product. Remember that the marketing environment is dynamic and that today's ideal product may be obsolete in the future due to changes in technology or public interest, for example. Just as the successful business marketer looks beyond the product being designed to forecast future needs and demands of the consumer, so too does the successful social marketer include strategic planning as part of product development. Pretesting the service/product, using a sample of the target market, will provide useful information on the appropriateness of the product's design.

Place

Place denotes the location where tangible goods are offered and also includes the product's distribution system (the channels through which the product is offered to the target market, including storage, transport, sales, and delivery). For intangible products, place may denote the location where a service is offered, including the channels through which the target market will be reached (restaurant, cafeteria, clinics, hospitals, daycare centers, congregate meal sites, shopping malls, etc.). When considering *place*, remember to ensure that the product will be accessible to the target market and to ensure the quality of product delivery.

Price

Price is perhaps the most critical component of the marketing mix for both traditional business and social marketing, because *price* is the component most evident to the consumer in the target market. In business marketing, *price* is often a competitive tool and can assist a business in developing product image.[37] In most cases, business marketers establish a product's price so that the business will profit and the consumer will be happy with the value received. Social marketers are not usually interested in generating a profit (remember that the ultimate objective in social marketing is to effect

> **Learning Point:** Because of the obesity crisis in the United States, some restaurateurs have attempted to combine traditional marketing and social marketing. This combination would allow the marketing of good food and service but would also take into account the need to limit saturated fat and portion size. This is the new challenge for twenty-first century foodservice managers: being profitable while selling meals that are equated with being healthy.

a behavioral change that will benefit the individual, the community, or the society).

Promotion

Promotion is the means to introduce the product to the targeted audience. Promotion involves communicating a message through a variety of mediums to create awareness and promote action. The 5 A Day campaign, for example, is a promotion to encourage the public to eat five or more servings of fruits and vegetables per day. As mentioned earlier, the campaign is a joint venture between the NCI and the industry group, Produce for a Better Health Foundation. The 5 A Day promotion includes a fruit and vegetable of the month with corresponding recipes.[39]

Advertising

Advertising is an important part of a promotional campaign. Advertising can take many different forms, from print to radio to television. Advertising is expensive; therefore, choosing the correct medium is important. *Reach* and *frequency* are important to consider when selecting the advertising medium. Reach refers to the number of people exposed to a message during a given period of time (how many people the message will "reach"). Frequency is the number of times an individual will be exposed to the message.[21] Paying for expensive advertising when it does not reach the targeted audience is a costly mistake. Sometimes, lower-level ad campaigns, such as flyers, are more effective than television advertising. Flyers can saturate a particular neighborhood from bulletin boards, health fair handouts, car windshields (check local ordinances), or packed with groceries at a local supermarket. Advertising of any kind needs to be more than a one-time event.

In the case of social marketing, the targeted population must be reminded of the action to take, and reinforcement is needed for behavior change to occur. Advertising, as part of a social marketing campaign, may promote social/nutritional services such as school breakfast or Meals on Wheels. Table 4.3 outlines a social marketing campaign to increase participation in the School Breakfast Program.[40]

Advertising must be accurate, its message clear and consistent, and the main points repeated. The message must be relevant to the target population. An advertisement can be amusing, frightening, a testimonial, or use a celebrity spokesperson. Whatever tone the advertisement takes must be acceptable to the targeted population.[41]

Public Service Announcements (PSA) are advertisements for a social action or cause. Television and radio stations set aside free airtime for PSAs to meet Federal Communications Commission requirements. However, most PSAs are aired during non-primetime hours, limiting the reach of the PSA.[42]

Web Sites

How do you get consumers to use Web sites? Web sites can be referenced in your print advertisements or your radio and television PSAs. Consumers should be given the site's Uniform Resource Locator (URL) so that they may log on to the Web site for more information. If a consumer has not seen your promotional materials, but uses the Internet to find information, the dietitian or health organization needs to make sure that the Web site is included in the major search engines' referencing systems. A fee will be charged by a search engine for a business or organization to be included in its database.[43] Some search engines do not charge to be in their database but do charge for a primary position. For example, where a URL appears in a search engine's results is important. Is the Web site the first one listed or the fiftieth? How many times a Web site is visited ("hits") is valuable information and should be tallied using readily available automatic counters.

Table 4.3 The Campaign

The Food for Thought campaign uses a cost-effective combination of live delivery, publicity, public relations, and advertising techniques to maximize the potential for exposure and success. This richly interdependent mix is best represented as follows:

Audience	Students	Parents	Education Professionals
Message to each audience	"Breakfast at school is cool."	"Your child needs breakfast."	"Your students will do better if they eat breakfast."
Live Delivery Formats to Launch Campaign	• "Kickoff" Assembly • Give out Healthy Breakfast Pack (mini-box cereal, fruit, juice, nutrition tips booklet, bulletin for parents) • Jump Rope Demo/Contest • Health Teacher speaks	• PTO Meeting • Show samples of Healthy Breakfast Pack • Walk-thru nutrition tips & bulletin info • Give out new applications for $ aid	• Teachers' Meeting • School Committee Meeting • Show samples of Healthy Breakfast Pack • Give out educators' flyer & discuss points therein
Publicity	Poster • in schools • in libraries, civic centers • in city stores	Poster • in supermarkets • in libraries, • civic centers & in city stores	Poster • in schools • in libraries • in city stores

continues

Table 4.3   *(continued)*

Audience	Students	Parents	Education Professionals
Public Relations Activities	• TV PSAs (network & cable) • Radio PSAs • School newspaper articles (where available)	• TV & Radio Talk Shows • TV PSAs (network & cable) • Radio PSAs • Newspaper articles	• TV & Radio Talk Shows • TV PSAs (network & cable) • Radio PSAs • Newspaper articles
Advertising Activities	• :30 TV Spot (cable) • :60 Radio Spot • Print ad in school newspaper	• :30 TV Spot (cable) • :60 Radio Spot • Print ad	• :30 TV Spot (cable) • :60 Radio Spot • Print ad

Source: Massachusetts Department of Education, 1993.

The following steps are suggested for Internet marketing:

- Acquire a domain name
- Build a Web site
- Put the Web site on the server
- Promote the site
- Update the site[43]

Public Relations

Public relations are a means to gather free publicity for your product, business, service, or idea. Public relations are a valuable component of a marketing campaign. Although publicity is free, time and materials are not. It is important to develop publicity objectives for guidance to advance your marketing agenda. Examples of public relations that can garner restaurant publicity include:

- Fairs and community gatherings
- Events (walkathons, road races, golf tournaments)
- Food contests, such as cook-offs, cooking demonstrations, and taste testings

Other means to achieve publicity objectives for a dietitian's services may include:

- Public speaking at community events, schools, senior centers
- Writing nutrition columns for local newspapers
- Providing short nutrition messages for local radio stations
- Acting as a nutrition resource expert for the media on late-breaking nutrition news[44]

Evaluation

An important component of any marketing effort is evaluation and how to estimate success. Evaluation is an ongoing process and should not be left until the entire project is complete. Evaluation should start with the inception of the idea and the problem to study. The following questions are important to consider at the beginning of the evaluation process:

- How do we define the goal/problem?
- What are our objectives?
- Who is the market we want to reach?

- What information do we have about the target market?
- What is our message?
- What communication media will we use?
- Will it be cost-effective?
- What is the timing?
- How will we measure our goals and objectives?
- How will we evaluate the marketing program?[45]

There are three types of evaluation to consider when assessing your marketing campaign: *formative evaluation, process evaluation,* and *outcome evaluation.*

Formative Evaluation

Formative evaluation begins during the development of the marketing program and helps to define the problem and to refine possible interventions. It includes pretesting of ideas, procedures, and materials, and using focus groups, surveys, and interviews.[21] For example, you may ask, "Did the target market understand the PSA message?" "Was the print material at a readability level appropriate to the audience?" "Was the action requested of the target market realistic?" This type of information allows revisions to be made before the full marketing program is implemented.

Process Evaluation

Process evaluation assesses the implementation of the social marketing program. Did the plan proceed as outlined? Did the PSA air during the appropriate month? Were print materials delivered in adequate quantities to the correct locations? Are activities occurring according to schedule? Did the program reach the target market?[21] Process evaluation uses **continuous quality improvement** (CQI) to monitor progress. CQI is a tool that is constructed on the premise that there is always room for improvement.[46] Customers are asked how satisfied they are with the services, materials, venues, and costs associated with a program. CQI has been used in health care, including nutrition services, since the 1990s.[47-50]

Outcome Evaluation

Outcome evaluation (sometimes referred to as **summative evaluation**) determines whether the goals and objectives of the social marketing campaign are met.[21] It is important that the goals and objectives are well-defined at the inception of the social marketing process; otherwise it is difficult to measure the success of meeting them. Goals and objectives should be specific in order for them to be evaluated effectively. An example of an objective that can be measured is: "20% of the target audience/market will increase fruit and vegetable consumption by 1 serving within 3 months of initiating the campaign."

Marketing Ethics

The opening years of the twenty-first century were marked by several major business scandals in the United States and other countries.[51-54] In this climate, it is important to revisit the topic of business ethics, in general, and of marketing ethics, in particular.

Whether engaging in business or social marketing, the marketer must begin with a strong code of personal ethics. With a good sense of the moral principles and values that govern individual and group behavior within a society, one can reliably choose the right and just action when faced with a moral dilemma. Ethics courses may be found in colleges and universities, and ethics may be incorporated into the curriculum in elementary and high schools. However, the elementary school curriculum is not consistent across the country, and there is debate about the best approach for teaching ethics, otherwise known as "building character,"[55] as well as debate over where and when ethics can be taught. Many believe that codes of personal ethics are already formed by the time a person enters college,[56] and there is evidence that geographic and cultural variables affect the process.[57, 58] Others hold that ethics can be taught at the college level.[59, 60] It is evident that the process of ethical development is multifactorial and that some elements of truth may be found in each of the disparate views.

Kerin and colleagues[61] hold that in marketing, ethics are concerned with personal morals and values in juxtaposition with organizational, legal, and societal morals and values. Situations present themselves in an ethical, legal matrix in which technically legal actions could be viewed as unethical or in which ethical actions may not be seen as legal. In such an environment, the dietitian must learn to think and plan like a marketer, under the guidance of personal ethics informed by sociocultural, business/industry, and corporate ethical guidelines.

Traditional business ethics in the last century were largely guided by the principle of **caveat emptor** (the principle in commerce that the buyer *alone* is responsible for assessing the quality of a purchase before buying). By the 1990s, consumer interests had overtaken those of business, ushering in an era of "**consumer sovereignty**," which eludes to the power consumers have in directing market economies because goods and services are produced and exchanged mostly to satisfy consumer desires.[62] Although exceptions exist, today most traditional business marketing ethics are guided by the principle that the customer's wants and needs are paramount and profit-generating activities are aimed at customer satisfaction. Social marketers, too, are focused on the customer, but with the ultimate aim of improving their personal welfare and that of their society.[4] Thus, the social marketer faces ethical challenges that are not seen in traditional business marketing, challenges that are only now being identified and studied.[63] As the dimensions of marketing ethics in both traditional business and social marketing contexts are explored and debated, the dietitian, drawing on a strong personal code of ethics, will do well to follow the guidelines of the American Dietetic Association's Code of Ethics.[64]

In closing this overview of marketing ethics, we must point out that many of the ethical dilemmas that a public health dietitian is likely to face will arise from cultural differences between the dietitian and the client or the population being served. The United States is a multicultural land with minority ethnic populations from most parts of the world. When serving those whose ethnic backgrounds are different from yours, make an effort to understand the societal culture and norms that govern them and underlie the prevailing U.S.

Truth in Menu Law

A part of marketing ethics is the *Truth in Menu Law*. This means that foodservice managers cannot misrepresent menu items. The law was designed to protect consumers from fraudulent food and beverage claims and is currently overseen by dozens of agencies and administrative entities. The key is honesty in menu claims, both with regard to the price that is charged and the food that is served.

societal culture and norms. When entering into partnerships with multinational or global organizations, be sure to consider the often extreme differences in marketing ethics of the cultures represented.[65-70]

Student Activities

1. Discuss how a dietitian should approach partnerships with multinational, fast food, and toy companies to promote healthful eating practices for children.
2. Design a pretest instrument or program for a new nutrition service, food product, or business.
3. Research some examples of social marketing that exist in foodservice promotions.
4. Research restaurant menus that include social marketing.
5. Research restaurant menus and how the Truth in Menu Law was demonstrated.
6. Give several examples of how the 4 Ps have been used for a restaurant business.
7. Give an example of how the 4 Ps have been used for a dietitian's private practice.
8. Give an example of how the 4 Ps have been used for a clinic or nonprofit business.
9. Discuss a possible moral or ethics dilemma that can exist in wanting business for a restaurant and marketing language.
10. Discuss a possible moral or ethics dilemma that can exist in wanting business for a private practice or nutritional food product and marketing language.

References

1. National Public Health Leadership Institute. (2002). Retrieved June 7, 2004, from http://www.phli.org:9018/Marketingconference/.
2. Pride, W. M. & Ferrell, O.C. (2003). *Marketing: Concepts and strategies* (12th ed.). Boston, MA: Houghton Mifflin.
3. Kotler, P. & Zaltman, G. (1971). Social marketing: An approach to planned social change. *Journal of Marketing, 35*(5).
4. Andreasen, A.R. (1995). *Marketing social change: Changing behavior to promote health, social development, and the environment.* San Francisco: Jossey-Bass.

5. Andreasen, A.R. & Kotler, P. (2003). *Strategic marketing for nonprofit organizations* (6th ed.). Englewood Cliffs, NJ: Prentice-Hall.
6. Andreasen, A.R. (2002). Marketing social marketing in the social change marketplace. *Journal of Public Policy and Marketing, 21*(3).
7. Kotler, P. & Roberto, E. (1989). *Social marketing.* New York: The Free Press.
8. Andreasen, A.R. (1994). Social marketing: Definition and domain. *Journal of Public Policy and Marketing, 13*, 108.
9. Maibach, E.W. (2002). Explicating social marketing: What is it, and what isn't it? *Social Marketing Quarterly, 8*, 7.
10. Kotler, P. & Roberto, E. (1989). *Social marketing: Strategies for changing public behavior.* New York: The Free Press.
11. California Department of Health Services. (2004). *California project LEAN: Leaders encouraging activity and nutrition.* Retrieved May 21, 2004, from www.californiaprojectlean.org/programs.
12. U.S. Department of Agriculture, Food, and Nutrition Service. *TEAM nutrition.* Retrieved May 21, 2004, from http://www.fns.usda.gov/tn.
13. Sloan, E.A. (2002). The *top* 10 functional food trends: The next generation. *Food Technology, 56*, 32.
14. Gruber, A.J., Pope, H.G, Jr., Lalonde, J.K., & Hudson, J.I. (2001). Why do young women diet? The roles of body fat, body perception, and body ideal. *Journal of Clinical Psychiatry, 62*, 609.
15. Kris-Etherton, P.M., Harris, W.S. & Appel, L.J. (2002). American heart association nutrition committee: Fish consumption, fish oil, omega-3 fatty acids, and cardiovascular disease. *Circulation, 106*, 2747.
16. National Restaurant Association. Retrieved June 8, 2004, from http://www.restaurant.org.
17. Marconi, J. (2001). *Future marketing.* Chicago: American Marketing Association, NTC Business Books.
18. Reyes, S. (2002). Shopping list: Quick, classic, cool for kids. *Brandweek. 43*, 52.
19. Bogumil, C. (2002). *Humoral theory in cultural food beliefs.* Retrieved June 8, 2004, from http://food.oregonstate.edu/ref/culture/humoral.html.
20. Beijing Medboo Health Center. *Traditional Chinese dietotherapy.* Retrieved June 8, 2004, from http://www.ontcm.com/healthy/foods.htm.
21. U.S. Department of Health and Human Services. (1992). *Making health communication programs work: A planner's guide.* Washington, DC: National Cancer Institute, NIH Pub No. 92-1493.
22. Yussman, S.M, Auinger, P., Weitzman, M. & Ryan, S.A. (2002). Complementary and alternative medicine use in children and adolescents. *Journal of Adolescent Health, 30,* 105.
23. Tharp, M.C. (2001). *Marketing and consumer identity in multicultural America.* Thousand Oaks, CA: Sage Publications.
24. Ibid., 113.
25. Ibid., 263.
26. Wong, A.M. *Target: The U.S. Asian market.* (1997). Palos Verdes, CA: Pacific Heritage.

27. Perez-Escamilla, R., Himmelgreen, D., Bonello, H., Peng, Y. Mengual, G. Gonzalez, A., Mendez, I., Cruz, J., & Phillips, L. (2000). Marketing nutrition among urban Latinos: The !salud! campaign. *Journal of the American Dietetic Association, 100,* 698.

28. Whitaker, L. (1999). A tasty business. *Psychology Today, 32,* 52.

29. Gurber, S. & Berry, J. (1993). *Marketing to and through kids.* New York: McGraw-Hill.

30. Kotler, P. & Turner, R.E. (1995). *Marketing management: Analysis, planning, implementation, and control* (8th ed.). Scarborough, ON: Prentice Hall Canada.

31. Weinreich, N.K. (1995). *Hands-on social marketing: A step-by-step guide.* Thousand Oaks, CA: Sage Publications.

32. Mississippi Urban Research Center, Jackson State University, Southern Prevention Intervention Center. (Fall 2001). What is social marketing? Social marketing tools promote health issues. *Adinkra Newsletter* 2. Retrieved June 8, 2004, from http://www.apinonline.org/Pubs/Newsletters/Adinkra.SPIC-Fall2001Issue2.pdf.

33. Alcalay, R. & Bell, R.A. (2000). *Promoting nutrition and physical activity through social marketing: Current practices and recommendations.* Davis, CA: Center for Advanced Studies in Nutrition and Social Marketing, University of California.

34. Social Marketing Institute. *Success stories: National WIC breastfeeding promotion project.* Retrieved June 9, 2004, from http://www.social-marketing.org/success/cs.

35. U.S. Department of Agriculture, Food, and Nutrition Service. *Fathers supporting breastfeeding.* Retrieved June 9, 2004, from http://www.fns.usda.gov/wic/Fathers/SupportingBreastfeeding.HTM.

36. Szcodronski, H., Dobson, B., Losch, M.E., & Bryant, C. (2002). Iowa's implementation of the WIC national breastfeeding promotion project report and findings. *Loving Support Makes Breastfeeding Work.* Des Moines, IA: Iowa Department of Public Health.

37. Spears, M. (2000). *Foodservice organizations: A managerial and systems approach* (4th ed.). Upper Saddle River, NJ: Prentice-Hall.

38. Weinreich, N.K. (2003). *What is social marketing?* Weinreich Communications. Retrieved May 23, 2004, from http://www.socialmarketing.com/whatis.html.

39. U.S. Department of Health and Human Services. National Cancer Institute. Five a Day Recipe Box. Retrieved June 8, 2004, from http://www.5aday.gov.

40. Massachusetts Department of Education. Food for Thought Campaign. (1993). Get a jump on the day.

41. Baltas. G. (2001). The effects of nutrition information on consumer choice. *Journal of Advertising Research,* 57.

42. Small Business Association. Women's Business Center, Public Service Announcements. Retrieved June 4, 2004, from www.onlinewbc.gov/docs/market/mk_psa pr.html.

43. Marconi, J. (2001). *Future marketing.* Chicago: American Marketing Association, NTC Business Books.

44. Kaufman, M. (1990). *Nutrition in public health.* Rockville, MD: Aspen.
45. McDonald, M.H. & Keegan, W.J. (1997). *Marketing plans that work.* Boston, MA: Butterworth Heinemann Publishers.
46. Leebov, W. & Ersoz, C. (2003). *The healthcare manager's guide to continuous quality improvement.* Lincoln, NE: iUniverse, Inc., Authors Choice Press.
47. McLaughlin, C.P. & Kaluzny, A.D. (1999). *Continuous quality improvement in healthcare: Theory, implementation and applications* (2nd ed.). Boston, MA: Jones and Bartlett Publishers.
48. Knapp, M.L. (1998). Applying continuous improvement to community health. Collaborative effort by the American society for quality and the institute for healthcare improvement identifies components of model for community health improvement. *Quality Progress, 31,* 43.
49. Behrens, R.. & Blocker, A.K. (1993). *Continuous quality improvement and nutritional care planning: A manual for long-term care facilities.* Rockville, MD: Aspen.
50. Jackson, R. (1992). *Continuous quality improvement for nutrition care.* Amelia Island, FL: American Nutri-Tech, Inc.
51. Keeping an eye on business. (2004). *The Economist, 371,* 68.
52. Verschoor, C.C.(2004). Unethical workplace is still with us. *Strategic Finance, 85,* 15.
53. Tsianiar, B. & Shannon, E. (2003). Cooking the books. *Time, 162,* 55.
54. Colvin, G. (2002). Scandal outrage, part III. *Fortune, 146,* 56.
55. Davis, M. (2003). What's wrong with character education. *American Journal of Education, 110,* 32.
56. Carroll, A.B., & Scherer, R.W .(2003). Business ethics in the current environment of fraud and corruption. *Vital Speeches of the* Day, *69,* 529.
57. Mayer, D. (2001). Community, business ethics, and global capitalism. *American Business Law Journal, 38,* 215.
58. Barker, T. S., & Cobb, S.L. (2000). A survey of ethics and cultural dimensions of MNCs. *Competitiveness Review, 10,* 123.
59. Lawson, R.A. (2004). Is classroom cheating related to business students' propensity to cheat in the "real world"? *Journal of Business Ethics, 49,* 189.
60. Alsop, R. (2003). The top business schools (a special report): Right and wrong: Can business schools teach students to be virtuous? In the wake of all the corporate scandals, they have no choice but to try. *Wall Street Journal Eastern ed,* p. R9.
61. Kerin, R.A., Berkowitz, E.N., Hartley, S.W., & Rudelius, W. (2003). *Marketing* (7th ed.). New York: McGraw Hill.
62. Smith, N.C., Lawler III, E.E., & Berndt, E.R. (1995). Marketing strategies for the ethics era. *Sloan Management Review, 36,* 85.
63. Brenkert, G.G. (2002). Ethical challenges of social marketing. Journal of Public Policy and Marketing, *21,* 14.
64. Code of ethics for the profession of dietetics. (1999). *Journal of the American Dietetic Association, 99,* 109.

65. Palazzo, B. (2002). U.S.-American and German business ethics: An intercultural comparison. *Journal of Business Ethics, 41,* 195.
66. Pitta, D.A., & Fung, H-G. (1999). Ethical issues across cultures: Managing the differing perspectives of China and the USA. *Journal of Consumer Marketing, 16,* 240.
67. Singhapakdi, A. & Rawwas, M.Y.A. (1999). A cross-cultural study of consumer perceptions about marketing ethics. *Journal of Consumer Marketing,16,* 257.
68. Taka, I. (1997). Business ethics in Japan. *Journal of Business Ethics, 16,* 1499.
69. Izraeli, D. (1997). Business ethics in the middle east. *Journal of Business Ethics, 16,* 1555.
70. Stajkovic, A.D. & Luthans, F. (1997). Business ethics across cultures: A social cognitive model. *Journal of World Business, 32,* 17.

PART II

HUMAN RESOURCES

## CHAPTER 5

EMPLOYEE DISCIPLINE AND GRIEVANCE PROCESSES AND PRACTICES

Patrice L. Spath, BA, RHIT

Reader Objectives

After studying this chapter and reflecting on the contents, you should be able to:

1. Identify techniques to help people become better employees.
2. Define the positive discipline process.
3. Describe the key elements of effective employee counseling.
4. Identify strategies for minimizing the legal risks associated with employee discipline and termination.
5. Describe the common causes of employee performance problems.

Key Terms

Behavior issues: problems with acting or controlling oneself.

Disciplinary action: reducing, restricting, suspending, or revoking the rights or privileges.

Employee counseling: consists of interviewing and counseling employees by utilizing policies, procedures, and rules concerning grievances, disciplinary actions, performance evaluations, and career development.

Employee performance: the way an employee is accomplishing the goals of the organization, a department, or a service.

Initiate-Focus-Problem-Plan discussion technique: a technique for reducing an employee's defensiveness when approaching him or her about his performance.

Performance feedback: part of a developmental plan to monitor whether the employee is accomplishing the goals of the organization, department, or service.

Performance problems: when an employee is not meeting the minimum standards as outlined in the job description or handbook.

Performance standards: the guidelines which an employee must follow in order to accomplish the goals of the organization, department, or service.

Positive discipline: describes a way to reduce undesirable behavior, and increase desirable behavior, by rewarding the positive rather than punishing the negative.

Progressive degrees of discipline: is a system of discipline where the penalties increase upon repeat occurrences.

Suspension: a temporary debarment (from a privilege or position).

Termination: a coming to an end of a contract period.

Wrongful termination: when an employee is discharged without a proven cause, that employee has the right to sue the employer for damages such as loss of wage and "fringe" benefits, and, under certain circumstances, for punitive damages.

Introduction

People working in foodservice must work together to get the job done. Employees rely on one another for information, supplies, and support. A problem employee creates a weak link that can threaten the quality of services and the safety of coworkers and customers. The longer management tolerates substandard work and negative behaviors in employees, the worse those behaviors tend to become. Worse yet, other employees notice that some people are getting away with things and, in time, everyone begins adjusting their performance downward to the lowest level tolerated. Before long, the majority of employees are simply doing just enough to stay out of serious trouble and collect their paychecks. Even potentially excellent workers function at less than half of their capacity in such an environment. The way to stop this downward spiral is for managers to recognize, confront, and resolve staff performance problems as quickly as possible. Overlooking marginal performance can lead to further declines in performance.

In this chapter you'll learn techniques for avoiding the common causes of poor employee performance and strategies for handling problem situations that require coaching, counseling, or disciplinary action.

Common Employee Problems

Dealing with employee **performance problems** is perhaps the most difficult and unpleasant task that managers must perform. Confronting problematic situations and employees takes time and energy. It may seem easier to just ignore a problem employee. Ignoring situations and employees is not as uncommon as one might think in organizations where firing an employee is a multi-step process. Yet, lack of action sets up everyone for lower performance and creates morale problems. Regardless of how well you manage the people in your department, performance problems will occur from time to time. Some of the more common types of problems are:

- Habitual tardiness
- Missed deadlines
- Doing just enough work to get by
- Frequent errors
- Inability to perform a task, even after repeated training
- Being slower than others when completing tasks
- Avoiding unpleasant jobs

Obvious performance problems, such as an employee showing up for work in an impaired physical state, must be addressed immediately. Passive performance problems, although sometimes more difficult to recognize, must also be addressed. If an employee seems to be having trouble getting the job done or you are receiving complaints about the employee from other staff, look for a pattern:

- Does the employee frequently "forget" policies or procedures?
- Are there regular misunderstandings that get in the way of the job being completed correctly?
- Does the employee continually ignore supervisory directives?

- Is the employee frequently giving reasons why a task cannot be done properly?

Taken case by case, these behaviors may seem inconsequential, but a pattern of such behaviors is a symptom of employee insubordination. It is important that you identify and deal with passive performance problems in the same manner as you would for more obvious problems. Some questions you can ask to help diagnoses employee performance problems are listed in Table 5.1.

Table 5.1   Diagnosing Performance Problems

Questions to Ask

- Does the employee know what is expected of him or her? In exact, non-ambiguous, did-or-didn't, cannot-argue-about-it language?
- Does the employee know the five Ws/two Hs (who, what, when, where, why, how, how much) of performance expectations?
- Can the employee repeat back to you performance expectations, and have you say, "That is right!"
- Does the employee know how well he or she is doing against the performance expectations?
- Is the information about the employee's unwanted conduct accurate (and would everyone agree it is)?
- Is the performance feedback to the employee understandable to him or her?
- Is the performance feedback tied to something over which the employee has control (i.e., personal performance)?
- Does the employee have all the items he or she needs need to do the job?
- Is the environment helping or hindering the employee's performance?
- Are incentives contingent on the employee's performance?
- Are the departmental systems conducive to the employee's good performance?
- Do supervisors support effective employee behavior (through modeling, counseling, etc.)?
- Could the employee do it right for 1 million dollars? (If so, they already have the skills and knowledge—they don't need training.)

Why an employee does not meet **performance standards** can be generally categorized into one or more of four causes:

Cause 1: Standards Are Not Clearly Communicated

It is the manager's job to establish performance standards and communicate these standards to employees on an ongoing basis. Remember to be specific when setting standards. Below is an example of performance standards for a diet technician employed in a residential senior care center. The standards describe clear and specific performance expectations.

- Observe resident food intake and report dietary problems to dietitian.
- Prepare meals, following recipes and determining group food quantities.
- Analyze menus and recipes, standardize recipes, and test new products.
- Assist the dietitian in food service supervision and planning.
- Obtain and evaluate dietary histories of residents to identify special nutritional needs.
- Plan menus for residents with special dietary needs based on established guidelines.

Performance standards should not be simply posted or given to employees. During a new hire's probationary period and at regular performance evaluations, the standards and performance expectations should be reviewed with employees. Make sure employees understand the performance standards for their job. To check if an employee understands the standards, one technique is to simply ask him or her to summarize the expectations. Remember, employees are not mind readers; they may not know what's important or critical. Be sure to prioritize tasks and responsibilities. It is also helpful to communicate the big picture and how the employee fits in it.

Cause 2: Employee Hasn't Received Feedback

All of your staff members need to know on a regular basis how they are doing. Give as much time to praising the good performers as you do to counseling those needing improvement. When an employee excels, even in the smallest ways, point it out. If an employee exhibits poor or marginal performance, don't wait until the next formal evaluation to point out the problem. As close as possible to the poor performance, talk with the employee about the problem and jointly explore ways to correct it.

Cause 3: Employee Lacks Knowledge, Skills, or Resources

An employee's work may be hampered by a lack of knowledge or skills to do the job. This can be especially problematic if the employee is given new job responsibilities or expected to work with new equipment or assist with new procedures. If an employee hasn't been adequately trained on how to do his or her job, it's unlikely he or she can meet performance expectations. Resolving this cause requires providing instruction in how to do the job. Another obstacle may be existing processes, methods, or systems that interfere with the employee's ability to do the job. These underlying root causes must be addressed to lessen the impact on staff job performance.

Cause 4: Motivation and Attitude

If employees have clear and understandable performance standards, know how they are doing, and have been appropriately trained, there may be another reason why an employee isn't meeting performance standards—*his or her motivation or attitude.* To determine if motivation or attitude is a problem, ask yourself, "Has the employee been able to do the job well in the past?" If performance has rarely been a problem, look for other factors.

Whatever the reasons for poor or marginal performance, you need to address problems when they occur. Not addressing the issue sends the message to everyone in the department that the manager doesn't see the performance as a problem. Often, silence is interpreted as condoning the behavior. Managers who want to be seen as nice tend to ignore employee problems. These managers often hope problem employees will improve without any intervention, and when they do not, they drop hints. Instead of *coaching, counseling,* and *terminating* employees who do not improve, some managers ignore the problems or encourage the employee to transfer to another department. What do these managers get for being nice? They lose their employees' respect. Staff members know that their manager is shirking responsibility by not dealing with performance problems.

Because the reasons for employee problems can be broad and varied, and each factor plays on the others, the exact cause may at first be hard to see. But, whatever the cause, the good news is that most times it is curable. Feedback, coaching, and counseling, as well as performance evaluations, are tools managers can use to correct poor performance. All employees should be receiving ongoing *feedback* and *coaching* throughout the year as a regular part of their performance cycle. If, after feedback and coaching, the employee is still performing below expectations, the manager should move to counseling.

Learning Point: There are four common causes of employee performance problems:

1. Standards are not clearly communicated.
2. Employee hasn't received feedback.
3. Employee lacks knowledge, skills, or resources.
4. Motivation and attitude.

When a positive, nonpunitive approach to improving an employee's performance does not work, managers must take a more forceful approach.

Help People Become Better Employees

One of a manager's key roles is to help employees learn how to become better employees. When a problem arises that requires a manager to have a discussion with the involved employee, the manager must become a coach and a counselor. The role of a manager is to assist the employee in understanding the issue at hand, listen to the individual's feedback, and provide input that will help the employee deal with the issue.

Employee problems fall into two categories: **behavior issues** and substandard performance. Sorting out the underlying cause is an important first step in the **employee counseling** process. To determine whether you have a staff member with a performance problem or a behavior problem, ask yourself:

- Is this something the person can do but won't?
- Is it a condition, circumstance, or behavior over which this person has complete control?

If you answer "yes" to either question, you are probably dealing with an individual who has a behavior problem. Although it may be uncomfortable to address an employee's behavior, it is possible to do so effectively. Begin by considering exactly what behaviors you want changed. Write them down and assign a degree of importance to each. A bad attitude can mean many things, so clearly define what behaviors constitute a bad attitude. Just as important, define the impact on the department. Does the attitude cause morale problems? Inefficiencies? Mistakes?

Hold a counseling session with the staff member to discuss the changes you want and provide the rationale for the changes. Ask the employee what he or she needs in the way of training or support to make these changes. Explain how you'll be monitoring the employee's future performance and what will happen if his or her behavior does not change. Be sure you don't ignore any future behavior problems or you'll just reinforce the problematic behavior. Also, make sure to praise the staff member for any progress you see.

While there may appear to be barriers to changing a problem behavior, these may simply be excuses. Listen carefully to what the employee has to say and probe to determine the difference between an excuse and a truly extenuating circumstance. Before meeting with the staff member, it is important to plan your entire course of action. This includes the types of disciplinary actions that you can and are willing to carry out if the behavior does not improve.

To illustrate the importance of preplanning, consider the following situation. A manager once had an employee who began to arrive late almost every morning. When asked the reason she was late, she said her husband just started working the night shift and often did not get home on time with the car. The manager reiterated why it was critical for her to be on time and asked what ideas she had for solving the problem. She said she couldn't control when her husband got home, so there was nothing she could do. Several possible solutions were discussed, including riding the bus or carpooling with neighbors or other employees. No matter what solution was suggested, she had a reason why it wouldn't work.

The manager had no choice but to tell her that her job required her being to work at 7:00 AM. However, if that could not be worked out, there was a part-time afternoon shift position that she could have. Of course, it would pay less than she was currently making due to the shorter hours. The next Monday, the employee had figured out a way to get to work on time and never had another problem getting to work on time.

An employee behavior problem will be most easily resolved if it is dealt with as soon as it appears. It must be observed and documented specifically and accurately. Third-hand information is hard to prove and only leads to finger pointing, excuses, and blaming. This means you must spend time around your employees and check out complaints personally.

The issue of performance relates to an employee's ability to apply knowledge and skills in actual practice. Performance may relate to specific standards of practice or procedures or more general aspects of the job such as managing time and communicating with others. If a worker routinely fails in performing job responsibilities, you are probably dealing with a performance problem. Start your investigation of the problem by confirming that the employee knows what is expected and knows the 5 Ws and 2 Hs (*who, what, when, where, why, how, and how much*) of your expectations. If the individual can't understand that he or she is doing something wrong, the performance problem may be an easily correctable miscommunication or orientation oversight.

If a performance problem is confirmed, discuss the concern with the individual. Draw out the employee's views of his or her performance and plans for improvement by asking questions. You can always add points later in the discussion if the employee doesn't raise them first. If performance does not improve within the agreed upon time frame, then a more formal counseling session is necessary.

Ensure that the employee is prepared to talk about his or her performance by scheduling the counseling discussion ahead of time. Ask the individual to prepare for the meeting by considering his or her own actions in the areas of concern. The staff member should already be aware of what is needed to improve and, if given the opportunity, the person may be able to constructively criticize his or her own performance.

Begin your counseling meeting with a general question about the employee's performance in the areas of concern. For example, ask the employee to rate his or her performance during the last 3 months. If you get a general response like, "Pretty good," follow-up with a more focused question, such as, "What in particular seems to be getting in the way of the plans for improvement that we discussed previously?" or "Why do you think we are having this meeting?" Probe further by asking what the employee has already done to improve performance and provide feedback to substantiate the continued performance problems. Assist employees in reevaluating their improvement actions by asking what they would do differently, knowing what they do know or what changes they would make if they worked on this problem again. By using an **Initiate-Listen-Focus-Probe-Plan** discussion technique, you can reduce some of the employees' defensiveness.

Addressing behavior or performance problems with an employee is a difficult discussion because it is very personal. "Constructive criticism" is a phrase commonly associated with employee counseling. Many managers struggle to find a way to tell employees that they are performing a job responsibility poorly and need a different approach, a training course, or something else. Unfortunately, many workers feel personally criticized and become defensive.

Managers must clearly communicate to an employee that a problem exists, provide constructive feedback, and do it in a caring manner. How a manager handles problems as they arise can have a significant impact on employee morale. If an employee is not made well aware of behavior or performance problems, it is more difficult to terminate the individual should that become necessary. To effectively coach and counsel an employee, keep these things in mind:

- Talk about what you perceive, what you feel, and what you need. Be extremely clear.
- Restate the employee's remark by paraphrasing to be sure you fully understand what has been said as the person provides input to the process.
- Talk about what the employee does. Stay away from personality traits. Address behavior, not the personality; don't become a psychologist.
- Zero in on observed or known behavior or performance. Be very careful about how you approach an employee about hearsay. Try to avoid dealing with hearsay unless you have a strong reason to suspect it is true.
- Be specific and discuss only one issue at a time.
- Provide some positive feedback in addition to the negative feedback. Try to start the conversation in a positive manner.

- Allow the employee to give feedback freely. But be careful to not get caught in a repetitive conversation that goes nowhere or dwells on excuses.
- And most importantly, listen, listen, listen!

Following the counseling session, make sure that what you've discussed doesn't fall through the cracks. This is especially critical if you're coaching someone for the first time. Make a note in your calendar or computerized tickler file that will remind you of the reevaluation date. Then step back and give the employee a chance to improve; don't interfere unless asked for assistance.

It is safe to assume that the majority of the people working in foodservice want to do their best, work hard, make good impressions, and get along well with co-workers, managers, and customers. Although poor performers are not the norm, they are bound to emerge on occasion. The majority of employee problems can be resolved if confronted as soon as possible by the manager. The worst thing you can do is to ignore the problem, hoping it will go away on its own. Effective employee coaching and counseling can help to ensure that small, easily reconciled problems don't grow into larger, unmanageable ones.

> **Learning Point:** Poor performance by an employee generally falls into two categories: behavior issues and substandard performance. To resolve the problem, begin by sorting out the underlying cause. Next counsel the employee about the undesired performance and jointly develop strategies for improvement.

When Counseling Fails

If you have a problem employee, you'll want to take the extra steps to help the person improve performance. That may make more economic sense than terminating the person and training a replacement. There are times, though, when you face an employee whose problems are unmanageable, and stronger action is needed. Discipline, although inevitable, is part of a manager's most difficult and stressful leadership tasks. Faced with problems with people, management often goes into a state of paralysis. Nonetheless, when coaching and counseling fail, no matter how difficult, the manager must initiate **disciplinary action**.

A pink slip for poor performance should never surprise its unfortunate recipient. It may disturb, dismay, or dishearten the employee, but it should never come from out of the blue. That's why most organizations use **progressive degrees of discipline**. This gives the employee the opportunity to correct his or her performance.

There is no set standard for how many oral warnings must be given prior to a written warning or how many written warnings must precede **termination**. Factors to consider are:

- How many different offenses are involved
- The seriousness of the offense
- The time interval and employee response to prior disciplinary action
- The employee's previous work history

In general, the steps consist of several oral warnings, followed at the next infraction by a written warning, followed at the next infraction by termination. This is especially true in cases where the time between offenses is short and the employee demonstrates a lack of desire to improve performance. Most employers have defined disciplinary procedures to protect employees' rights from arbitrary dismissal and lack of feedback. *These procedures should always be consulted before initiating action, because employers have policies that must be followed prior to any termination.*

A model known as **positive discipline** emphasizes giving staff reminders rather than reprimands or warnings. The positive discipline approach, a three-step process, is summarized in Table 5.2.

Step 1: The manager and employee meet to discuss a solution to the employee's performance problem. The outcome is the employee's oral agreement to improve performance. At this first meeting, refrain from reprimanding the employee or threatening further disciplinary action. After the meeting use your notes from the session to write a memo or other documentation that summarizes the conversation. A written record of this first conference may not be placed in the employee's personnel file but keep the notes in your own files. Here's an example of verbal reminder documentation:

"I talked to [employee] today about her attendance record and gave her a verbal reminder. Since July 1, [employee] has

Table 5.2 Steps in Positive Discipline

Step 1
- Give the employee a verbal explanation of the errant behavior.
- Reiterate your department's performance standards regarding that behavior.
- Advise the employee of the consequences of further infractions of the standards in question.
- If no further problems occur with the issue raised at the verbal reminder stage, no further disciplinary action needs to be taken.

Step 2
If the problem persists:
- Give the employee a written explanation of the errant behavior.
- Reiterate your department's performance standards regarding that behavior.
- Advise the employee that if the problem continues, the employee will be suspended or terminated.
- As before, give the employee an opportunity to change the unwanted behavior. If the behavior does not recur, no further disciplinary action is taken.

Step 3
If verbal and written reminders fail to bring about a change in the undesired conduct, the employee is suspended or immediately terminated without additional reminders.

been absent from work on 12 occasions for a total of 17 days. [The employee] response was, 'You can't make people work when they are sick,' and she argued about the verbal reminder. I told her that she could request a medical leave of absence if she needed it, but that I expected her to be here every day unless a doctor says otherwise.

[Signature]
[Date]

Step 2: If the performance problems continue, schedule another meeting with the employee to discuss the cause of the continued problems. Jointly determine why the solution agreed upon during the first meeting did not work. Give the employee a written reminder stating the new or repeated solution to the problem. Place a copy of this reminder in the employee's file. You may also ask the employee to sign an affirmation acknowledging responsibility for improving performance, with the understanding that this is a condition of continued employment. After this meeting, you will want to make some documentation based on your notes. Use the checklist in Table 5.3 to make sure you include everything you need in your verbal and written reminder documentation. *Any manager who has been accused of* **wrongful termination** *by an employee will tell you how important documentation is to supporting the manager's decision.*

Table 5.3   Documentation Checklist

Verbal Reminder

Be sure that all verbal reminders are documented in writing. They are a building block to more formal reminders in the future. All documentation should include:

- the employee's name
- the date of the verbal reminder
- the specific offense or rule violation
- a specific statement of the expected performance
- any explanation given by the employee or other information that is significant

Written Reminder

A written reminder is more serious than a verbal reminder and represents a progression in the progressive discipline process. When documenting a written reminder, include:

- the employee's name
- the date of the conversation
- the specific offense or rule violation
- references to previous conversations and verbal reminders about the problem
- a specific statement of the expected performance
- any explanation given by the employee or other information that is significant
- a statement indicating your confidence in the employee's ability to perform properly in the future
- the employee's signature (if the employee refuses, include a note on the signature line indicating your attempt to get the employee to sign and his or her refusal to do so)

Step 3: This step occurs if the second manager-employee conference fails to produce the desired result. At this point, some companies give the employee a paid, one-day decision-making leave, during which time the employee is asked to decide whether he or she wants to continue working for the facility. Employees are instructed to return the following day with a decision—either commit to improving his or her performance or resign. If no commitment is made, then the employee is terminated. Another option is **suspension** with pay for a stated period, depending on the policies of your employer.

At this point, it is not uncommon for an employee to resign, just as you are ready to discharge the person. This is not just a way for the employee to save face but also a way to avoid a nasty confrontation and an employment record that includes a termination. If the employee does not resign, and you've established that verbal and written reminders haven't brought about a change in conduct, the person should be terminated without additional reminders. In most companies when an employee is discharged as the final step after warning notices have been given to an accumulation of infractions, the employee is terminated for cause instead of being given the option to resign, be laid off, or retire.

It is often easier to deal with employee behavior problems than performance problems. Workers who are disruptive, break key rules or standards, or hide their mistakes often make a manager so angry that disciplinary action becomes easier. However, it is best to start with discussions and attempts to resolve the matter before pulling the plug entirely. Many managers have had to fire employees in their career and always find the behavior problems easier to deal

---

Learning Point: When counseling fails to change an employee's unwanted performance, progressive corrective action serves as a means of positive reinforcement—the manager and staff member engage in joint problem solving to gain early correction of employee misconduct. The process serves as a warning to the employee of further repercussions if undesirable behaviors or actions continue. Plus, by carefully documenting the corrective actions the manager can show "just cause" in the event the employee must be terminated.

with. Firing someone for poor performance, even after counseling, reviews, and warnings is never easy.

Minimize Legal Risks

Contending with nonperforming employees can provide the basis for potential legal risks. The terminated employee may feel unfairly treated or discriminated against. Though you have complied with the law, unfortunately some employees may seek restitution through the courts. Even when employees lose their lawsuits, defending cases can be costly to your employer and consume hundreds of hours of your time. Very few employee disciplinary actions or terminations result in the filing of a lawsuit, although by taking a few precautions you can help avoid employee trouble.

- Be sure all job descriptions are current and that performance is evaluated regularly against those job descriptions. Job-related requirements should be specifically defined; generalities such as "good attitude" are too vague. A more objective way to address "attitude" is the way an employee treats co-workers and customers.
- Tell an employee who is not performing up to standard what is needed to achieve standards, how to correct the problem, and how much time he or she has to correct the problem. Don't give people an unjustified glowing appraisal that you'll later need to rescind. An inflated evaluation could be used in court by the employee's attorney to establish a claim of discrimination.
- The hardest lesson for managers to learn is the importance of documentation. Without adequate documentation of counseling and warnings, an employee can successfully claim the actions never took place. The employee should receive a copy of any write-ups and be asked to sign a copy for the file, indicating receipt and the opportunity to discuss the contents. The employee should be told that signing the write-up is not an indication of agreement and the employee should be given the opportunity to write a rebuttal to be included in the file. Table 5.4 is a form that managers can use to document formal discussions with employees.

Table 5.4   Form Used to Document Formal Discussions with
Employees

Employee Name: _____ Title: _____

> This conversation is intended to be: ____ During 90-day
> Probation; ___ Recognition; ___ Coach & Counseling ___
> Formal Level of Discipline: (Verbal Warning, Written Warning,
> Objective Met, Suspension, Terminations, etc.) or other
> Describe:
> _____
> _____

(A) Facts: Be specific and focus on behavior. Provide date, time,
     what you observed, etc.

_____
_____
_____

(B) Objectives: Refer to the job description to set specific, realistic,
     and measurable expectations?

_____
_____
_____

(C) Solutions: What solutions will you and/or the employee take to
     meet the objectives?

_____
_____
_____

(D) Actions: Specify timeline, next meeting date, and what actions
     could be taken if the employee does not meet the objectives.

_____
_____
_____

Prepared by: _____ / _____ _____
                    Printed Name   Signature   Title
Employee: _____ / _____
                        Signature   Date

- If a new employee appears to be a problem very early in his or her employment, terminate the employment before the end of the usual probationary period. There is no need to wait until the end of probation when it is obvious early on that it is not working out. You are asking for trouble if you extend the probationary period in hopes of improvement.

- When there is a recommendation for discipline, be sure you can articulate the reason in writing before that discipline is imposed. Also be sure the discipline has been consistently applied without regard to race, gender, age, national origin, religion, disability, or any other protected class.

- Before imposing any serious discipline, especially suspension or termination, consult your human resources department and/or legal counsel. They can help facilitate the process and make sure there is consistency. It is also useful to have someone from human resources participate in imposing the discipline.

- When terminating an employee, never apologize. The employee may view this phrase as an admission of unfair treatment. Help the employee retain dignity by wishing him or her well and saying that, although this situation did not work out, he or she can perhaps find a situation more fitting.

- Be totally consistent in your reason for terminating an employee. Tell the employee the precise truth, put the same reason on the separation notice form used in your local jurisdiction, and tell the Equal Employment Opportunity Commission the same thing if a charge is filed. Inconsistency almost always leads to trouble if there is litigation, because it can be used to show that your reason is merely a pretext for discrimination or wrongful termination. Not telling the employee the reason for the termination is an open invitation for that employee to seek legal recourse.

- Don't try to intimidate an employee into quitting. That practice is considered unfair. If a wrongful termination case gets to a jury, that jury will be concerned with the perception of fairness. If the employer's version of the facts suggests the employee was treated unfairly, the jury will likely find liability. Good communication with employees is the key to avoiding problems, as is honesty in that communication.

Following these tips will not guarantee an end to all employee-generated workplace problems, but it will help decrease the number and the ultimate cost. Following these tips will also help create a more productive workplace and help both the employee and the employer meet their goals.

Summary

Effective managers communicate their expectations to employees and provide ongoing feedback on performance. Occasionally **employee performance** problems arise that must be confronted and resolved. Many of these problems can be resolved through supervision, employee counseling, and progressive discipline. It is important that managers identify the root cause of unwanted employee performance and minimize the legal risks associated with employee discipline and termination.

Successful foodservice managers insist on quality performance from every employee and create a positive work environment where productivity will be enhanced. Managers are obligated to identify the strengths and weaknesses of each employee, evaluate employees fairly and objectively on a regular basis, identify causes of performance problems, and initiate actions to eliminate any weaknesses. Coping with employee performance problems is one of the most difficult and stressful, yet essential parts of the manager's job. Managers should take an extra step to rejuvenate the problem employee. This extra step may prevent charges of wrongful discharge or employment discrimination. Also, it may be wise, economically, for a company to salvage a problem employee rather than to terminate the person and train a new replacement.

The discipline process involves more than just managerial instinct or intuition to resolve workplace performance problems. Most companies have human resource policies and/or union agreements to protect employees' rights from arbitrary dismissal and lack of feedback. Foodservice managers must comply with company requirements for providing fair, factual, and timely disciplinary feedback.

Most of your employee counseling sessions will be relatively easy. An employee breaks a rule, such as being late or does not meet a performance standard, such as not completing a task correctly.

The majority of employees try to follow the rules and exceed the standards. But, like you, they are human and make mistakes. The main reason for conducting employee counseling sessions is to get them documented. Then, if the employee's performance begins to deteriorate, you have it on record so that you can legally take the appropriate disciplinary action.

Foodservice managers should not tolerate poor performers. One of the advantages of positive discipline is that managers are more willing to address problem employees. In the short-run, it may be easier for managers to avoid confronting a problem employee. This may be due to the manager's need for affiliation with his or her employees or a lack of upper-management support in addressing the problem employee. Yet, when the problem performance is allowed to continue, managers risk losing credibility and authority with sub-ordinates. The long-term effects of ignoring poor performance can be much more devastating than the manager's short-term discomfort about confronting it.

Student Activities

1. Identify techniques or programs from other sources (texts, journals, or the web) that give assistance to help people become better employees.
2. Contact by telephone or in person a foodservice manager and ask about his or her discipline process. Evaluate the discipline process for its positive points.
3. Obtain an example of a court case that depicts a dispute between employer and employee that is representative of a complaint against a discipline process. How could this problem have been avoided?

CASE STUDY #1: STEP ONE OF PROGRESSIVE DISCIPLINE

The foodservice manager is faced with a dilemma. One of the diet technicians is a bright, energetic person who demonstrates excellent technical skills. The only problem is that she often arrives late to work and rarely, if ever, calls to let people know her whereabouts.

Other employees notice her absence and occasionally comment to the manager about how unfair it is that she is allowed that kind of flexibility. The manager discusses the tardiness problem with the human resources director to see what his options are. He receives information about the company's policies and procedures on employee discipline and some advice on how to document conversations he has with the technician. However, the human resources director encourages the manager to try to work out the problem in a more informal manner before turning to the formal proceedings.

The manager meets with the diet technician and indicates that it's important to address her tardiness in the mornings. He points out the negative impact that her absence is having on the work team. The subordinate responds that her babysitter is often late, which causes her to arrive late to work.

The manager acknowledges how difficult this situation is but also reiterates how disruptive her absence is to the work environment. After more discussion, the technician indicates that she understands that her behavior is having a negative impact on her work team and promises to arrive on time in the future. She also agrees to seek out the assistance of neighbors or family members to stay with her child until the babysitter arrives. The manager offers to help her identify alternatives to using the babysitter, such as daycare services that might provide discounts to the company's employees.

Discussion Questions

1. What aspects of this meeting make it more likely that the employee's behavior will change?
2. Would you have handled the situation differently? How?

CASE STUDY #2: EMPLOYEE PERFORMANCE COUNSELING

Sally has been an excellent employee who has not needed any performance counseling up to this point. But, when you review the time sheets for last week you notice that she clocked out 30 minutes early on Thursday. You check your records and find no indication that she requested to leave early on that day.

You arrange to meet with her in your office at 8:30 AM. You start the meeting by stating, *Sally I have been very pleased with your performance. But, you clocked out 30 minutes early last Thursday without giving the team any notice. This is in violation of our department policy. Could you please explain why you left early?*

Sally replies, *I'm so sorry, when I looked at my watch, I thought it was quitting time. It was not until I was on my way home that I realized I left early.* You respond by saying, *How do you plan to ensure this will not happen again?* Sally responds, *I will look at the time more closely to ensure I do not make the same mistake twice.*

Since this was not a serious violation, you decide that no further action is needed. You let Sally know this by saying, *Sally, I'm sure you will not let it happen again. Except for one mistake, your performance has been great, your tasks are always on par and on time, and this is the first rule you have broken.*

Discussion Questions

1. Would you have called Sally into your office for this discussion? If not, why not?
2. Would you have handled the situation differently? How?

CASE STUDY #3: ABHORRENT BEHAVIOR COUNSELING SESSION

Sam has been an excellent employee since he started working for you 2 years ago. However, in the last few weeks, he has not been performing up to standards:

- He has been late three times.
- His performance has been below standards on many occasions.
- Two of his co-workers have reported that he seems to be extremely agitated most of the time and on two occasions threw equipment at a fellow staff member. You checked this out with some other employees and found it to be true.

Today he was late for the fourth time. You have called him into your office for a performance counseling meeting.

You start off the meeting by saying, *Sam, I have called you in because there is a problem, and quite frankly the problem involves you. I have been going through the documentation on your performance over the last few weeks. Sam, you know that today is the fourth time you have been late, and your performance has not been up to department standards. Recently it was reported to me that you have not been getting along with other staff. Your unacceptable performance cannot continue. We are here to find out what you are going to do about it.*

Sam tries to interrupt by making an excuse why he was late today. He says, *My car had a dead battery this morning, and my neighbor had to help me jump start it.* You stop Sam from interrupting by saying, *Excuse me Sam, I want to give you the opportunity to respond, but I feel it is important for you to see the entire picture. Once I lay out the pattern of your deterioration over the past few weeks, then I certainly want to hear from you.* At this point you show and explain to Sam the documentation you have.

continues

Sam becomes very defensive, saying, *I cannot meet my job responsibilities because the other staff and some of the customers are getting in my way!* Although you start to feel defensive yourself, you maintain control of the situation by returning to the facts. *Sam, you may feel that is important to the meeting, but the primary issue is...* Now you go back to your documentation and show Sam the pattern of poor performance.

After the documentation and the issues have been covered, you move to closure. First, to get Sam to take responsibility for the problem, you ask, *Do you understand the problem I have just addressed?* Sam replies, *Yes, I understand the problem.* Next, you ask Sam to explain the reason for his decline in performance. Sam shrugs and says, I *don't know.* You show concern for Sam by then saying, *Is there a personal problem causing your performance to deteriorate? We have an employee assistance program where you might be able to find some help.* Sam replies that he does not have any personal problems; he has just been having a string of bad luck.

Now you let Sam make a personal choice between keeping his disruptive behavioral pattern or keeping his job by saying, *Sam, whatever the problem is that is causing your performance to deteriorate, there is help if you want to deal with it. I want you to know that we so value your potential here that you have a job if you want to deal with your personal issues. However, if there is no problem or you choose not to ask for help, then you leave me no choice other than to fire you strictly for your unacceptable performance problem. What is your choice?*

Discussion Questions

1. Would you have called Sam into your office for this discussion? If not, why not?
2. Would you have handled the situation differently? How?

Web Sites

1. Building human resource management skills: Leadership development for managers. http://www.nfsmi.org/Information/HR_modules/leadership_modules.htm.
2. Building human resource management skills training kit: Management skills for success. http://www.nfsmi.org/Information/HR_modules/management_modules.htm.
3. Business owners toolkit. http://www.toolkit.cch.com/.
4. Coaching employees: Will you make a difference? Retrieved month, day, year, from http://www.nfsmi.org/Education/Satellite/ss36/partic.pdf.
5. Conflict and challenge in the workplace. http://www.nfsmi.org/Education/Satellite/ss30/partic.pdf.
6. Employer-employee.com: Your workplace information portal. http://www.employer-employee.com/.
7. Employment law information network. http://www.elinfonet.com/.
8. Performance management and appraisal help center. http://performance-appraisals.org/.
9. Tools for hiring successful school foodservice assistants. http://www.nfsmi.org/Information/tools_for_hiring.pdf.

References

Chapter reprinted with permission from *OR Manager*:
1. Spath, P.L. (2005). Help! I have a problem employee. *OR Manager, 21*(3), 30–31.
2. Spath, P.L. (2005). Counseling to help problem employees. *OR Manager, 21*(4), 23–24.
3. Spath, P.L. (2005). When coaching and counseling fail. *OR Manager, 21*(5), 22–23.

## CHAPTER 6

PROFESSIONAL JOB DESCRIPTIONS AND PERFORMANCE APPRAISALS

Julie M. Moreschi, MS, RD, LDN

Reader Objectives

Upon reading the chapter and reflecting on the contents, the reader will be able to:

1. Understand the uses of job descriptions in managing a food and nutrition service operation.
2. Learn how to conduct a job analysis to create a job description.
3. Be able to list the critical elements to include in a job description.
4. Become familiar with where to locate and implement job description formats and samples.
5. Understand the uses of performance appraisals in managing a food and nutrition operation.
6. Be familiar with three types of performance appraisals.
7. Understand the connection between competency checklists and performance appraisals.
8. Be familiar with performance appraisal techniques.
9. Understand the steps in a performance appraisal process.
10. Understand the concept of performance management and how it differs from performance appraisals.
11. Learn elements of diversity that should be considered when dealing with job description and performance evaluation development and processes.
12. Become familiar with the concept of the learning organization.

Key Terms

Ability: a present competence to perform an observable behavior or a behavior that results in an observable product.

Competency: a personal characteristic (skill, knowledge, trait, or motive) that drives behavior and leads to the ability to perform required job activities that meet acceptable levels of performance.

Credentials and experience: the acceptable level of education, experience, and certifications necessary for employment.

Job analysis: in-depth study of a job; provides information for job descriptions.

Job description: a document that is a descriptive summary of the responsibilities and required work completion of a position.

Job duty: a single specific task.

Skill: a present, observable competence to perform a learned activity.

Knowledge: a body of information applied directly to the performance of a duty.

Other characteristics: duties, knowledge, skills, and abilities that do not have a logical place in the job description.

Performance appraisal: a process, often combining both written and oral elements, that managers can utilize to provide feedback on employee job performance, including steps to improve or redirect activities as needed.

Performance management: a process for ensuring that the performance of employees is effectively managed and that employees' performances meet the organizational standards.

Physical characteristic: the physical attributes employees must have to perform job duties unaided or with the assistance of a reasonable accommodation.

Introduction

Employees with optimal skills and high levels of performance are essential to the efficient and profitable management of any food and nutrition service operation. A food and nutrition service manager who focuses effort at the outset on establishing sound job descriptions and performance measurement tools for his or her operation can avoid potential problems with poor performance and turnover in the long run. Quality employees at all levels of a food and nutrition service operation can be the building block that then leads to high levels in customer satisfaction, employee satisfaction, and financial performance.

Job Descriptions

What Is a Job Description?

A written **job description** is a document that is a descriptive summary of the responsibilities and required work completion of a position. Job descriptions are multipurpose documents that put into writing the content of any particular job. A job description provides information to the employer and employee regarding what the employee does, how it is done, and under what conditions it is done.

Purpose of Job Descriptions

Job descriptions serve many useful purposes for any organization. In his book, *The Handbook of Model Job Descriptions*, Barry Cushway outlines the purposes of job descriptions in the following manner:

I. Legal and Contractual

There is no legal requirement mandating that employees be given a job description. There is, however, a requirement to describe a job briefly, or indicate the job title, in the statement of terms and conditions of employment included in an employee contract. Depending on the type of foodservice operation, there may be regulatory agency requirements for job descriptions. Foodservice managers need to be aware of the standards and job description requirement for such governing bodies, such as the Joint Commission on Accreditation of Healthcare Organizations (JCAHO), state and local health departments, and/or union contract requirements. Job descriptions are also a useful tool in communicating job expectations clearly to employees, particularly if issues of disciplinary action or grievance occur.

Job descriptions can list any potential safety issues related to a position such as risks or hazards. They also help to identify the necessary safety training and precautions that need to be in place.

II. Human Resource Planning

An organizational chart assists an organization in determining the types of job needed in order to make the facility operational. Job descriptions then define these positions in terms of identifying the **knowledge**, skills, and experience required and then assist management in determining the number of jobs per position that are required to meet the objectives of the operation.

III. Recruitment and Selection

Job descriptions allow an operation to clearly define the qualifications, experience, and personal attributes that are required for a position, as well as establish fair and equitable salary levels. Managers can then use this information in matching job openings with the most qualified applicants.

IV. Training and Development

To begin, a job description is a good tool for a manager to use to explain and clarify reporting relationships, accountabilities, and expected deliverables of a job to a new employee during orientation training. If upon orientation training, an employee is found to lack a skill(s) necessary to perform optimally in a job, further training can be planned and scheduled immediately.

Managers can also use job descriptions to compare an employee's current skill level to more than one job description to uncover training opportunities to enhance cross-training of employees and/or promotional opportunities within the work force.

V. Job Evaluation and Performance Management

Job descriptions provide information regarding the requirements of the job, and this information is useful in providing employee feedback regarding their **ability** to meet the established objectives and tasks associated with their position.

Performance management is a process for ensuring that the performance of employees is effectively managed and that the employee's performance meets the organizational standards. A clear definition of the job requirements via the job description is an essential element in effectively measuring and appraising performance.

VI. Organizational Change and Job Redesign

Food and nutrition service managers can expect change to be a constant feature to any organization that they operate. With the increased difficulty in hiring qualified and dependable food and nutrition service personnel, managers must look to design jobs that meet the work force's desire and legal right to request flexibility. Also, change often results in organization structure and reporting lines being changed, and these adaptations may result in job content alterations. Job descriptions must be updated to reflect organizational and job redesign.

Job Analysis

In order to write job descriptions, jobs must be observed and analyzed. **Job analysis** is an in-depth study of a job and provides information for job descriptions. The job analyst will gather information about jobs through interviewing employees, observing performance of certain tasks, asking employees to fill out questionnaires and worksheets, and collecting information about a job from secondary sources that provide sample job descriptions, such as *Model Position Description: Restaurant Industry.* Information may also be obtained by reviewing job descriptions from similar food and nutrition services operations.

The job analyst records the results of the analysis and reviews them with the current employee. The documentation is then presented to the employee's supervisor for review (often the employee's supervisor is the job analyst.) The supervisor may add, delete, or modify duties, knowledge, skills, abilities, and **other characteristics.** After supervisory approval is obtained, the documentation is forwarded through channels for final approval. A signed and dated job description is then prepared. This job description becomes the official record for this particular job.

What Information to Include in the Job Description

When writing a job description, keep in mind that the job description will serve as the major basis for outlining job training or conducting future job evaluations. As with job analysis, it is helpful to include employees, supervisors, and managers when writing the job description. After the first draft of the job description is written, it is a good idea to step away from the process for a few days before making the job description final.

Some ideas regarding the information to include in a job description are as follows:

- Job title
- Job objective/summary or overall purpose statement is generally a summary designed to orient the reader to the general nature, level, purpose, and objective of the job. The summary should describe the broad function and scope of the position and be no longer than three to four sentences.
- List of duties or tasks performed contains an item-by-item list of principal duties, continuing responsibilities, and accountability of the occupant of the position. The list should contain each and every essential job duty or responsibility that is critical to the successful performance of the job. The list should begin with the most important functional and relational responsibilities and continue down in order of significance. Each duty or responsibility that comprises at least 5% of the incumbent's time should be included in the list.
- Description of the relationships and roles the occupant of the position holds within the company, including any supervisory positions, subordinating roles, and/or other working relationships.
- Job specifications, standards, and requirements are the minimum amount of qualifications needed to perform the essential functions of the job, such as education, experience, knowledge, licenses, certifications, and skills. Any critical skills and expertise needed for the job should be included.
- Job location is where the work will be performed.
- Equipment to be used in the performance of the job. For example, does the employee need to be able to operate certain types of foodservice equipment?
- Collective bargaining agreements are agreements and terms that relate to job functions, if applicable, such as when your company's employees are members of a union.
- Nonessential functions are not essential to the position or any marginal tasks performed by the incumbent of the position.
- Salary range is the range of pay for the position.

Once a job description is completed, this is only the beginning. Job descriptions are fluid documents that should be reviewed at least annually and used frequently. Job descriptions should be flexible enough to allow employees to utilize all of their skills and to encourage teamwork and collaboration. Job descriptions need to be well-written, because errors can cause problems if termination lawsuits are ever pursued by disgruntled past employees. Job descriptions should be available for use by all members of the foodservice operation, because once written the documents are only useful applied in the workplace. Managers should refer to them when ever working on a hiring or job redesign project, and managers should encourage employees to refer to them for job clarifications on a frequent basis.

Table 6.1   Sample Job Description Format

Job Title: _____

Department: _____

Reports to: _____

Position Summary:

_____

_____

Essential Job Responsibilities:

1. _____

_____

_____

_____ %

2. _____

_____

_____

_____ %

3. _____

_____

_____

_____ %

Other Functions:

1. _____

_____

continues

Table 6.1   (continued)

2. _____
   _____
3. _____
   _____

Minimum Job Requirements:
Education: _____
Experience: _____
Specific Skills:_____
Specific Knowledge, Licenses, Certifications: _____
Supervisory Responsibility (if applicable): _____
_____

Working Conditions: _____

APPROVALS:
Supervisor: _____   Date: _____
Acting HR Director: _____   Date: _____
Employee's Signature: _____   Date: _____

Performance Appraisal

An employee **performance appraisal** is a process, often combining both written and oral elements, that managers can utilize to provide feedback on employee job performance, including steps to improve or redirect activities as needed. Documenting performance provides a basis for pay increases and promotions. Appraisals are also important to help staff members improve their performance and as an avenue by which they can be rewarded or recognized for a job well-done.

An organization can have several goals for its performance appraisal system. Some of these goals include:

1. Improving the company's productivity.
2. Making informed personnel decisions regarding promotion, job changes, and termination.
3. Identifying what is required to perform a job (goals and responsibilities of the job).
4. Assessing an employee's performance against these goals.

5. Working to improve the employee's performance by naming specific areas for improvement, developing a plan aimed at improving these areas, supporting the employee's efforts at improvement via feedback and assistance, and ensuring the employee's involvement and commitment to improving his or her performance.

There are many different types of appraisals that managers can use in providing feedback to employees. The following are some of these types of appraisals.

Traditional Appraisal

In a traditional appraisal, a manager sits down with an employee and discusses performance for the previous performance period, usually 1 year. The discussion is based on the manager's observations of the employee's abilities and performance of tasks as noted in a job description. The performance is rated, with the ratings tied to salary percentage increases.

Self-Appraisal

The self-appraisal is used in the performance appraisal process to encourage staff members to take responsibility for their own performance by assessing their own achievements or failures and promoting self-management of development goals. It also prepares employees to discuss these points with their manager. It may be used in conjunction with or as a part of other appraisal processes but does not substitute for an assessment of the employee's performance by a manager.

360 Degree or Multiple Rater Feedback

360 degree feedback in the performance appraisal process refers to feedback on an employee's performance being provided by the manager, different people or departments an employee interacts with (peer evaluation), external customers, and the employee. This type of feedback includes employee-generated feedback on management performance (also known as upward appraisals).

360 degree feedback allows each individual to understand how his or her effectiveness as an employee, coworker, or staff member is viewed by others. The most effective processes provide feedback that is based on behaviors that other employees can see. The feedback provides insight about the skills and behaviors desired in the organization to accomplish the mission, vision, and goals and live the values.

Evaluating Competence

Soon after orientating a new employee to the food and nutrition operation, it is advisable for the manager to have systems in place to validate that the new hire is competent in all aspects of his job duties. Accreditation bodies, such as the JCAHO, mandate that organizations show proof of **competency** validation.

A simple method that can be used for this purpose is the creation of a competency checklist. The manager or supervisor observes the employee performing the required job elements and signs and dates when each competency is validated. These records are then placed in the employee's file. It is also advisable to incorporate random competency check systems to assess maintenance of skill level by all employees in the operation.

Performance Appraisal Techniques

There are many techniques that a manager can use when conducting a performance appraisal. W. Oberg discusses commonly used appraisal techniques and their strengths and weaknesses in his article "Make Performance Appraisal Relevant." Oberg contends that the organizations often apply a wide variety of performance appraisal techniques without really thinking how the techniques might best achieve the company's performance appraisal objectives.

The types of performance appraisal techniques include:

1. Essay appraisal. In its simplest form, this technique asks the rater to write a paragraph or more covering an individual's strengths, weaknesses, potential, and so on. This method can be variable in length and content.
2. Graphic rating scale. This technique uses a scale to rate an employee on various job functions. A scale that is typically used includes ratings of outstanding, above average, average, or unsatisfactory.

3. Field review. In a field review, additional personnel are asked to evaluate an employee. This approach is usually done when the rater is suspected of bias in evaluating an employee.
4. Forced-choice rating. This method is designed to minimize bias in evaluating. The evaluation is completed by only one rater, but the rankings are not weighted, thus minimizing the rater's ability to bias the outcome of the appraisal.
5. Critical incident appraisal. This type of evaluation requires a manager to record specific positive and negative employee performance incidents throughout the evaluation period. The evaluation then focuses on a discussion of the manager sharing his or her observations with the employee.
6. Management by objectives. Management by objectives requires the employee to establish and rate himself on a set of standards.
7. Work-standards approach. The work standards technique establishes manager written work and staffing targets aimed at improving productivity. When realistically used, it can make possible an objective and accurate appraisal of the work of employees and supervisors.
8. Ranking methods. This method ranks employee performance against other employees in the same job category. This method is more frequently used to determine merit and/or promotional decisions.
9. Assessment centers. This method is used to help determine an employee's ability for future performance. For example, an employee is put into a new position for a few days, and an evaluation regarding the employee's potential to remain at that job is reviewed.

Conducting the Performance Appraisal

The process of conducting a performance appraisal is more than a one-time meeting where the manager provides feedback to an employee via a written document. Managers can create cohesive models that encompass employee input and coordinate efforts of the work force toward optimal performance. A performance appraisal system not only includes the use of the review form, but should also include components that prepare and encourage staff participation and prepare management in skill development in providing both written and verbal performance feedback. See Figure 6.1 for a sample Performance Review Model.

When planning to conduct performance appraisals, managers can utilize the following steps:

1. Schedule a performance review meeting 1 to 2 weeks in advance to allow both you and the employee to prepare for it. Select a time that the employee is not busy and a quiet, yet public place.
2. Ask employees to appraise themselves 2 weeks prior to the evaluation meetings. Relevant questions a manager may ask

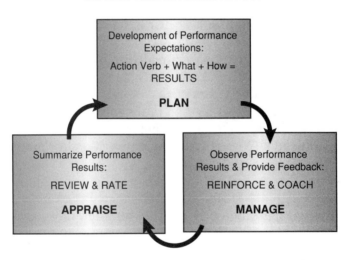

Creating Dialogue in Performance Evaluations
It's More Than an Annual Review!

Goal of Performance Reviews: Encourages employees to work to their potential!

1. Creates a dialogue between supervisor and employee.
2. Provides a written summary of feedback given to employee throughout the year.
3. Focuses on performance and job results.
4. May identify skill deficiencies that require improvement and suggest methods to improve.
5. Supports staff development plans.
6. Remains in the personnel file.

FIGURE 6.1   Performance Review Model

Reprinted with permission from: Hoddy, M. *Creating Dialogue in Performance Evaluations: It's More Than an Annual Review.* Available at: http://www.wisc.edu/improve/case/CSDialoguein%20erfEval.pdf.

the employee to answer include: What do you think you have achieved in the past year? What targets or achievement have you not realized? How do you think you could have improved your performance since your last evaluation? How do you think you get along with the other members of the team?

3. Gather and review information about each employee. Refer to attendance records, manager's notebook, and personnel records. The rating should reflect the employee's performance over the entire review period. Note specific examples in which the employee was either effective or ineffective in meeting organizational goals. Quote feedback from coworkers.

4. Be specific. In addition to giving numerical ratings, provide written comments—the more specific, the better. Use quantifiable data, such as volume of work completed, quality of work, innovative ideas, and ability to meet deadlines.

5. Be objective and fair. Avoid being too lenient, too tough, or giving everyone the same rating. Rate employees only on job performance; don't let other factors—such as their personality traits, race, sex, or age—affect you.

6. Set an approachable and professional tone for the evaluation meeting.

7. Plan ahead so that the appraisal meeting is not interrupted.

8. Take special care with an employee's first review. Give thorough explanations and allow extra time for employee questions. Conduct the first review after about a month.

9. End a review meeting by discussing employee goals. Make sure the goals are realistic and measurable, and be prepared to check on the employee's progress. Ask the employee what objectives he or she would like to achieve in the coming year.

Mary Hoddy at the University of Wisconsin-Madison created a model for the annual performance evaluations for Wisconsin Union Staff members. The purpose of her model was to make the evaluation process useful and positive and to encourage all employees to work to their potential. The process involves reviewing, analyzing, and planning, hence the acronym R-A-P. The model is focused on including employees in the review process and making sure that no information covered in the evaluation is a surprise.

The steps of the model include:

1. Review/update position description.
2. Conduct pre-evaluation interview (R-A-P worksheet below).

Table 6.2 RAP Worksheet

REVIEW

1. What actions did you take in the past year to further the Mission and/or the Strategic Plan?

ANALYZE

2. What went well and why? (Include highlights and successes.)

3. What things do you wish had worked better in the past year?

4. What have you learned from the experiences described above?

5. Think about your work environment, including department culture. What resources, tools, or improvements are needed to help you create an ideal work environment?

6. Considering the Mission, Strategic Plan, and your own goals, what are the most important things that you would like to accomplish in the next year?

PLAN

7. What first steps do you need to take to make those goals a reality?

8. What things can your supervisor and/or the Leadership Team do to help you accomplish these steps?

9. What job-related training or professional development would help you in your job or career progression?

10. What additional comments or observations would you like to make?

Adapted with permission from: Hoddy, M. Creating Dialogue in Performance Evaluations: It's More Than an Annual Review. Available at: http://www.wisc.edu/improve/case/CSDialoguein%20erfEval.pdf.

3. Write the performance review, including: goals/objectives, performance expectation/standards, performance results, development/future goals, and achievement/results of past year's development goals.
4. Conduct performance review.

Performance Management

Performance management deals with not only individual employees, but with how the company as a whole is shaping up. This includes everything from departments, groups, and teams to programs, products, projects, and processes. Performance management measures whether each of these systems or groups is working well within a company to meet an overall results-oriented goal.

Organizations can go beyond a performance appraisal system and enhance employee performance through use of a performance management system. The Office of Personnel Management of the Federal Government's Human Resources (HR) Agency has a performance management handbook that can assist managers in expanding their employee feedback systems.

Performance management is a system that focuses on the management of employee performance (planning, developing, monitoring, rating, and rewarding employee contributions) rather than performance-based or performance-oriented approaches to managing, measuring, and accounting for a company's performance.

The Office of Personnel Management uses an eight-step model for performance management. These steps include:

1. Look at the overall picture.
2. Determine work unit accomplishments.
3. Determine individual accomplishments.
4. Convert expected accomplishments into performance elements, indicating type and priority.
5. Determine work unit and individual measures.
6. Develop work unit and individual standards.
7. Determine how to monitor performance.
8. Check the performance plan.

Learning Point: Issues of Diversity

Food and nutrition operations must focus efforts on addressing the needs of a work force dominated by young people, women, and persons from diverse cultural backgrounds. Job descriptions and performance appraisals are systems that rely heavily on written and verbal communication, and managers would be well-served to examine if the messages they are conveying are being received accurately by employees. Managers must consider diversity issues related to gender, age, religion, disability, sexual preference, culture, etc.

Job descriptions and traditional staffing patterns may need to be challenged to meet the needs of a diverse workforce.

Some questions that managers may ask include:

1. What policies, practices, and ways of thinking within our organizational culture have differential impact on different groups?
2. What organization changes should be made to meet the needs of a diverse work force as well as to maximize the potential of all workers?
3. Organizations may share similar values, such as respect or need for recognition, but how we show those values through behavior may be different for different cultures. Does saying hello making eye contact when speaking mean the same thing to all members of your staff?

Ignoring diversity issues costs time, money, and efficiency. Tensions in the workplace can result in loss of productivity due to increased conflict; inability to attract and retain talented people of all kinds; complaints and legal actions; and inability to retain women and people of diversity, resulting in lost investments in recruitment and training.

Boston College Dining Service (BCDS) received an award for Diversity Programs. Among the BCDS initiatives cited were its active recruitment throughout area high schools, vocational schools, and community colleges, and of senior citizens in Boston neighborhoods, as a means of promoting age diversity. BCDS also drew praise for giving persons with special needs the opportunity to work in kitchens and dining rooms and for supporting community-assisted living programs that help men and women rehabilitate their personal lives.

> Other BCDS programs include culinary training for those seeking careers in foodservice but lacking formal education; developing multi-ethnic menu items; English as a second language classes; and formal diversity training programs to broaden cultural awareness.

The goal of performance management is not simply to do an employee review or to touch base on a project for the sake of doing it. It's all about making sure that your employees, projects, processes, services, departments, and so on, are actually producing results. Employees can be busy all day but still may not get anything done. Departments can seemingly function well, but are they really getting the job done in an effective and efficient manner? Performance management assists an organization in assessing if individual and team efforts are efficient in attaining organizational objectives.

Summary

Job descriptions and performance appraisals are essential elements of any food and nutrition services organization. Through job analysis, job descriptions can be created that assist an organization in recruiting, hiring, training, and maintaining employees with superior skills. Performance appraisal systems that involve employees and are deemed an essential element to the organization's success can make the difference between an average operation and a GREAT one. Knowledge, skill, and ability to implement job description and performance appraisal systems are an essential requirement for any leader in the area of food and nutrition services.

Student Activities

Student Activity #1

Job Description Analysis

Analyze a job description to determine if it contains the components listed below. Check those items that are included in the job description. In the space provided, write suggestions for improving the job description.

1. Are the following subtitles included within the job description?
   - Position Title
   - Position Setting
   - Qualifications
   - Rationale/Purpose for the Person
   - Orientation/Training Requirements
   - Duties and Responsibilities
   - Time and Hours
   - Evaluation/Supervision Methods
2. Is the title appropriate and reflective of current trends in food and nutrition nomenclature?
3. Does the job description include enough detail about expectations for the position, such as what the food and nutrition employee will be doing?
4. Does the job description show a true relationship to what employees in this type of area are currently doing?
5. Does the supervision section adequately inform the employee of how he/she will be supervised?
6. Does the job description provide direction for the development of employee goals?
7. Is information included on the methods of evaluation of the employee?
   Additional Comments and Suggestions:

Student Activity #2

Redesign Scenario

You are working as a food and nutrition manager in a healthcare facility. The organization has decided to redesign the food delivery system from a traditional decentralized trayline system to a host/hostess service model. You have been placed in charge of determining staffing needs for the project.

Work in a small group and answer the following questions:

1. Describe the steps you might take to update the food and nutrition department job descriptions.
2. What personnel might you ask to assist in updating the job descriptions?
3. Where might you locate information that could assist in updating the job descriptions? Include sources that are internal and external to the foodservice operation.

Student Learning Activity #3

Performance Appraisal Session

Read and discuss the following scenario with your group.

Manager M has been extremely busy. Employees have been calling in sick with some flu bug the last few days, the produce supplier brought the wrong size peppers for the stuffed pepper recipe, and the dishmachine keeps clogging. To add to the pressure, Employee E's performance evaluation is a week overdue, and HR is calling to insist that the appraisal be completed ASAP.

Manager M just wants to get the performance appraisal off his desk. He thinks "What difference does it make anyways? Employee E works hard. No problem." He goes out to the production area and finds Employee E. "Hey, Employee E, we need to finish your evaluation ASAP. HR is breathing down my neck. Plan on coming to my office during lunch so we can get this over with, OK?"

So Manager M proceeds to get out the forms HR sent him about 3 months ago. Hmm, he thinks, there are two forms...what's the deal with that?

Manager M proceeds to go through the rating system. Employee E is above average, I'll just give him a rating of 3 on all of the elements. He knows I think he does a good job. I'll give him a few examples when I talk with him, but I'm not wasting my time writing down any essay examples on the form. Who looks at it anyway? There's a goal section. Oh well, Employee E can fill it out when he gets here. He's happy in this job, so I doubt there will be anything new he wants to learn.

A few minutes later, Employee E knocks on Manager M's door. "Boss, I have about 15 minutes—should we do my evaluation now?" Manager M gives the evaluation form to Employee E. "Here, read this while I make a quick phone call." Employee M reads the form. Manager M gets off the phone, he tells Employee E that "he does a good job and to keep up the fine work." He tells Employee E that he really likes how he's been keeping the production tables so clean lately and asks if he has any questions?

Employee E has no questions. Manager M asks him to write down a goal. Otherwise HR will send the stupid form back down to them. Employee E writes down that he will continue to keep the work tables clean, signs the form, and goes to eat a quick lunch.

Answer the following questions:

What did Manager M do well? What could Manager M do to improve this scenario? Be specific.

Other Resources

360 degree feedback. http://www.360-degreefeedback.com/.

Addressing the needs of a diverse work force. (1997). Retrieved July 6, 2006, from http://www.restaurant.org/rusa/magArticle.cfm?ArticleID=427.

Archer North's performance appraisal: The complete online guide. http://www.performance-appraisal.com/home.htm.

Barry, C. *The Handbook of model job descriptions.* (2006). Wales: Creative Print and Design.

Beginners guide staff: How is this different from conducting an annual employee review. (2005). Retrieved June 25, 2006, from http://beginnersguide.com/assessment/performance-management/how-is-this-different-than-conducting-an-annual-employee-review.php.

Beginners guide staff: What is performance management. (2005). Retrieved June 25, 2006, from http://beginnersguide.com/ assessment/perform-ance-management/what-is-performance-management.php.

Bread and butter: Defining an employee's duties. (2000). Retrieved July 6, 2006, from http://www.restaurant.org/business/bb/2000_05.cfm.

Bread and butter: Using evaluations to guide employees to greatness. 1999. Retrieved July 6, 2006, from http://www.restaurant.org/business/bb/1999_08.cfm.

Business and legal reports (BLR). http://hr.blr.com/.

Clark, N. How to write a job description. (2003). Retrieved June 5, 2006, from http://www.uman.com.au/Articles/jobdesc.html.

Create the job description. Retrieved June 25, 2006, from http://www.uvm.edu/~farmlabr/?Page=recruitment/create.html&SM=recruitment/submenu_recruitment.html.

Donohue, G. Creating SMART goals. Retrieved June 25, 2006, from http://www.topachievement.com/smart.html.

Gale, T. Employee performance appraisals. (2006). Retrieved June 5, 2006, from http://www.referenceforbusiness.com/small/Di-Eq/Employee-Performance-Appraisals.html.

Gawlik, S. BC dining service earns award for diversity programs. (2000). Retrieved July 9, 2006, from http://www.bc.edu/bc_org/rvp/pubaf/chronicle/v9/s8/bando.html.

Guide to managing human resources. Chapter 12: Managing diversity in the workplace. (2006). Retrieved July 9, 2006, from http://hrweb.berkeley.edu/guide/diversity.htm.

Heathfield, S. Job *descriptions: Why effective job descriptions make* business sense, part 2: Five warning signs about job descriptions. (2006).

Retrieved June 25, 2006, from http://humanresources.about.com/od/
policiesproceduressamples/l/aajob_descrip2.htm.

Hoddy, M. Creating dialogue in performance evaluations: It's more than an
annual review. Retrieved June 5, 2006, from www.wisc.edu/improve/
case/CSDialoguein%20erfEval.pdf.

How to develop job descriptions. (2006). Retrieved June 25, 2006, from
http://www.cmfweb.org/PersonnelJobDescriptions.asp.

Lindner, James R. Writing job descriptions for small businesses. Retrieved
June 25, 2006, from http://ohioline.osu.edu/cd-fact/1376.html.

Job description writing made easy. (2005). Retrieved June 5, 2006, from
http://www.hrtoolkit.gov.bc.ca/compensation/job_description/Job_
Descriptions_Made_Easy.pdf.

Job description writing made easy. http://www.hrtoolkit.gov.bc.ca/
compensation/job_description/Job_Descriptions_Made_Easy.pdf.

(2000). *Model position descriptions: Restaurant industry*. National Restaurant
Association.

Oberg, W. Make performance appraisal relevant. Retrieved June 30, 2006,
from http://www.unep.org/restrict/pas/paspa.htm.

Office of Personnel Management: The Federal Government's Human
Resources Agency. A handbook for measuring employee performance.
(2001). Retrieved June 30, 2006, from http://www.opm.gov/perform/
wppdf/2002/handbook.pdf.

Office of Personnel Management: The Federal Government's Human
Resources Agency. http://www.opm.gov/perform/index.asp.

Performance appraisal PowerPoint™ tutorial. http://www.uni.edu/
~hitlan/chapter7_spring2005_io.pdf.

Performance appraisal. Retrieved June 30, 2006. http://filebox.vt.edu/
users/dgc2/staffinghandbook/perfappraisal.htm.

Sayed, D. Why job descriptions are important. (2006). Retrieved June 5,
2006, from http://office.microsoft.com/en-us/FX011894721033.aspx.

The Performance Management and Appraisal Help Center. http://
performance-appraisals.org/index.htm.

Writing effective job descriptions. Retrieved June 5, 2006, from
http://www.business.gov/phases/managing/manage_employees/
effective_job_descriptions.html.

Wright, K. *Performance management: Beyond appraisals*. (1997). Retrieved
June 5, 2006, from http://www.ciras.iastate.edu/publications/ CIRAS-
News/summer97/performance.htm.

## CHAPTER 7

IN-SERVICE EDUCATION AND MEETING REGULATIONS: SANITATION, SAFETY, AND HACCP

Jacqueline S. Gutierrez, MS, RD, CDN

Reader Objectives

After studying this chapter and reflecting on the contents, you should be able to:

1. Understand why you should provide in-service education to your kitchen staff on a regular basis.
2. Name at least two federal agencies that monitor food safety.
3. Know what the Food Code is and why it is relevant to your facility.
4. State the reason that controlling food temperatures is important.
5. Name the seven principles of HACCP.
6. Recognize how to implement HACCP in your foodservice establishment.
7. Know what a critical control point is and how to find one in your kitchen.
8. Name at least two ways of keeping foods safe from bacteria.

Key Terms

Cross contamination: the act of infecting clean food with microorganisms by placing the food on dirty surfaces through carelessness in cleaning and hygiene.

Food Code: collaboratively created by the Food and Drug Administration (FDA), Food Safety and Inspection Service (FSIS), and

Centers for Disease Control and Prevention (CDC) to monitor retail and commercial food safety. The Food Code is revised every 2 years and is one step that the U.S. government is taking to monitor and prevent foodborne illness.

Hazard Analysis and Critical Control Point (HACCP): the process of analyzing food handling to identify where a food may become unsafe for consumption. The points of possible food contamination are identified, and procedures are written and followed to prevent potential foodborne illness.

Holding temperatures: designated temperatures in which food can be held for a designated amount of time to prevent growth of microorganisms.

In-Service Education

Effective properly conducted employee training could make the difference between a well-run foodservice facility and a facility that could be the breeding ground for hidden bacteria. In 2004, FoodNet identified 15,806 laboratory-diagnosed cases of foodborne infections. Although the observed incidences of most foodborne illnesses actually decreased between 1998 and 2004, the decrease was largely due to increased diligence of foodservice managers nationwide and improved compliance with **Hazard Analysis and Critical Control Point (HACCP)**. Also, better training of food handlers, improved investigations of outbreaks, better knowledge of bacteria growth patterns, and more information about proper food handling helped decrease the incidences of foodborne illness. However, many cases of foodborne illness continue to remain unreported each year.[1]

All new employees need to be instructed on the importance of proper sanitation. They should be taught about common foodborne bacteria, how these can grow, potential types of foodborne illnesses, the importance of keeping food at proper temperatures, and the importance of proper hand washing and hygiene. This information should be given on the first day of employment, preferably as part of the new employee's orientation. When a new employee starts, safe food handling techniques should be discussed and demonstrated. Proper equipment, needed supplies, and training on how to get the job done safely and properly are needed to have a safe and clean work environment.

> **Learning Point:** Try to catch your employees doing the right thing and commend them for performing techniques properly and safely.

Well-trained employees will have the needed knowledge and skills to keep food safe. However, it is ultimately the manager's responsibility to make sure that foods are being handled safely and that employees are doing what they should to maintain a safe and healthy workplace. Although the training process is associated with some cost and time requirements, the cost of training your employees to properly handle food is much less than the cost of dealing with the legal and medical expenses from an outbreak that originated from your facility. In addition, the cost of lost business due to a damaged reputation is much greater than the cost of proper training.

Managers need to be well-informed about the possible sanitation hazards that could occur in the facility during all phases of food production and serving. Also, they should know about the proper use of cleaning detergents and sanitizers, which microorganisms may grow in foods, and the importance of temperature control.

There are several steps involved in an effective training program. First, determine the training needs of your staff. A training need is the knowledge difference between what employees need to do their jobs properly and what they already know. The training needs may include food safety, personal hygiene, such as proper hand washing, how to use thermometers to monitor potentially hazardous food, proper cleaning and sanitizing procedures, proper ways of dealing with chemicals, pest prevention, and/or what to do about pests. Second, set learning objectives that state what the employees should be able to do or understand after the instruction. Third, decide which delivery methods would be best to get the message across. Delivery methods for training include hands-on demonstrations, lectures, role playing, computer-based training, group inservices. Fourth, select an instructor. The instructor may be the manager, supervisor, designated employee in charge of training for the whole organization, or outside consultant. There are many available materials to choose from, such as written handouts, flip charts, and audiovisual materials.

Training should not be scheduled when the kitchen is busy. Training can either be done in the kitchen or at a location where employees can sit down and take notes. The trainer should make an outline, practice, be prepared to answer any relevant questions, and make sure any needed materials are available for the training. A length of approximately 20 to 30 minutes is recommended. The training should not cover too many topics at once and should make the employees understand how they can benefit by learning how to work more efficiently, faster, easier, and better.[2]

Many foodservice employees are of low socioeconomic status or have low levels of formal education. They may speak a different language than you do. This sociocultural gap may contribute to

Learning Point: For those employees who do not speak English, training should either be conducted partially in their native language or handouts in their native language should be supplied. Demonstrations and audiovisuals can also help bridge the gap in the language barrier because these teaching delivery methods rely on visual and tactile cues instead of on language.

employee job dissatisfaction and insecurity. Each employee must be made aware that his or her role is vital and important to food safety. For example, the dishwasher has one of the most important jobs in the establishment because he or she is cleaning and sanitizing all the dishes so that the customers do not contract foodborne illness. This position is often taken by those who have the highest language barriers because the job does not involve reading or customer contact. In addition, employees from foreign countries are often accustomed to food-related practices that might be very different than what is expected in the United States. Therefore, make sure that your employees clearly understand what is expected of them.

For training to be effective, it should be made relevant to your employees' lives, enjoyable, and informative. To motivate employees, you must be able to understand their needs. Well-trained staff should have knowledge of food safety and knowledge of procedures for keeping food safe. Staff should have the motivation to carry out the procedures properly without taking dangerous shortcuts and should work in an environment where proper procedures and policies are expected of them, encouraged, reinforced, and enforced.

The instructor who in-services the foodservice staff can be the manager or an outside contractor. However, training is ultimately

> **Learning Point:** Since most foodborne illnesses can be prevented with proper procedures and methods in place, training of all employees is of paramount importance. Potentially hazardous foods held at danger zone temperatures are a major, but preventable, cause of food-related illness. See Figure 7.1 for a pictorial of the danger zone.

the manager's responsibility even if an outside consultant is used for the training.

According to the National Restaurant Association, the U.S. Department of Labor's Bureau of Labor Statistics report a decline in injuries and illnesses in 2004 at foodservice establishments. These totaled 4.2 per 100 full-time equivalent employees (average of all industries is 4.8) with 66.7 of these cases involving no lost workdays. This is attributed to the industry considering employee safety to be an important priority.[3]

In-service requirements vary from county to county and from state to state. However, in general, an institution such as a hospital may have to in-service its kitchen staff once a month. Managers need a certification from an approved food safety course. They also will need

> **Learning Point:** In addition to food safety, as the foodservice manager you must consider accident and injury prevention to be a top priority. The employees will know that you care and that procedures need to be properly followed and safety rules should not be ignored.

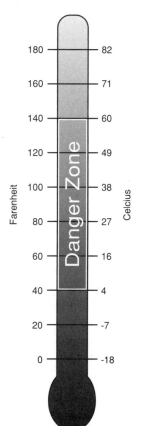

FIGURE 7.1 Danger Zone Temperature Range

to renew their certifications based on the requirements of the county in which they work, as opposed to where they live. This can range from every 3 to 5 years, depending on location.

ServSafe®

The National Restaurant Association Educational Foundation developed the ServSafe® Program, which can be taken online or in person. This program has an excellent reputation and is highly recommended by managers in this field. A manager who attended ServSafe® training would generally know more about food safety and ways of preventing foodborne illness than a manager who only took a course that met the minimum requirements mandated by his county. The program focuses on the role of the foodservice manager in determining risks, creating policies, and training and supervising staff. ServSafe® certification lasts a maximum of 5 years, but requirements vary by county. For example, in Nassau County, New York, the manager must have at least 10 hours of instruction, and certification must be renewed every 3 years.[4,5]

The ServSafe® Program is a well-recognized food safety training program. It covers the range of food preparation and serving safety knowledge and how to implement it. ServSafe® graduates become members of the International Food Safety Council, started by the National Restaurant Association in 1993.

Other Food Manager Training Programs

There are several programs that focus on proper foodservice safety and sanitation. Programs are offered at various locations and at various levels. Some are at the college level, some are from professional organizations, and some are from federal, state, and local agencies.

The National Assessment Institute operates nationwide and runs the National Certified Professional Food Manager (CPFM) program. The CPFM certification is a well-recognized credential that certifies that the recipient knows how to protect public health through food safety. This certification also makes the recipient more marketable for future positions.[6]

The Dietary Managers Association is a nationwide non-profit organization established in 1960. There are almost 15,000 members who strive to provide the best nutrition care using foodservice management. This organization offers several continuing education opportunities, some of which are available online.[7]

The Food Safety Training and Education Alliance for Retail, Food Service, Vending, Institutions, and Regulators were founded in response to the President's Food Safety Initiative of 1997 to encourage cooperation between the government and foodservice establishments. This organization also offers several training programs and materials.[8]

In a healthcare facility, a Dietetic Technician (DTR) or a Registered Dietitian (RD) may be responsible for both foodservice management and monitoring of nutritional status. Both RDs and DTRs are certified nationally in the United States by the Commission on Dietetic Registration. They need to complete continuing education hours to remain certified and have a responsibility to follow the foodservice related journals and attend meetings to stay current.

Meeting Regulations

The Federal **Food Code** is published collaboratively by the FDA, FSIS, and CDC. It applies to agencies that monitor retail and commercial food safety. The Food Code is revised every 2 years and is one step that the U.S. government is taking to monitor and prevent foodborne illness. The Food Code states that HACCP plans should be implemented and kept on file in the foodservice establishment. Therefore, if a manager or an owner feels that he needs to bring records home, only copies of these should leave the facility. The purpose of the Food Code is to protect the public health and provide the consumer with safe, unadulterated food. It covers a wide range of topics including employee hygiene, such as covering open infected cuts and proper hand washing, wiping cloth use, and food handling. The entire list would be too exhaustive to include in this textbook, but it would be worthwhile to review the Food Code online at http://vm.cfsan.fda .gov/%7Edms/foodcode.html.[9]

The CDC tracks emerging pathogens that could be spread globally due to imported foods with low levels of contamination. In 1993, the CDC developed PulseNet to detect clusters of foodborne disease outbreaks using pulsed-field gel electrophoresis, a technique that gives scientists a DNA profile of each type of infecting bacteria. This process helps with early identification of common outbreak sources, helps in outbreak investigations, lets scientists differentiate cases associated with outbreaks from sporadic cases, helps to identify the sources and strains of outbreaks, and helps facilitate communication between public health laboratories.[10]

The FDA and its parent, the U.S. Public Health Service (PHS), both fall under the U.S. Department of Health and Human Services. The FDA works to protect the public against unsafe and impure food, drugs, and cosmetics. It is the main agency that regulates food safety in the United States. These agencies work to protect human health in the United States. The CDC, also in the PHS, tracks reported foodborne illnesses and tries to determine their causes. The agency also does this for diseases and other hazards.

FoodNet is the Foodborne Diseases Active Surveillance Network of CDC's Emerging Infections Program. This agency gathers information from 10 locations on foodborne diseases caused by enteric pathogens. The locations are in Connecticut, Georgia, Maryland, Minnesota, New Mexico, Oregon, and Tennessee, as well as some counties in California, Colorado, and New York. Incidence is monitored using population-based examination for laboratory-diagnosed related diseases. When FoodNet started in 1996, cases of Campylobacter, Escherichia coli (E. coli) O157, Listeria, Salmonella, Shigella, Vibrio, and Yersinia were tracked. In 1997, FoodNet started monitoring for Cryptosporidium, Cyclospora, and hemolytic uremic syndrome, and in 2000, FoodNet started monitoring non-E. coli O157. From 1996–2004, FoodNet increased its surveillance population from 14.2 million people in five states to 44.1 million people (15.2% of the U.S. population) in 10 states.[1]

In 2004, FoodNet identified 15,806 laboratory-diagnosed cases of foodborne infections. There were declines in foodborne infection incidence caused by Campylobacter, Cryptosporidium, Shiga toxin-producing E. coli O157, Listeria, Salmonella, and Yersinia. The overall incidence per 100,000 people was 14.7 for Salmonella, 12.9 for Campylobacter, 5.1 for Shigella, and 0.9 for E. coli O157. In addition, incidence per 1 million people was 13.2 for Cryptosporidium, 3.9 for Yersinia, 2.8 for Vibrio, 2.7 for Listeria, and 0.3 for Cyclospora.[1]

Bioterrorism Preparedness

On June 12, 2002, the U.S. Congress passed the Public Health Security and Bioterrorism Preparedness and Response Act of 2002

Learning Point: Customers can sue a foodservice establishment for food safety violations, as covered in USDA AER-799. Each state deals with food-related liabilities according to the Uniform Commercial Code, which is standardized between the states. To have a case for a lawsuit, a dissatisfied customer must be able to show that the food was not fit to be served, that the food caused harm, and that the foodservice establishment did not handle food in the safe and proper manner expected. There can be a failure due to *negligence* or due to a *failure to warn* customers about potential hazards. For example, if you have rare steak on your menu, it is a good idea to put a warning note on your menu that this may contain bacteria that can harm the very young, very old, and pregnant women. If the lawsuit is successful, the customer can be given compensatory damages for lost work time, lost wages, or medical expenses, as well as punitive damages to punish the establishment for neglect.

If there is an outbreak of food poisoning, and if your facility is diligently following HACCP guidelines and keeping the required documentation, the reasonable care defense can be used. This means that you can prove that everything possible was done to keep food safe and to protect your customers from potential foodborne illness. *Save your written rules and regulations, training logs, HACCP flow charts, HACCP temperature charts, health department inspection reports, and internally done inspection reports to show that your facility was diligently following food safety guidelines.*[11]

(Public Law 107-188). This was developed in response to the attacks on September 11, 2001, which underscored the need to further protect our food supply. "TITLE III—Protecting Safety and Security of Food And Drug Supply" of this act focuses on ensuring that the food supply is safe and secure. This act amends the Federal Food, Drug, and Cosmetic Act. The FDA can test for possible food adulteration due to biological, chemical, or radiological agents more rapidly under this act. Food imports received from a "debarred" supplier will be held and prevented from arriving at their destination. A person who is not "debarred" may establish at his or her own expense that the item meets federal requirements and may receive the item. *This is another good reason to order from reputable, approved suppliers.* It is noted that many foreign suppliers are now seeking and obtaining U.S. FDA HACCP certification. The Secretary of Health and Human Services now requires any facility that manufactures, processes, packs, or holds food for consumption in the United States must be registered with the secretary. In addition, an imported food from a source not registered with the secretary may be held at the port; thus it will not be allowed to enter the United States. The Secretary has the right to review written and electronic records relating to the manufacture, processing, packing, distribution, receipt, holding, or importation of such article maintained by or on behalf of such person in any format and at any location, excluding farms and restaurants, and this documentation must be held for at least 2 years at the facility. *Although the act says this does not directly apply to restaurants, it can only be to your benefit to hold on to HACCP related items such as temperature logs and shellfish tags for 2 years.*[12]

The Center for Food Safety and Applied Nutrition oversees the U.S. food supply and conducts research on possible emerging food safety threats to public health. This agency tests a variety of foods for biological and chemical agents. The Center for Veterinary Medicine oversees food and food additives intended for animal consumption. This agency can detect substances such as drug residues in food. The Office of Regulatory Affairs deals with FDA activities, including inspections at ports of entry into the United States. This agency is working on research to develop tools that can quickly analyze large numbers of samples and to test foods for many substances at once. The FDA's National Center for Toxicological Research conducts scientific research based on the future needs of the FDA. This agency is working to define mechanisms of action associated with the potential toxicity of FDA-regulated foods (U.S. Food and Drug Administration, Report to Congress, 2005). Read more about bioterrorism and the food supply in Chapter 16.

Sanitation and Safety

The United States is composed of myriad consumers who have changing eating habits and an increased taste for ethnic and exotic menu items. This leads to an increased use of imported foods and foods obtained from a variety of sources. Also, more people are relying on readily available foods such as cold cuts, take out foods, and fast foods, to cut down on cooking time due to busy schedules.

Learning Point: The Food Code says that fish which will not be thoroughly cooked must either be blast frozen to −31° F or below for 15 hours or frozen to −4° F or below for 168 hours (7 days). The manager must keep records of the product and temperature treatment of such raw fish for at least ninety days. This is an example of how the Food Code can give guidance for HACCP implementation at your facility.

Because we now are able to consume foods that are brought to us from all over the country and all over the world, transit time for deliveries has increased. The increased traveling time also increases the possibility of *danger zone* temperatures during transport (most bacteria grow best between 41°F (5°C) to 135°F (57°C).

Learning Point: More Americans than ever before are becoming susceptible to foodborne illness. This is due to the aging population, increase in average lifespan, and increase in lifespan of those with chronic diseases such as cancer or HIV/AIDS due to better medications. Other vulnerable groups include the very young, pregnant women, and those on immunosuppressants.

Safety, sanitation, and maintenance are equally important. Receiving and storage areas should be checked after deliveries to make sure that items were put away properly and in a timely manner. These areas need to be cleaned on a daily basis. This will help prevent vermin such as rodents or cockroaches from using these areas as nesting grounds. The receiving and storage areas should be considered when developing your foodservice establishment's HACCP program.

Foodborne illness can be caused by a variety of *microbiological, chemical, or physical* reasons. Foodborne illness is the term used to describe any disease carried by food or contracted from food. According to the CDC, an outbreak of foodborne illness occurs when two or more people have the same illness after consuming the same food. This is confirmed by laboratory analysis of the food in question.

Continuous cleaning throughout the day is required and safe food handling should be given top priority. Maintenance issues are important. These include prompt cleanup of spills, which could prevent a slip or fall, and removal of grease buildup on hoods, which can prevent fires and remove grease that attracts pests.

Cockroaches, flies, rodents, and other animals or insects that enter your foodservice establishment are considered to be vermin. These can spread disease. If an infestation is found during a health department inspection, it can lead to closure of your facility. Vermin hide in small openings in walls, boxes, or furniture and come out at night. You should patch holes, cracks, and areas around pipes to decrease the number of available hiding areas.[13]

Spoilage is the term used to indicate that food is no longer fit for human consumption due to microbiological, biochemical, physical, or chemical contamination changes in the food. Spoiled food may be difficult to detect using our senses alone. The food item may have a normal appearance, smell, or taste. However, more obvious signs of contamination are easily detected by our senses if the food has obvious signs of mold, discoloration, foul odors, or bad flavors.

Foodborne illness does not always come from bacteria. Some foodborne *parasites* are trichinae, tapeworms, and roundworms. Consuming undercooked meat, such as pork, may lead to trichinosis (characterized by fever, muscle weakness, and diarrhea).

It is recommended to cook pork to 145°F (63°C) or 165°F (74°C) in a microwave oven. Beef or pork may be infested with tapeworms, which are intestinal parasites. Undercooked or raw seafood may contain tapeworms or roundworms.

Prions are the newest category of potential foodborne illness. They are small glycosylated protein molecules. They are best known for causing Bovine Spongiform Encephalopathy, commonly called Mad Cow Disease, and can be found in brain, spinal cord, spleen, and lymph tissues of infected animals.[14]

There are many different types of bacteria that can lead to illness. *Protozoa* may cause foodborne illness when ingested. They are unicellular organisms present in seawater, lakes, streams, and soil. Protozoa in food or water can spread amoebic dysentery.

Bacteria need time, a hospitable temperature range, enough moisture, some form of food, a range of pH (measure of acidity or alkalinity), and many (but not all bacteria) need oxygen to grow. A good way to remember this is the acronym FAT TOM—*food, acidity, time, temperature, oxygen, and moisture.*[2] As mentioned earlier, most bacteria grow best between 41°F (5°C) to 135°F (57°C). Any food left out in the danger zone more than 4 hours should be discarded. Food should really not be left between 70° (21°C) to 125°F (52°C) for more than 2 hours. Both time and temperature need to be considered to keep food safe from microbiological growth. Table 7.1 lists those bacteria and viruses that cause foodborne illness, and Table 7.2 delineates the correct food temperatures to follow.

When bacteria first enters a food, their growth is in the lag phase, meaning they are not growing rapidly. At this stage, decreasing the time the food is held, properly controlling temperatures, cut-

Table 7.1 Foodborne Illness Chart

Name of Bacteria/Virus	Potential Sources	Symptoms
Campylobacter (bacteria)	raw or undercooked poultry meat	causes fever, diarrhea, and abdominal cramps
Ciguatoxin (toxin)	contaminated fin fish Heat, cold, gastric juices, drying, salting, or marinating does not deactivate the Ciguatoxin-1 toxin.	gastrointestinal, neurological, and sometimes cardiovascular symptoms
Clostridium botulinum	improperly canned products, honey given to infants < 1 yr	nerve toxin causes rare, serious paralytic illness; blurred vision, slurred speech, impaired swallowing, dry mouth, and muscle weakness; infants may seem lethargic, feed

continues

Table 7.1   (continued)

Name of Bacteria/Virus	Potential Sources	Symptoms
		poorly, be constipated, have a weak cry, and poor muscle tone. If untreated, it may lead to paralysis of the arms, legs, trunk and respiratory muscles.
Hepatitis A (virus)	improper hand washing and uncleanliness	fever, jaundice, and abdominal pain, possible liver failure or even death
Listeria monocytogenes (bacteria)	leafy vegetables, unpasteurized cheeses, soft cheeses, hot dogs, luncheon meats, cold cuts, poultry, refrigerated smoked seafood, and refrigerated meat spreads	meningitis and other infections
Noroviruses (Norwalk-like viruses and caliciviruses) (viruses)	undercooked seafood, any contaminated foods or beverages, contaminated surfaces, or transmitted due to poor hygiene	nausea, vomiting, diarrhea, and some stomach cramping potentially accompanied by fever, chills, headache, muscle ache, and tiredness
Salmonella (bacteria)	undercooked poultry or eggs	fever, diarrhea, and abdominal cramps

Table 7.1 (continued)

Staphylococcus aureus (bacteria)	food handlers with runny noses or sore throats or with infected cuts. The toxins remain after the foods are cooked and the bacteria is killed	gastrointestinal illness
Toxoplasma gonii (a parasitic infection)	undercooked meat	Although usually asymptomatic, maternal toxoplasmosis infection may lead to congenital impairments including hearing loss, visual impairment, and mental retardation and chronic toxoplasmic encephalitis affects those who have impaired immune systems.

Source: Department of Health and Human Services, Centers for Disease Control and Prevention, Disease Listing. (2006, March 29). Retrieved July 19, 2006 from http://www.cdc.gov/ncidod/dbmd/diseaseinfo/default.htm and Gutierrez, J. (2005). Food Safety for Restaurants and Institutions. CEU Module, Level I, 2 contact hours, CEU4U.com.

ting down on moisture content, and decreasing pH (more acidic) can help prevent the rapid growth of bacteria in the next phase, which is the log phase. In the log phase, bacteria grow at exponential logarithmic levels, potentially doubling in population every 20 minutes. Foods containing bacteria in this phase have a great potential to cause foodborne illness. When the bacterial population gets too crowded, uses up much of the available nutrients, and produces wastes, it reaches the stationary phase. In this phase some bacteria

Table 7.2   Guidelines for Safe Food Temperatures

Frozen food: keep < 0°F (–18°C)

Refrigerated food: keep < 41°F (5°C)

Dry storage: keep between 50°F (10°C) and 70°F (21°C)

Items being chilled: go from 70°F (21°C) to 135°F (57°C) in 2 hours or less, and should be chilled to 41°F (5°C) in less than 4 hours in small batches and shallow containers.

Items being reheated: reach 165°F (74°C) within 2 hours.

Cold items: held at 41°F (5°C) or below

Hot items: held at 135°F (57°C) or above

Cooked Items:

Food Item	Internal temperature
Hamburger	155° F
Ground beef, veal, lamb, or pork	155° F
Beef, Veal, or Lamb Roasts & steaks	
medium	145° F
well-done	145° F
Pork, medium	145° F
Pork, well-done	145° F
Ham/Sausage, fresh	145° F
Chicken, whole & pieces	165° F
Duck	165° F
Turkey (without stuffing)	165° F
Whole	165° F
Breast	165° F
Dark meat	165° F
Stuffing (prepared separately)	165° F
Egg Casseroles	145° F
Egg sauces and custards	145° F
Fin Fish	Flesh opaque & flakes easily with fork; 145°F
Shrimp, Lobster & Crabs	Shells red and flesh pearly & opaque
Clams, Oysters & Mussels	Shells are open

Source: USDA (2006). Retrieved on 11/3/2006. Available at: www.fsis.usda.gov/thermy.

are dying while others grow. Eventually, when more bacteria die than grow, the bacterial population is in the death phase. See Figure 7.2 for a pictorial of the Bacterial Growth Curve. Therefore, the chicken salad left out at room temperature since 10:00 AM could have quite a population of salmonella residing in it by the time the 3:00 PM lunch stragglers come in.

As per the Food Code, foods including eggs, fish, meat, pork, and some game animals should be cooked to an internal temperature of 145°F (63°C) or higher for 15 seconds. Other foods including fish, injected meats, and some game animals, should be cooked to 155°F (68°C) for 15 seconds. Poultry, some wild game animals, stuffed fish, stuffed meats, stuffed poultry, and stuffed pasta should be cooked to 165°F (74°C) or higher for 15 seconds. These cooking times were established because the offending bacteria are generally killed off at these temperatures.[15]

Foods with a water activity (A_w) of less than 0.85 do not easily support bacterial growth. This is because they do not hold sufficient moisture for bacterial growth.[16]

Dented or swollen cans should never be accepted during a food delivery. This is because cans may become dented or bulge due to gas formation caused by bacterial growth, indicating the contents are spoiled or may contain the deadly bacterium called *botulism*. Rust can damage the seals and allow the food to become contaminated.

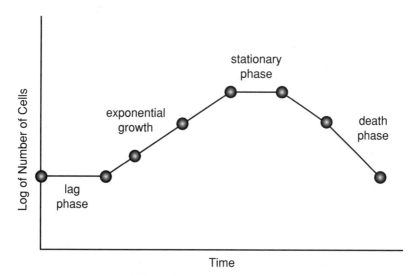

FIGURE 7.2 Bacterial Growth Curve

Learning Point: Potentially hazardous foods include milk, milk products, eggs, fish, shellfish, potatoes, tofu, soybean products, garlic in oil, cooked vegetables, raw seeds, bean sprouts, sliced melons and meat, such as beef, pork, lamb, and poultry. In general, any protein containing food is a potentially hazardous food. Potentially hazardous food should be defrosted under cool running water. The cool running water helps to minimize the amount of time the product is in the danger zone. Stagnant water easily comes to room temperature, thus promoting bacterial growth. Another good way of defrosting is to put the item overnight in the refrigerator to defrost. Although placing the item into the microwave for a few seconds is permissible if the food is to be cooked immediately; this method is not preferable. Never defrost at room temperature, as this encourages bacterial growth near the outside of the item, which defrosts quicker than the inside.

Cross contamination can occur when bacteria transfers from one surface or food to another. For example:

1. Raw, contaminated ingredients are added to a dish that will not be cooked further.
2. Food contact surfaces are not properly cleaned and sanitized between uses.
3. Raw, contaminated foods drip onto foods that do not require further cooking.
4. Employees touch contaminated foods and then touch ready-to-eat items without first washing their hands.
5. Wiping cloths that have not been sanitized are used.
6. Employees return to work without washing their hands after using the restroom, coughing, or sneezing or they have open cuts or sores.

Examples of Cross Contamination

Example #1: Raw meats should be stored below any vegetables in the walk-in refrigerator. For example, if raw steak is placed above raw onions in the refrigerator, when the meat juice drips down onto the onions, the onions can easily be contaminated with E. coli. A few hours later, the salad person then takes out the onions needed to add to the garden salads. These onions now have many E. coli growing in and on them, just waiting to get a customer sick.

Example #2: Acidic foods should not be prepared or stored in metal containers because brass, copper, galvanized metals, cadmium, enamel, or lead can leach into the food products. Metal poisoning, or chemical hazards, has been contracted from acidic foods including sauerkraut, tomatoes, lemonade, and fruit punch.

Example #3: Almost 20% of poultry imported into Finland in 2005 contained Salmonella. The National Food Agency Finland found Salmonella in 9 out of the 54 randomly inspected poultry shipments from Poland, Hungary, France, and Brazil despite certificates issued from the originating countries saying they were salmonella-free. Because of a more recent effort for careful monitoring, now less than 1,000 people get salmonella poisoning in Finland per year.[17]

Example #4: Raw milk (milk that has not been processed via pasteurization or homogenization before consumption) obtained using cow shares, a practice in some rural areas where someone could rent the cow for a certain period of time, is associated with an outbreak of E. coli. The milk is actually unregulated because the consumer is renting a cow, not purchasing the milk. Fifteen children became sick and five needed hospitalization, three in critical condition, because they drank raw milk instead of pasteurized milk. According to the Washington State Department of Agriculture, raw milk is hazardous and may contain several bacteria such as Enterotoxigenic Staphylococcus aureus, Campylobacter jejuni, Salmonella species, E. coli, Listeria monocytogenes, Mycobacterium tuberculosis, Mycobacterium bovis, Brucella species, Coxiella burnetii, or Yersinia enterocolitica.[18,19]

Example #5: Salad bars can be hazardous places for several reasons. Foods in the salad bar may be held at improper temperatures. This may not be readily obvious unless a variety of foods in the salad bar are measured for temperature on a regular basis because one side of the salad bar may be cold enough, but the other not cold enough due to a malfunction of the internal fan. There should be sneeze guards to reduce the possible spread of bacteria. Customers may spill food, touch food items with their fingers, or refill soiled plates with second helpings. Extra plates should be kept near the salad bar and any employee observing such behaviors by customers

Learning Point: Food storage should be given an important priority in your facility. Use the *first in, first out* (FIFO) method and be sure to label and date all food items. All items that require refrigeration should be kept at 41°F (5°C) or below. All potentially hazardous food should be below 41°F (5°C) or above 135°F (57°C). Storage areas should be clean and dry and cleaned on a regular basis. All food should be stored 6 inches off the floor.

should discourage them and redirect them to the proper course of action, such as taking a new plate.

Foodborne illnesses generally have an incubation period. Customers likely will not develop symptoms until they get home. Many foodborne bacteria lead to diarrhea, stomach cramping, nausea, and vomiting after the incubation period.[13]

If your foodservice location is involved in an outbreak, the increased costs include higher insurance premiums, lawyer and court fees, expenses to test foods and employees, time and money for retraining employees, time lost to re-sanitize the equipment, and money lost due to discarded questionable food supplies. There also may be lower employee morale, increased absenteeism, a feeling of embarrassment due to bad publicity, lost sales, and a decreased reputation for your establishment.[2]

If a consumer does complain about foodborne illness, the person

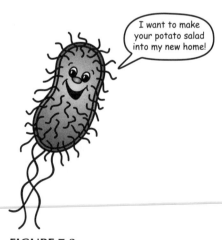

FIGURE 7.3

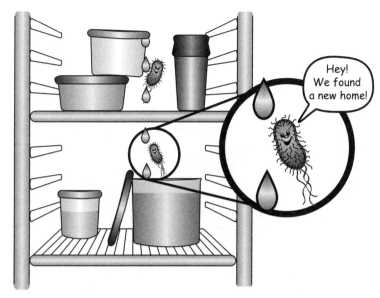

FIGURE 7.4

should be asked to complete a complaint report form that asks appropriate questions and a record of the incident should be kept in the foodservice establishment. The complaint form should include the names and addresses of all customers in the party, the name of the waiter/waitress, date and time of the meal, and items ordered/consumed. You should write down the onset time of symptoms, and obtain a list of other foods eaten before and after the meal. A sample form is included in Table 7.3.

HACCP

HACCP was first envisioned in the 1960s by the National Aeronautics and Space Administration (NASA) along with the Pillsbury company to make sure that the food given to the astronauts was safe, because foodborne illness in space could devastate the entire space program. HACCP was actively used in 1971 to provide microbiologically safe food to the astronauts and in 1973 by NASA for the Skylab laboratory. The goal was to provide safe, convenient, nutritious, and appetizing foods for the astronauts. HACCP's main thrust is identifying *critical control points* (CCPs) that could affect

Table 7.3   Foodborne Illness Complaint Record

Name: _____   Date: _____

Address: _____

_____

Phone: (work)_____   (home) _____

Others Dining With You:

Name: _____   Date: _____

Address: _____

_____

Phone: (work)_____   (home) _____

Name: _____   Date: _____

Address: _____

_____

Phone: (work)_____   (home) _____

Name: _____   Date: _____

Address: _____

_____

Phone: (work)_____   (home) _____

Symptoms: _____

Onset (date) _____   (time) _____

Medical Treatment: Doctor/Hospital Name: _____

Address: _____

_____

Phone: _____

Foods in Meal Eaten: _____

_____

Table 7.3 (continued)

Meal: (date) _____ (time) _____
Location of Meal: _____
Identifying Factors: _____
Description: _____
Leftovers: _____
Other foods or beverages eaten before or after this meal: _____
Other Agencies Notified: Agency: _____
Contact Name: _____ Phone: _____
Signature of Employee Collecting Information: _____
Date: _____ Time: _____
Referred To: _____

quality or safety of the food during procurement and processing as well as standards for the delivery of the finished food products. These standards were developed with *clean room standards* in mind where microbiologically tests are conducted on the foods.[20]

Formal HACCP rules were established for the seafood industry on December 18, 1995 and for the juice industry on January 19, 2001, which took effect between January 2002 and January 2004. In 1998, the U.S. Department of Agriculture also made HACCP a requirement for meat and poultry processing plants, which had to implement HACCP by January 1999 although very small plants had until January 25, 2000.[21]

Your facility's HACCP plans should be unique due to the unique aspects of your establishment as well as properties of the raw ingredients. Preliminary steps to developing an HACCP plan outlined by the FDA are to first assemble the HACCP team by including knowledgeable management and production personnel. Next, describe the foods used at the location, their ingredients, and their methods of processing and distribution. Decide on the purpose of the food, for instance as dinner items at an airport or meals served to sick or elderly people in a hospital or nursing home. Next, the team develops

---

Learning Point: HACCP involves seven main principles:

1. Hazard analysis—what can go wrong?
2. Determine the CCPs.
3. Establish critical limits.
4. Establish a system to monitor CCPs.
5. Decide upon a corrective action.
6. Verify that HACCP is working properly.
7. Document and demonstrate that it works.

---

a flow diagram that shows a basic outline of all the steps needed in food production. The team should review the flow diagram to check it for accuracy and completeness, and make and document any needed modifications to it.[22]

First, potential hazards need to be identified. Potential hazards are associated with a food and ways of controlling hazards need to be identified. The hazard could be biological, such as E. coli, a chemical, such as the botulinum toxin, or physical, such as broken glass in the ice machine. Additional risk factors to consider include: water content and pH of food items, actions taken at each step of the recipe, quantity of food prepared, and the type of customer normally served (young, old, chronically ill, those who may be pregnant). Larger quantities of food need more time for heating, cooling, and reheating.

A food item's water A_w is defined as being the ratio between its own vapor pressure when it is completely undisturbed and the vapor pressure of distilled water under identical conditions. If an item's A_w is 0.80, its vapor pressure is 80% of the vapor pressure that pure water exerts. A_w increases with temperature, because more water vapor is produced at higher temperatures.[23] Since most foods have an A_w greater than 0.95, they contain enough moisture to support the growth of bacteria mold. If the amount of available moisture is reduced to 0.85 or less, microorganisms will not find the food a very hospitable place to grow. This is because bacteria need nutrients and waste dissolved in water to pass through their cell walls, and not enough water is available at lower A_w values. Although most microorganisms grow best at A_w between 0.91 and 0.99, Clostridium botulinum can grow and produce deadly botulism toxin in items with a pH above 4.6 and an A_w above 0.85.[23,24]

Table 7.4   Water Activity (A_w) of Some Common Foods

Food Item	Aw
Liverwurst	0.96
Cheese Spread	0.95
Red Bean Paste	0.93
Caviar	0.92
Fudge Sauce	0.83
Soft Moist Pet Food	0.83
Salami	0.82
Soy Sauce	0.80
Peanut Butter 15% total moisture	0.70
Dry Milk 8% total moisture	0.70

Source: USDA. (2006.) Compiled from: http://www.nal.usda.gov/fnic/foodcomp/ Data/ SR18/nutrlist/sr18a255.pdf

Second, CCPs need to be identified. These points can be determined anywhere in the production process or recipe of a food item where controlling the food or action could prevent, eliminate, or reduce the potential hazard to levels that are acceptable. These include points in time from when the item is raw and still is with its producer or grower to the time it is consumed by your customers. At each step during the workflow of food production, there is a risk or chance that the hazard of unacceptable contamination can occur. CCPs include cooking, holding hot foods, chilling foods, or storing chilled foods and packaging. Also included are sanitizing cutting boards between products, **cross contamination**, personal hygiene (including proper hand washing), receiving deliveries, thawing, mixing together of ingredients, changing pH, and making sure that approved vendors who handle the food properly before it gets to your facility are used.

Preventive measures with critical limits need to be set for each control point. A critical limit can be either the greatest or smallest measurement or a biological, chemical, or physical condition. Critical limits need to be controlled to prevent, eliminate, or reduce the chance of a food safety hazard to an acceptable level. Critical limits must be based on scientific data. These include temperature, time, physical dimensions, humidity, moisture level, water content, pH/acidity, salt concentration, chlorine concentration, viscosity, preservative content, and sensory data including aroma and appearance. For example, one critical limit is that the chlorine concentration for the automatic dishwasher should fall between 50 to 100 parts per minute. This concentration is needed to properly sanitize dishes and silverware. Another critical limit is that chicken needs to be cooked to an internal temperature of at least 165°F (74°C).[23,25]

CCP steps should be identified separately for each menu item and each corresponding recipe. After establishing the CCPs, establish measures with critical limits to prevent contamination and foodborne illness at each control point. These should include temperature and time requirements.

Procedures need to be established to monitor the CCPs. These include monitoring cooking and **holding temperatures**. Temperature must be properly monitored and recorded. Also, deep containers should not be used for hot foods, which would take longer to cool in deeper containers. If for some reason a critical limit is not met, establish a corrective action. For example, if the food was in the steam table for 1 hour and dropped below 135°F (57°C), it can be reheated. However, if it was out four hours, it should be discarded.

Once the CCPs are established, monitoring procedures are needed to focus on the areas that may be the most problematic. HACCP requires good record keeping procedures. Records such as temperature logs, any needed laboratory tests for bacteria, and the concentration of sanitizer for the dishwashing machine should be kept. There should be procedures that verify that HACCP is working properly in your facility. These include regular use of temperature logs. Keep all HACCP records, including your HACCP plans, monitoring forms including temperature logs, any corrective actions taken, and any verification activities on file in your facility. Time required to keep the records varies by county.[21]

Corrective actions for each CCP need to be specified ahead of time and included in the facility's HACCP plan. Corrective actions are taken when routine monitoring shows a critical limit has not been met. Procedures should verify that HACCP is working properly. All HACCP records such as HACCP plans, monitoring forms including temperature logs, corrective actions plans, and any verification activities should be kept on file in your facility. Time required to keep the records varies by county.

Corrective action plans should state, determine, and correct the reason for noncompliance. Include the fate of the product that does not meet standards, and keep track of any corrective actions that have been taken. The plan should include the date the violation was noted, the date that repair was ordered for the apparatus or that the first remedial action was taken, and the date and time of the actual problem resolution.[22]

To verify that HACCP is working as planned, the manager should review logs, including those for times and temperatures. Any personnel who cook should use pocket, refrigerator, freezer, dry storage, hot holding, and meat thermometers regularly. The manager, chef, or other trained employee should take food items' temperatures at various time points during the day. The purpose of verifying and validating the HACCP plan is to prove that it is scientifically and technically sound, that possible hazards were recognized, and that if the plan is used properly these will be controlled. Data used may come from expert advice and scientific studies, observations, measurements, and evaluations. For instance, validation of the cooking process for hamburgers needs to include the scientific justification of the heating times and temperatures needed to destroy pathogenic bacteria and research studies to confirm that the cooking conditions will provide the needed amounts of time and temperature to each hamburger. Documentation should include a summary of the hazard analysis, the facility's complete HACCP plan, validation records, and quality control-related records.[22,25]

The Role of the Manager and HACCP

A well-educated manager should be able to implement HACCP and train employees on their roles in any size foodservice operation. Even with HACCP properly in place, the risk of foodborne illness is not completely eliminated although it is substantially reduced. There is always the possibility that food can be mishandled or contaminated food ingredients could be received during a delivery. An analysis is the careful study of all aspects of the food preparation process.

The only items purchased that should have microbiological or mold counts are the ones that are supposed to contain these microorganisms such as yogurt, blue cheese, and tempeh. Ideally, a manager should visit the warehouses and check the transportation systems of potential suppliers before selecting one. For example, how do you know if a supplier's refrigerated trucks are keeping foods at 41°F (5°C) or below? Good suppliers be able to deliver foods at proper temperatures, have clean refrigerated trucks, also be aware of food safety, use packaging that protects the food, allow you to inspect the food deliveries, and be able to deliver when you or your employees are available to handle the delivery.

A HACCP flowchart should be used for each multistep process that involves food production. This will help to keep track of the most hazardous parts of the procedure and the controls in place that could help prevent the hazards. A blank sample form is included in Table 7.5, and Table 7.6 provides a form filled out using fried chicken as an example.

More and more supervisory job postings state that they are looking for people with strong knowledge of HACCP and regulatory requirements. In addition to learning about HACCP to improve conditions at your current location, the skills and knowledge that you acquire will make you more marketable for future positions.

Summary

Effective, properly conducted employee training can make the difference between a well-run foodservice facility and a facility that can be the breeding ground for hidden bacteria. It is ultimately the manager's responsibility to make sure that foods are being handled safely and that employees are acting within accordance of the rules and regulations set forth by the Federal Food Code. The Federal Food Code discusses rules and regulations about food safety that are monitored and enforced on the local level. Other government agencies are also involved in food testing and protecting the health and safety of the public, including food safety. Foodborne illness is the term used to describe any disease carried by food or contracted from food. Foodborne illness can be caused by a variety of microbiological, chemical, or physical reasons. HACCP involves seven main principles—perform hazard analysis, determine CCPs, establish critical limits, establish a system to monitor CCPs, decide upon a corrective action, verify that HACCP is working properly, and document and demonstrate that HACCP works.

Table 7.5 HACCP (Hazard Analysis and Critical Control Points) Worksheet

Date: _____ Start Time: _____

Product: _____ End Time: _____

Ingredients: _____

_____

_____

Sources: _____

_____

_____

Steps	Potential Problem or Hazard	CCP	Control or Solution

Comments: _____

Signature: _____

Adapted from National Assessment Institute, 1994, pp. 47–50.

Table 7.6 HACCP (Hazard Analysis and Critical Control Points) Worksheet

Date: ___Jan 7, 2006___ Start Time: ___10 AM___

Product: ___Fried Chicken___ End Time: ___11:15 AM___

Ingredients: ___frying chicken, bread crumbs, eggs, water___

Sources: ___USDA inspected poultry, generic bread crumbs,___
___eggs from an approved source___

Steps	Potential Problem or Hazard	CCP	Control or Solution
Received poultry	It may not be from an approved source or may have salmonella contamination	YES, a CCP	Do not accept the shipment if not 41°F or below or not USDA inspected from an approved source.
Storage	Spoilage. Raw contact/drip		Keep at 41°F or below. Check the cooler temperatures. Store raw foods below cooked foods. Use FIFO.
Portion	Contact with dirty equipment or dirty hands		Handwashing. Clean/sanitize equipment. Return excess to refrigerator.
Batter/ Bread	Bacterial spores in breading/batter ingredients	YES, a CCP	Do not reuse flour or batter.
Fry	Bacterial spores survive.	YES, a CCP	Cook to a minimum internal temp. or 165°F, as measured in the center of the meat.
Hot-Hold	Bacteria may multiply unless high temperatures are maintained.	YES, a CCP	Product temperature checks 140°F internal temperature. Measure center every 2 hours. Return to stove and reheat to 165°F.
Serve			
Storage	Must cool to 45°F internal temp. within four hours. Do not touch with bare hands.	YES, a CCP	Shallow pans, measure depth. Measure temperature of refrigerator daily. Discard contaminated pieces.
Reheat Leftovers	Slow, inadequate reheating.	YES, a CCP	Reheat to 165°F internal temp. in less than 2 hours with proper equipment. Measure internal temp.

Comments: _____

Signature: _____

Adapted from National Assessment Institute, 1994, pp. 47–50.

Student Activities

1. Select a recipe. Determine the possible food safety-related hazards that could go wrong with this recipe. Decide what controls can be used to minimize or prevent these hazards. What corrective action would you use? Use the HACCP worksheet as a guide.
2. As the owner of an expanding restaurant chain, you want to hire a manager for a new location that you are about to open. What training and knowledge should you look for in the applicants for this position? Why is hiring an HACCP trained manager a good idea?
3. There is frequently a pool of water on the floor near the ice machine. You observe employees carelessly using the scoop and waiting several hours to clean up the water. As the manager, you decide that it would be a good idea to in-service your staff about proper use of the scoop and the importance of keeping the floor dry to prevent injuries from falls and to discourage pests. How would you proceed?
4. A customer orders baked ziti at your restaurant. He does not finish and takes the remainder of the meal home in a "doggie bag." The next evening, he calls your restaurant and tells the manager that he had a case of foodborne illness, with diarrhea and vomiting. What is your restaurant's liability? What should you ask the customer?
5. The chef at your restaurant starts to defrost a bag of calamari under cool running water in the sink. The salad prep employee passes the sink and shuts off the water. As the manager, you notice the bag of calamari sitting in a bowl of water in the sink, but there is no running water on. What would you do?

CASE STUDY #1

After Hurricane Katrina hit the southeast coastline of the United States in late August 2005, there was considerable damage to businesses and massive flooding in the affected states. The Southern Shrimp Alliance, comprised of shrimp fishermen and processors from eight southeastern states, urged the government to promptly provide test results of food and water supplies to the public. This organization wanted to assure the public that wild-caught U.S. shrimp remained safe for consumers. The organization is required by law to follow HACCP plans. Therefore, any caught shrimp that contacted the floodwaters or that were kept at or above 45°F (7°C) for more than 3 hours had to be destroyed. FDA inspectors inspected the processing plants before work resumed. In addition, the National Oceanic and Atmospheric Administration tested shrimp for contamination.[26]

Your restaurant routinely orders shrimp from a vendor who is located in Louisiana and is a member of the Southern Shrimp Alliance. How would your business have been affected in October 2005? The shrimp fishermen properly followed HACCP protocols. What was their main motivation?

CASE STUDY #2

Marmum, subsidiary of Dubai Investments, is a dairy based in Dubai. It recently received HACCP certification from the U.S. FDA. Alan Comyn, Marmum's General Manager said, "The size and diversity of the regional food industry calls for a rating method that can signify product quality and safety to the consumer. Marmum's HACCP certification is testament to our stringent quality control and premium dairy products. There is a growing trend in international trade for worldwide equivalence of food products and HACCP as the international standard for food safety. Marmum's certification will allow us to compete at a global level with other international players. Not only does our HACCP let us focus on identifying and preventing hazards from contaminating food, it also permits more efficient management and governmental oversight as detailed recordkeeping allows investigators to see how well a firm is complying with food safety laws over a period of time. Acquiring this much sought after certification is an important milestone in Marmum's growth."[27]

Why is the General Manager of Marmum, a company located in Dubai, so proud that his company received HACCP certification? What does it mean for his company? What does this mean for your facility?

References

1. Vugia, D., MD, et. al. (2004). Preliminary foodnet data on the incidence of infection with pathogens transmitted commonly through food–10 Sites, United States. *Morbidity and Mortality Weekly Report 54*(14), 352-356.
2. *ServSafe® coursebook.* (1999). Chicago, IL: Educational Foundation of the National Restaurant Association.
3. Hensley, S. & Stensson, A. (2006). National restaurant association news release. Retrieved February 21, 2006, from http://www.restaurant.org/pressroom/print/index.cfm?ID=1186.
4. National Restaurant Association Educational Foundation. (2006). ServSafe® food safety training. Retrieved February 20, 2006, from http://www.nraef.org/index.asp.
5. National Restaurant Association Educational Foundation. (2003). New York state food safety requirement summary. Retrieved February 20, 2006, from http://www.nraef.org/reg_require/rr_state_juris_summ.asp?flag=lcd&level1_id=7&st=Ne w%20York&tid=120.
6. National Assessment Institute. (1994). *Handbook for safe food service management* (2nd ed.). Upper Saddle River, NJ: Prentice-Hall, Inc.
7. Dietary Managers Association (DMA) Online. (2006). About dietary managers association. Retrieved February 19, 2006, from http://www.dmaonline.org/about/main.html.
8. Food Safety Training and Education Alliance (FSTEA). (2005). Retrieved February 19, 2006, from http://www.fstea.org/.
9. U.S. Food and Drug Administration, Center for Food Safety and Applied Nutrition, *Food* Code, U.S. Department of Health and Human Services, Public Health Service, Food and Drug Administration. (2005). Retrieved February 27, 2006, from http://www.cfsan.fda.gov/~dms/fc05-toc.html.
10. Department of Health and Human Services. (2005). What is pulsenet/CDC pulsenet. Retrieved on February 20, 2006, from http://www.cdc.gov/pulsenet/whatis.htm.
11. Buzby, J., Frenzen, P., & Rasco, B. (2001). Food and rural economics division, economic research service/USDA, product liability and microbial foodborne illness/AER-799. Retrieved February 21, 2006, from http://www.ers.usda.gov/publications/aer799/aer799.pdf.

12. Public Law 107-188, 107th Congress. (2002). *Public health security and bioterrorism preparedness and response act of 2002.* Retrieved February 27, 2006, from http://www.fda.gov/oc/bioterrorism/PL107-188.html.
13. Gutierrez, J. (2005). Food safety for restaurants and institutions. CEU module, Level I, 2 contact hours, CEU4U.com.
14. (2005). Illness can make BSE prions appear in more organs than originally thought. *Medical News Today.* Retrieved February 20, 2006, from http://www.medicalnewstoday.com/medicalnews.php?newsid=19169.
15. U.S. Food and Drug Administration. (2005). Testing for rapid detection of adulteration of food. Report to Congress. Retrieved February 27, 2006, from http://www.fda.gov/oc/bioterrorism/report_adulteration.html.
16. McSwane, D., Rue, N., & Linton, R. (1998). *Essentials of food safety and sanitation.* Upper Saddle River, NJ: Prentice-Hall, Inc.
17. Sanomat, H. (2006). Spot-checks show a fifth of poultry import shipments contain salmonella. *Food HACCP News.* Retrieved February 19, 2006, from http://foodsafetyinfo.org/phpbb/viewtopic.php?t=1208.
18. Johnson, E. (2006). E-coli outbreak prompts consideration of 'cow-share' rules. Retrieved February 19, 2006, from http://www.publicbroad casting.net/opb/news.newsmain?action=article&ARTICLE_ID=8 71123.
19. Washington State Department of Agriculture. (2005). Dairy, raw milk. Retrieved February 20, 2006, from http://agr.wa.gov/FoodAnimal/Dairy/RawMilk.htm.
20. Heidelbaugh, ND., Smith, MC, Jr., DVM., MS, Rambaut, PC. (1973). Food safety in NASA nutrition programs. *Journal of the American Veterinary Medical Association, 163*(9), 1065-1070.
21. FDA. (2001). FDA backgrounder–HACCP: A state-of-the-art approach to food safety. Retrieved February 21, 2006, from http://www.cfsan.fda.gov/~lrd/bghaccp.html.
22. U.S. Food and Drug Administration, U.S. Department of Agriculture, National Advisory Committee on Microbiological Criteria for Foods. Hazard analysis and critical control point principles and application guidelines. Retrieved July 15, 2006, from http://www.cfsan.fda.gov/~comm/nacmcfp.html.
23. U.S. Food and Drug Administration, Office of Regulatory Affairs. (YEAR?). ITG subject: Water activity (a_w) in foods. Definition, Date: 4/16/84, Number: 39, Retrieved July 18, 2006, from http://www.fda.gov/ora/inspect_ref/itg/itg39.html.
24. Penn State University. (YEAR?). Water activity of foods. Retrieved July 18, 2006, from http://foodsafety.cas.psu.edu/Foodpreservation/Water_activity_of_foods.htm.
25. Gutierrez, J. (2006). HACCP-hazard analysis and critical control points—foodservice implications. CEU module, CEU4U.com.
26. (2005). Southern shrimp alliance: Shrimpers call for tests to ensure continued food safety in Katrina's wake. *Health Insurance Week.* Retrieved February 28, 2006, from NewsRx.com and NewsRx.net.
27. AME Info FX, LLC. (2005). Marmum dairy awarded FDA's HACCP quality certification. *Middle East Company News Wire.* Retrieved February 28, 2006, from NewsRx.com.

Enrichment Web Site Resources

Association of Health Facility Survey Agencies (AHFSA) State Web Sites:
http://www.ahfsa.org/statesites.htm
American Public Health Association: http://www.apha.org
Centers for Disease Control and Prevention and The National Center for
Infectious Diseases: http://www.cdc.gov/ncidod
Department of Health and Human Services and Centers for Disease Control
and Prevention: http://www.cdc.gov
Ecolab: http://www.ecolab.com
Everclean Services: Food Safety and Sanitation Trainers: http://www.ever-
cleanservices.com
FoodHACCP.com and General Food Safety Daily News: http://www.food-
haccp.com/0106.html
Food Marketing Institute: http://www.fmi.org
Food Safety Links and HACCP food service: http://peaches.nal.usda.gov/
foodborne/fbindex/HACCP.asp?subtopic=food%20service
National Environmental Health Association: http://www.neha.org
National Restaurant Association Educational Foundation: http://www
.foodsafetycouncil.org
North American Association of Food Equipment Manufacturers:
http://www.nafem.org
Partnership for Food Safety Information: http://www.fightbac.org
Product Liability and Microbial Foodborne Illness:
http://www.ers.usda.gov/publications/aer799/aer799ap.pdf
U.S. Food and Drug Administration: The Bioterrorism Act of 2002:
http://www.fda.gov/oc/bioterrorism/bioact.html
Food Products Association: http://www.nfpa-food.org
USDA, Food Safety and Inspection Service: http://www.fsis.usda.gov

## CHAPTER 8

FOODSERVICE AND CLINICAL EMPLOYEE STAFFING

Julie Jones, MS, RD, LD

Reader Objectives

After reading the chapter and reflecting on the contents, the reader will be able to:

1. Describe key staffing terms and apply them in schedules and case studies.
2. Describe the skill mix of staff and the impact on employee schedules.
3. Identify key productivity or staffing effectiveness measures for foodservice.
4. Identify specific food production's and foodservice delivery models' impact on employee staffing requirements.
5. Assess and evaluate clinical nutrition staffing.

Key Terms

Benchmarking: a comparison of key statistics for similar organizations using consistent data gathered for each of the participating organizations.

Cross training: the process of training staff members to perform more than one job function.

Fixed time: time that must be spent by employees regardless of the activity level of the operation. It includes time spent in meetings, training, or orientation.

Flexible FTE targets: uses time standards to determine projected staff members required for a particular workload volume.

Full-time employees: employees who work at least 32 to 40 hours each work week.

Full-time equivalent employees (FTE): a calculation that takes the total number of labor hours per year and divides by 2,080, which is the number of hours for an employee working 40 hours per week, 52 weeks per year. This calculation standardizes the reporting of part-time employees.

Living wage: raise the minimum wage requirements to provide a more adequate living to the lowest paid employees.

Minimum wage: the lowest level of pay that can be offered to employees.

Nutrition demographic: defines the number of patients in your facility at different levels of nutrition risk from low risk for nutrition problems to high risk for nutrition problems.

Part-time employees: employees who usually work 20 or less hours each work week.

Productivity: evaluates the activity and efficiency of staff members performing work.

Rate of pay: the amount of money employees are paid to perform their job duties. Can be an hourly wage or a set salary per year or pay period.

Skill mix: defines the mix of job functions necessary to complete all of the work of the department or area.

Staffing effectiveness: an evaluation of the organization staffing to ensure:
- Service levels to customers are consistent with organization goals.
- The labor cost paid meets the financial targets set by the organization.
- All regulatory requirements for staffing are met.

Total paid hours: includes both worked hours by the employee and nonworked benefit hours such as vacation, ill leave, or holiday pay paid to the employee.

Work schedule: the total staffing requirements for a foodservice operation during a given period—weekly, biweekly, or monthly.

Worked hours: the total number of hours employees are working in the operation.

Workload statistic: an indicator used to describe the amount of activity in an organization.

Introduction

Employee labor is the single largest expense in foodservice operations. The challenge for managers is to match the number and skill set of employees to the level of services needed to best utilize the labor resource.[1] Foodservice also experiences significant changes in meal volume during peak meal time periods. This tests the manager's ability to create effective employee schedules. Since foodservice jobs tend to be entry level, it can also be challenging for managers to find the right staff to do the right job.[2] Additionally, the foodservice industry has varied foodservice production and delivery methods. New technology and equipment are developed routinely in this industry. Managers must evaluate the current production and delivery models but also closely monitor the changing industry to find the best mix of equipment and labor for their operation.

For managers employed in healthcare settings, they will be expected to evaluate labor for clinical nutrition practitioners. Regulatory and licensure requirements impact staffing levels as well as the type of facility and patients or clients served, the role of the nutrition professionals in the facility, and the nutrition care process and model in place at the organization.[3]

Employees, Staffing, and Schedules

Why is labor such a strong consideration in foodservice? The typical person employed in foodservice is female, less than 30 years of age, a high school graduate or less, single, works part time, and has a short tenure in the job according to recent National Restaurant Association workforce overview.[2] More than 20% of foodservice employees are foreign-born, and employee literacy impacts operations. These characteristics are important considerations as you create and evaluate staffing plans.

Do you have the right skill level in your staff for the position? Does the employee need to communicate with customers? Are there any language barriers to training employees, and can they learn and develop new skills? Is employee turnover high, leaving gaps in schedule requiring overtime? **Cross training** of staff to serve more than one job function is expected today in foodservice jobs.[4] This cross training helps increase **productivity** because more employees can share the workload. Cross training also correlates with better employee satisfaction because it provides better opportunity for promotions and offers more variety in the jobs employees perform.[4]

To create employee **work schedules** and budgets, there are key terms and concepts that every manager should know. They are the building blocks of labor calculations, budgets, and productivity systems. These include *full-time and part-time employees, rate of pay, minimum wage, living wage, overtime, full-time equivalent employees, work schedules,* and *skill mix.* **Workload** statistic or *unit of service,* **worked hours,** and **total paid hours** are used to evaluate productivity or activity of the operation.

> **Learning Point:** The manager must consider:
>
> - Budget
> - Productivity needs
>   - *Full-time and part-time employees*
>   - *Rate of pay*
>   - *Skill mix*

In 2005, the typical foodservice employee worked almost 25 hours per week, which was far below than U.S. standard of the 40-hour work week.[2] An employee is usually considered full-time when she work 40 hours each workweek.[5] However, the designation of full-time or part-time can be dependent on the organization. Some businesses require only a 32-hour workweek to qualify as full-time to receive employee benefits. Part-time denotes working less than full-time hours. **Part-time employees** can be employed from 1 hour per week through 39 hours per week but are usually employed 20 or fewer hours, depending on the organization. Frequently, in foodservice, part-time employees work variable schedules and hours, depending on the need of the operation.

Employees are paid based on their **rate of pay**. Pay can be calculated hourly for most foodservice staff. Professional and management employees are salaried employees if they meet standards established by the Fair Labor Standards Act (FLSA).[5] Salaried employees receive the same base salary for a pay period that could be weekly, biweekly, or monthly. For example, a dietitian may be salaried at $52,000 per year and, therefore, paid $1,000 per week regardless of the number of hours worked. There are also **minimum wage** standards that employers must meet. Minimum wage describes the lowest level of pay that can be offered to employees. Minimum wage standards can vary by state. More recently, some municipalities and governments have adopted **living wage** standards, which raise the minimum wage requirements to provide a more adequate living to the lowest paid employees. These guidelines increase the minimum wages of employees so they have adequate money to pay for housing, food and insurance.

For employees who work greater than 40 hours per week, employees usually earn overtime unless they are salaried or exempt from overtime. Overtime is a premium wage that can be 1.5 times the employee's hourly rate of pay. The federal government has posted overtime regulations, including the job titles or classifications that earn overtime or those exempted from receiving overtime pay, on the Department of Labor Web site.[5] Additionally, the Department of Labor Web site lists the most current regulations for overtime pay and minimum wage standards for each state. Overtime is a significant consideration because it can drive up the labor cost significantly if overtime or premium pay is not well-managed through the work schedule.

For budgeting purposes, a full-time employee works 2,080 hours per year; that is, 40 hours per week, 52 weeks per year. Budgets will be based on the number of **full-time equivalent employees (FTEs)**. The full-time equivalents in an operation are the total number of labor hours per year divided by 2,080. Converting staff to FTE's standardizes the reporting of part-time employees. An organization may have 10 FTEs but employ 14 different people because of part-time status. As an example, the 10 FTEs include 8 full-time cooks, 2 cooks employed 20 hours per week, and 4 foodservice workers employed 10 hours per week.

> **Learning Point:**
> - Salaried employees receive the same base salary for a pay period which could be weekly, biweekly, or monthly. Salaried employees are usually exempt from earning overtime pay.
> - Hourly employees are paid only for the hours they actually work; minimum wage standards must be met. Hourly employees can earn overtime pay.
> - Overtime is a premium wage that can be 1.5 times the employee's hourly rate of pay.

Table 8.1   FTE Calculations

FTE Calculations:
8 Full-time Cooks: 8 × (40 hrs × 52 weeks/year) = 16,640 hours
2 Cooks at 20 hrs/week: 2 × (20 hrs × 52 weeks/year) = 2,080 hours
4 Foodservice Workers at 10 hrs/week: 4 × (10 hrs × 52 weeks/year):
    2,080 hours
Total Hours: (16,640 + 2080 + 2080)/2080 hours = 10 FTEs

Employee Work Schedules

A work schedule describes the total staffing requirements for a foodservice operation during a given period—weekly, biweekly, or monthly. Employee assignments typically follow a master schedule or rotation. Creating a master schedule is one of the most challenging tasks in foodservice. A master schedule defines the positions that need filled each day and balances the workload and required skills of employees to meet the peak demand at mealtimes. Unionized foodservice operations may also mandate specific scheduling procedures. Managers must be familiar with the contract language as it relates to rates of pay, scheduled shifts, and guaranteed hours. Additionally, the master schedule must also be consistent with the approved budget.

Scheduling is easy in an operation that is open only 8 hours per day, 5 days per week. Each employee represents a position, and the manager's primary concern is matching job skills for each position. In an operation that works 7 days per week with employees working 8 hour shifts, 1.4 FTEs are required to cover each 8-hour shift. The 7-day week increases the hours that must be paid to 56 hours per week, or 1.4 FTEs, per shift that must be covered instead of the usual 40-hour full-time workweek.

Scheduling 7 days per week increases the scheduling complexity because managers must balance days off and weekends worked for employees. Because most foodservice operations are open on weekends, there may be policies in the organization that define mandatory weekend work requirements for staff. Employees may also receive additional pay when working weekend or late hour shifts.

Because many foodservice jobs are entry-level, operations rely on teenagers to fill their schedule. Foodservice is the largest employer in the private sector and more than 4 out of 10 adults have worked in a restaurant during their lifetime.[2] Because foodservice jobs will continue to increase through the next decade,[2] it is important for managers to be familiar with the youth employment requirements in the FLSA because youth employees may fill some of these positions. Teenagers who are less than 18 years of age can be employed in foodservice jobs if they are performing nonhazardous work and those less than age 16 also have specific work hour rules to follow. The Department of Labor has an assessment tool on its Web site for foodservice employers to use as they determine tasks that youth can perform because some duties in foodservice operations are restricted.[6]

The master schedule defines the positions that need to be filled on a given shift or day. What employee titles fill the positions are equally important. **Skill mix** defines the mix of job functions necessary to complete all of the work of the department, operation, or area. Skill mix affects the rate of pay for positions. Higher skilled employees will have a higher rate of pay than less skilled employees.

Foodservice managers should balance the work to maximize the skill of the employees. For example, a manager wouldn't want to pay a chef to work in the stockroom putting goods away. The job duties of the chef and stockroom clerk are significantly different in both skill and pay. When higher paid employees do the work of lower paid staff, the overall costs of the organization go up.

As discussed previously, *cross training* is also a valuable tool to improve staff skill so employees can fill more than one job function when necessary. However, the manager must achieve the best balance of skill mix by having the right staff doing the right jobs for the right cost. Consistently using lower paid staff with fewer skills will impact customer satisfaction, and using higher paid and skilled staff to do lower paid work will result in lower staff satisfaction. Cross training is essential in smaller operations because fewer staff members are available and employee skill levels will need to be more consistent.

The commitment to ongoing training so staff can cover additional work is a key factor to successfully manage employee schedules. Employees may be able to perform the work required in different jobs with additional training. However, completing this

Able Kitchen—A Scheduling Example

How does a manager create a master work schedule? The process combines the number and skill of staff required to run the operation. Able Kitchen cooks food to order and plates cold foods, such as salads and desserts, that it sends to a resident cafeteria in a nursing home. The job functions the employees must perform are cooking foods from scratch, following recipes closely to meet residents' nutritional needs, making and plating cold salads, and plating desserts that are purchased in bulk. There is a separate sanitation crew who performs general cleaning and washes dishes for this area.

The duties of the required jobs determine the skill of the employee performing the job. Cooking foods from scratch is a skilled position and, in this case, would be filled by a cook. Plating foods and making cold salads is a lesser skilled position and is filled by food preparation workers. The manager of Able Kitchen must consider how best to utilize staff to complete the daily work. After reviewing the required duties and work, Able managers determined that three cooks are needed each day, and one cook is assigned to complete a meal for that day and to complete any preparation for the next day's meal. An additional 2 food preparation workers are requird each day. Each food preparation worker completes cold food lunch or dinner preparation and the employees share any breakfast duties. See Table 8.1 to view employees, their skills, and rates of pay. See Table 8.2 to view sample work schedules for Able Kitchen which operates seven days per week employing four full-time cooks and a total of three FTE food preparation workers. Each cook and food preparation worker can do all of the jobs in their respective title.

training can be challenging when English is a second language or staff only work part-time variable hours.

This master schedule shown in Table 8.3 defines each employee's scheduled shifts. However, the actual schedule will vary based on employee's request for time off or illness. In foodservice operations, most use part-time employees to cover full-time employees' time off. For example, it is better to use Carey to cover Vanessa's vacation than to pay Juanita overtime. Juanita would

Table 8.2 Employees and Skills, Able Kitchen

Employee Name	Title — FT/PT	Skills	Hourly Rate
Eric	Cook, full-time	8 years experience	$15.00 per hour
Debbie	Cook, full-time	6 years experience	$12.50 per hour
Juanita	Cook, full-time	1 year experience food prep worker for 15 years	$13.25 per hour
Wesley	Cook, full-time	5 months experience	$11.45 per hour
Linda	Prep, full-time, has trained for cook position	22 years experience	$13.00 per hour
Vanessa	Prep, part time, has	8 years experience	$10.50 per hour
Ralph	Prep, part time, has trained for cook position	3 years experience	$10.00 per hour
Carey	Prep, part time	2 months experience, college student	$9.50 per hour

Table 8.3 Employee Master Work Schedule, Able Kitchen

	Sun	Mon	Tues	Wed	Thurs	Fri	Sat
Eric	C1	D	C1	C1	C1	C1	D
Debbie	D	C1	C2	D	C2	C2	C1
Juanita	D	C2	D	C2	C3	C3	C3
Wesley	C2	C3	C3	C3	D	D	C2
Linda	C3	D	FP1	FP1	FP1	FP1	D
Vanessa	FP1	FP1	FP2	D	FP2	FP2	D
Ralph	D	FP2	D	D	D	D	FP1
Carey	FP2	D	D	FP2	D	D	FP2

C1 = Cook 1: works 4:30 AM – 1:00 PM – Breakfast cook
C2 = Cook 2: works 7:30 AM – 4:00 PM – Lunch cook
C3 = Cook 3: works 11:30 AM – 7 PM – Dinner cook
FP1 = Food Prep Worker 1: works 4:30 AM – 1:00 PM – Breakfast/Lunch
FP2 = Food Prep Worker 2: works 11:30 PM – 7 PM – Dinner/Breakfast

earn $19.88 per hour, 1.5 times her hourly rate, for the hours she works for Vanessa. In this case, the operation is paying a higher paid staff member for a lower level job as well as paying premium overtime wages to Juanita. Overtime is routinely paid in foodservice operations because of the variability in meals served. The manager must balance the overtime paid to the budgeted or planned amount.

Productivity and Staffing Effectiveness

How do schedules, skill mix, budgets, and FTEs come together? One of the answers is through productivity measurement. Productivity compares the worked hours to budgeted FTEs, positions, or workload volume. It evaluates the activity or level of work for staff members. Employee staffing should relate to the volume of work in the operation. A workload statistic is an indicator of the activity. Common workload statistics in foodservice are the number of meals produced or served, the number of individual sales or cash transactions, sales dollars earned, and patient or resident days in health care.

Workload statistics should predict staff required to serve this level of activity. For example, the number of students enrolled might not be the best workload statistic in a school that has an open lunch policy. While numbers of students can describe total available customers, it might not predict staffing requirements on an individual day. The total number of meals served, the sales dollars, or the number of individual transactions are better indicators to determine the staffing requirement. Some operations will have very sophisticated productivity systems in place because labor is the single largest expense in a foodservice budget. Managers can use these indicators to evaluate their staffing more effectively.

One of the indicators, full-time equivalents, can be further described by worked hour FTEs and paid hour FTEs. Worked hours are the total number of hours employees are working in the operation. Total paid hours include both worked hours by the employee and nonworked benefit hours such as vacation, ill leave, or holiday pay. Worked hours are a key statistic that drives productivity and staffing effectiveness. The number of worked hours per unit produced such as meals, customers, or sales plays a key role in evaluating the staff scheduling process. As a manager, it can be difficult to control total paid hours at times because of benefit pay, but worked hours are usually in the manager's control.

Math example . . .

Lunch Tray Assembly
Start Time: 10:20 AM Finish Time: 12:15 PM Total Time in Minutes: 115 minutes
Employee Worked Hours: 7 employees × 115 minutes per employee = 805 minutes
Patient Meals: 425 meals
805 minutes worked / 425 meals = .53 minutes/meal

Productivity can be further broken down into parts. Sometimes, time and motion studies are undertaken to determine the amount of time it takes to complete a task. This is used to evaluate speed or efficiency in completing the task. Time studies could also be used to determine the amount of time it takes to complete a certain workload volume. One of the easiest areas to review is a tray line assembly producing patient meals. By determining the number of trays produced divided by the total number of hours worked by tray line employees, an average time per meal can be calculated. By calculating this statistic many times, the average time per meal is determined. The average time per meal can be then used to compare productivity by day, shift, or meal.

Learning Point:

Productivity compares
• Worked hours to budgeted FTEs
• Positions to workload volume
• Activity or level of work to staff

Common workload statistics in foodservice
• Number of meals produced or served
• Number of individual sales or cash transactions
• Sales dollars earned
• Patient or resident days in health care
• Number of trays produced divided by the total number of ours worked by tray line employees can calculate an average time per meal.

Fixed time is also considered when evaluating productivity. Fixed time is time that must be spent by employees regardless of the activity level. For example, staff members participate in a 20-minute meeting each day. Employees are not creating any units of service during this time. The time is spent each day regardless of whether they have 500 meals to produce or 800 meals to produce. Some common tasks that represent fixed time for employees are employee training, orientation, or meetings. Another example of fixed time is setting up and tearing down foodservice stations in a cafeteria. In this operation, these duties must occur before and after each meal period regardless of the volume. This is a fixed task; the time must be spent each day or meal period.

In many foodservice operations today, flexible targets for FTE staffing are established to control workload volume. Flexible targets use time standards and determine projected staff for a particular volume level. They can be used to predict staffing needs or to evaluate staffing efficiency after the fact. For example, Liberty High School cafeteria served 10,000 meals during a workweek using 10 FTEs. The salary cost for the 10 FTEs this workweek was $4,550. This cafeteria had previously established a time standard of .045 worked hours per meal.

To calculate flexible FTE target

10,000 meals × .045 hours/meal = 450 hours
450 hours / 40 hours/week = 11.25 FTEs

This operation used 1.25 fewer FTEs than projected for the volume of work. The productivity of the staff was high during this workweek.

A manager can compare the worked FTEs to the **flexible FTE target** by using a productivity percentage calculated from these key

---

To calculate productivity percentage

(Flexible target FTEs /actual worked FTEs) × 100%
11.25 flexible target FTEs/10 actual worked FTEs = 1.04
1.04 × 100% = 104% productivity

> **To calculate labor cost per unit of service:**
>
> Labor cost/total units of service = cost/unit of service
> $4,550/10,000 meals = .46 cents/meal

statistics. A productivity percentage can be calculated by dividing the flexible target FTEs by the actual worked FTEs and then multiplied by 100%.

Productivity percentages greater than 100% use fewer staff than expected, and productivity percentages less than 100% use more staff than expected.

Labor cost can also be evaluated by standardizing cost using the workload statistic. The skill mix and overtime wages can impact the total cost of the operation by using higher paid staff to perform lower skilled positions or by using more overtime than the budgeted amounts. In this case, the manager can create a cost per unit of service. At Liberty High School cafeteria, the labor cost per meal is 46 cents. Labor costs can be calculated using either worked hour cost or total paid hour cost.

Productivity and labor cost occur on a continuum. The manager must routinely review the established plan for staffing and compare to actual staffing in terms of employees' hours paid and cost for the organization. Productivity comparisons are internal to the organization, and trending the information guides better decision making.

Managers should complete productivity assessments and then evaluate quality indicators like customer satisfaction to determine the staffing effectiveness for a foodservice operation. In other words, staffing effectiveness is an evaluation that ensures service levels to customers are consistent with organization goals, the labor cost paid meets the financial targets set by the organization, and all regulatory requirements for staffing are met. Staffing effectiveness will be evaluated differently in each organization depending on their specific goals.

Conversely, foodservice operations can compare externally as well through **benchmarking**. Benchmarking is the financial comparison of key statistics for similar organizations using consistent data gathered for each of the participating organizations. There are a variety of external benchmarking options for foodservice operations, and they are specific to the type of foodservice program. Chain restaurants will calculate key statistics in a similar fashion and there will be a process to benchmark each restaurant with others in the chain. This is similar to contracted foodservice programs, schools, extended care, or integrated health networks where there may be a district or corporate office that can facilitate comparisons of each other to gauge performance.

Companies can also participate through external agencies for benchmarking. In health care, Healthcare Foodservice Management (HFM) offers a benchmarking program for on-site foodservice programs for ites members.[7] Because healthcare operations typically offer many types of foodservice, HFM Express™ has established a uniform method for calculating meals. Therefore, all operations who participate in this program use the same methodology to calculate meals in their facilities.

External benchmarking is a valuable tool to evaluate labor performance against similar organizations. Peer organizations can sometimes offer the most insight into better ways to utilize labor. Benchmarking is a formal process that provides a forum to discuss action plans with best performers. Best performers are described as those with the best financial performance for a given set of indicators. Recently, HFM Express™ has added customer satisfaction to its benchmarking programs to include a quality indicator.[7]

Menu, Food Production, and Service

In the earlier sections, the nuts and bolts of employee scheduling were discussed. However, in foodservice operations, the menu that is offered, the food production methods used, and the delivery service all combine to create the specific staffing needs for the operation. Like other industries, technology and manufacturing enhancements offer more options for managers to control labor expenses.[8] The common theme in foodservice operations—it's all about the food—also holds true for the type and amount of labor needed to support the menu.

Each organization will have a philosophy that guides menu selection and foods offered. During the 1990s, it was challenging for foodservice operators to fill vacant positions. The improvements in ready-made food choices from manufacturers and equipment technology allowed foodservice managers to leverage the menu selections to utilize staff effectively. Foods made from scratch required significantly more staff time to produce. Two new concepts emerged, speed scratch and convenience cooking, which allowed foodservice managers to provide quality food choices without producing all of the foods on-site by themselves. Speed scratch cooking utilizes some ready made components to eliminate some steps in the food production process. Baking mixes, diced, cooked chicken and cleaned, processed produce are examples of items commonly used in speed scratch cooking.

Convenience cooking relies on ready-made foods that can be used to replace on-site food production. These foods, including prepared entrees, precooked vegetables, and premade desserts, can be purchased from food distributors or central food commissaries to support a foodservice program. Central food commissaries have been developed to centralize food production for integrated health systems, schools, and prisons to decrease labor requirements but to also maximize the use of food production equipment.

Today, most organizations rely on a combination of made from scratch, speed scratch, and convenience items as menus are drafted. Managers should craft the best balance of menu items to maximize labor efficiency while creating menus that satisfy customers.

The next step in the cycle from the menu and purchasing is foodservice production. Commonly used production terms are cook-serve, cook-chill, batch cooking, and made-to-order. Cook-serve is a traditional production format used in many institutional foodservice operations. It refers to the production of food, in bulk, which is held hot during a serving period. Foods can be held and served from a steam table in individual portions in either cafeteria or tray line operations. In healthcare operations, it can require more staff in cook-serve operations because more staff are needed during meal periods. Foods can't be made too far in advance and held because of quality and food safety issues. Today, there is improved equipment technology that allows for bulk reheating of foods in full-size pans. This process could supplement the cook-serve model where convenience foods could be heated in bulk without staff oversight for a meal service period.

The cook-chill model emerged in the 1980s as technology developed that allowed advanced food production and rapid chilling of foods. This technology helped maintain food quality and increased the time foods could be held safely.[9] Cook-chill production methods such as Cryovac™, tumble-chill, sous vide, and blast freeze help balance the workload throughout the day. Since foods are prepared in advance of service, from 1-day to 14-day lead times and quickly chilled, these foods can be held cold for longer periods prior to service. Cook-chill methods can also involve reduced oxygen packaging or vacuum sealing to preserve the quality of the food even more. Additional production staff members aren't needed at peak meal time since foods need only to be reheated. This process allows menu items to be produced in larger quantities so the recipe can be made fewer times in a cycle. However, due to the cost and space requirements of cook-chill equipment, it can be hard to justify the purchase.[9] Central food commissaries typically operate as a cook-chill model.

The batch cooking model is typically used to maintain quality of food when held in bulk for cafeteria style service. In batch cooking, smaller quantities of foods are prepared for service and held for shorter periods of time. Batch cooking typically increases the cook staffing requirements since the recipes are made at predetermined intervals in the service cycle and not in one "batch" for the entire service period.

Made-to-order has moved from restaurants and hotels to all other areas of foodservice including health care, college and university foodservice, and corporate cafeterias. This model has a high degree of customer satisfaction because the service is personalized for the customer. Made-to-order impacts staffing because each customer's order is made individually. Sometimes, these services occur behind-the-scenes or they could occur in theatre style cooking stations. Theatre style cooking stations require the most staff because of their high visibility in front of customers. Made-to-order can utilize cook-chill for some of the items served, making this process less labor intensive.

Foodservice delivery methods also impact staff requirements. Typically, as the level of service and personalization of the service provided to a customer increase, the number of staff to provide the service increases proportionally. Room service or hotel style service is one of the newer trends in health care.[10] With room service, patients or residents can place food orders similar to room service in a hotel. Historically, most healthcare operations created patient meals on a tray line, and patients were served during a standard meal time period. Because of the individualization with room service, the level of staff to support the program is higher than the more efficient tray line set-up.[10]

In retail areas, kiosks or grab and go stations are becoming more popular. Foods are packaged ready to eat for foods such as salads, sandwiches, and pastries. Customers have a much faster service time, so this concept has gained popularity as customers demand quick service. Because meals are made in advance, it requires fewer staff in the restaurant, deli, or café to sell the product—an added bonus.

These different models also need to be evaluated against skill mix of the employees. For example, made from scratch cooking, cook-chill processing, and made-to-order methods require higher skills than convenience and speed scratch cooking. The improvements in technology and food manufacturing have created more options for both food and foodservice equipment to better distribute labor. Ultimately though, customer satisfaction and financial targets will be key determinants in the models selected.

Dietitian-to-Patient Ratios

Staffing productivity and effectiveness is easier to measure in foodservice applications. There is a defined workload statistic, such as meals served or customer transactions, as well as quality indicators such as patient or customer satisfaction that are typically gathered in an organization. Clinical nutrition staffing with registered dietitians or dietetic technicians can be harder to quantify because of the difficulty identifying a single workload statistic that measures productivity. The challenge for a nutrition manager is to balance the level of staffing where positive patient outcomes are achieved using the right quality and quantity of staff.[11]

The earliest indicator or workload statistic used to determine clinical nutrition staffing was number of dietitians (FTEs) per licensed bed.[3] This was concise and easy to understand, but it didn't quantify the work that clinical nutrition staff needed to perform. Subsequent nutrition care models have sought to establish dietitian ratios based on the nutrition risk of the patient and the care setting of such medical service versus intensive care beds.[3]

Each organization must create a workload statistic that is meaningful to its operation. It could be nutrition interventions either in total number or based on time intervals such as every 15 minutes, inpatient admissions, or patient days. The workload statistic should be easy to capture and predict staffing needs. It is the equivalent of measuring meals or cash sales for foodservice.

Clinical Staffing Requirements

Because clinical nutrition services vary greatly among operations, it is helpful to complete a staffing assessment. This assessment process should evaluate five different areas—the facility, the department, legislation, accreditation, and professional practice issues and guidelines.[3]

The facility evaluation should account for things such as the mission and vision of the organization, the types of services offered, and the clients seen in the facility or community.[3] For example, a facility evaluation for an acute care cancer hospital with a research mission would be completely different than an assisted living facility serving only regular diets. The need for clinical nutrition services would be significantly higher for the facility treating acutely ill cancer patients and performing research. In this case, the mission of the organization is impacting the level of clinical nutrition staffing.

Likewise, it is critical to establish an overview of the nutrition department, its operations, and the specific requirements for clinical nutrition staff such as training dietetic interns.[3] There are different approaches to clinical nutrition staffing. Some departments use an integrated approach with foodservices. In these departments,, clinical nutrition staff might provide support for the foodservice activities for patients or retail operations. They could be involved with menu selection, call center operations, or menu preference. These duties are similar to fixed duties described earlier in this chapter. Other clinical nutrition providers could be employed directly by patient care units, be a part of a clinical nutrition department with no foodservice responsibilities, or be a combination of any of the listed options. Because of the variability in department set-up, it is essential to establish the non-clinical duties the registered dietitians and technicians are performing.

It is also important to establish the roles of the nutrition staff within the department evaluation. For example, are care extenders such as dietetic technicians used to perform some of the clinical nutrition services or are there other service providers who can supplement the registered dietitians' services? To more fully understand the roles and responsibilities of registered dietitians and dietetic technicians, the American Dietetic Association has established standards of practice that delineate the scope for each care provider.[12]

The third criterion to evaluate is legislation that establishes any legal requirements for staffing or staffing levels.[3] This could include licensure and certification. Licensure regulates the qualifications of the care provider and defines the scope of practice for dietetics and may establish the scope of services that can be provided by nonlicensed personnel. Certification governs the use of certified titles to individuals meeting predetermined criteria. Certification doesn't limit the practice of dietetics, but it limits those who can use the specific title of dietitian or nutritionist. The Commission on Dietetic Registration maintains a listing of licensure and certification requirements by state.[13]

Accreditation guidelines also impact staffing requirements.[3] Many agencies regulate the provision of clinical care in acute-care hospitals and extended care environments. These guidelines will vary based on the accrediting agency. Most hospitals use the standards published by the Joint Commission on Accreditation of Healthcare Organizations (JCAHO).[14] Nutrition care services should be provided on a continuum with a process for nutrition screening, assessment, development of nutrition care plans, and reassessment for identified patients. The organization has the ability to set its own practice standards defining nutrition assessment and reassessment time, and these guidelines impact total staffing needs.[14]

Finally, the fifth area of focus is professional practice issues and guidelines.[3] These define the professional practice standards for quality services for dietitians and dietetic technicians as members of the healthcare team.[12] With a thorough review of these factors, the clinical nutrition manager can move forward in establishing or validating staffing plans.

Staffing Plans

To determine the best staffing plan for your organization, Biesemeier suggests determining your facility's **nutrition demographic**.[11] The nutrition demographic defines the number of patients in your facility at different levels of nutrition risk from low risk for nutrition problems to high risk for nutrition problems. See Table 8.4 to see a sample form creating facility profile information on nutrition status.[3] Using these data, managers can quantify the direct patient care activities such as nutrition screening and assessment and indi-

Table 8.4   Nutritional Status—Faculty Profile

Date of Audit _____

Unit	Total Number of Patients	Low or No Risk	Moderate Risk	High Risk
Totals				
%				

Instructions:
1. List the total numbers of patients on each unit in the facility and the number of patients in each category of nutritional risk by unit. Add additional lines in the table as needed for additional units.
2. Add each column to obtain the total number of patients on all units on the day of the audit and the total number of patients in each nutritional risk category.
3. Calculate the percentage of the patients in each risk category for the entire facility: (Total number of patients in risk category + Total number of patients hospitalized in facility on the day of the audit) x 100.

rect patient care activities including team rounds, meetings, or student education. See Table 8.5 for a direct care activity tracking form.[3] This process is similar to time and motion studies in foodservice applications.

Activity logs are kept from a variety of practitioners and averages for each type of activity calculated. The average time required for the different activities can then be determined using history or estimated patient volume. Total staffing needs then can be deter-

Table 8.5 Direct Care Activity Tracking Form

Dietitians and dietetic technicians use this form to record the number of activities completed each week. RD/DTR

Dates	Nutrition Screening	Nutrition Assessment MR	Nutrition Assessment HR	Reassessment MR	Reassessment HR	Calorie Counts HR/MR	Basic Education HR/MR	Complex Education HR/MR
Monday								
Tuesday								
Wednesday								
Thursday								
Friday								
Saturday								
Sunday								
Totals								

Abbreviations: HR: high risk; MR: moderate risk

Instructions: List the numbers of each activity by date. List the total number for each activity completed for the week in the last row.

mined by a simple formula taking the average time to complete each activity multiplied by number of required activities for a given time—weekly, monthly, or annually. This method is best suited to validate staffing models rather than evaluating the staffing effectiveness on a day-to-day basis because it is cumbersome for clinical nutrition staff to report all of the required data.

Evaluating Staffing Effectiveness

JCAHO standards require the organization to review staffing effectiveness as a key measure of quality.[14] Both productivity and quality measurements are required for this review.

Productivity can be determined using the organization's workload statistic. For example, clinical nutrition staff productivity is reported using nutrition interventions at the Ohio State University Medical Center (OSU). Table 8.6 is a reporting form used by clinical nutrition staff to report nutrition interventions. These interventions are tallied for each biweekly pay period, and the total number of interventions is reported for productivity calculations. These interventions are the direct care activities provided by staff. The productivity percentage measures the efficiency of the staff providing these services.

Staffing effectiveness must also evaluate the quality of the services provided. This may require an additional indicator. While foodservice operations routinely evaluate customer or patient satisfaction, there are typically no organization-wide statistics on patient or client satisfaction with clinical nutrition. Note that on the productivity tracking form used at the OSU Medical Center, the clinical staff report missed interventions. These numbers are used to determine percentage compliance with nutrition screening and assessment time standards in the organization. By reporting units of service and a quality indicator, missed interventions simultaneously, it is easier to evaluate staffing effectiveness. These indicators can also become part of a performance improvement plan for the department. External benchmarking also exists for clinical nutrition services. These include Action O-I database by Solucient® and Premier Clinical Nutrition Benchmarking Tool. These databases offer comparative information for members participating in these programs. (See Chapter 14 for more information on benchmarking.)

Table 8.6   Pay Period Summary Productivity Form

Registered Dietitian

# Outpatient Interventions	# Inpatient Interventions	# Inpatient Interventions Incomplete	# Risk Assignments	# Risk Assignments Incomplete
Subtotal:	Subtotal:	Subtotal:	Subtotal:	Subtotal:

Dietetic Technician

# Outpatient Interventions	# Inpatient Interventions	# Inpatient Interventions Incomplete	# Risk Assignments	# Risk Assignments Incomplete
Subtotal:	Subtotal:	Subtotal:	Subtotal:	Subtotal:

Risk assignment = nutrition screen
Intervention = nutritional assessment, education or follow-up

Adapted with permission from: Pay Period Summary Productivity Form, Ohio State University Medical Center.

Summary

Managers must be able to create effective staffing plans in their operations. To do so, they must have a good understanding of key staffing terms. Managers plan positions based on the volume of work to be completed considering the duties each employee must perform. The rate of pay for an individual employee is based on the skills or duties required and the organization guidelines. Most foodservice operations will use a combination of full-time and part-time employees; having flexible part-time staff members allows operations to meet the peak demands of foodservice.

Employee work schedules are challenging to develop and, covering 7 days per week and multiple shifts each day, add more complexity to this process. Managers must be aware of any scheduling requirements for weekends, labor contracts, or youth labor. Most operations will cross train staff for more than one job so there is more flexibility in covering open positions on the schedule.

Managers must be able to evaluate their scheduling process. Employee scheduling should match the number and skill mix staff members required to complete the workload volume. Each organization should create a workload statistic that predicts the number of staff members needed. Productivity measurements should be completed consistently. In addition, managers evaluate staffing effectiveness to ensure the financial, regulatory, and customer service goals are met. Operations can also participate in benchmarking programs to compare the financial performance of their operation with other similar organizations.

The menu, the type of food production, and delivery systems used in the operation will affect the operation's staffing plan. Advances in food manufacturing and equipment technology have allowed operators to decrease the number of required staff members. There have also been changes in foodservice delivery models that have increased the amount of required staff, including made-to-order food production, theatre style cooking, and hotel style room service in healthcare operations. Each operation determines the menu, food production, and delivery system based on financial targets and customer service standards for its own organization.

Managers employed in healthcare operations must evaluate clinical nutrition productivity. Identifying a workload statistic that predicts staffing requirements can be challenging. Some common workload statistics compare dietitians to the number of patient beds or census. Other models incorporate nutrition risk of the patient, time-based indicators, or types of patients seen.

A staffing assessment can be done to identify clinical nutrition staffing requirements. In this assessment, the manager evaluates the facility and nutrition department characteristics, legislation issues, accreditation guidelines, and professional practice issues and guidelines to determine the required work for clinical staff. Additionally, staffing effectiveness is evaluated for clinical services to ensure that the quality of care standards are met for patients.

Managers must combine multiple elements when creating their staffing plan and work schedules. Labor expense is the single largest expense in a foodservice budget. Like any other resource, it must be well-managed to meet the organization's customer service, financial, and regulatory goals.

Student Activities

1. Telephone or interview in person a foodservice manager about how he or she cross trains foodservice employees to cover a schedule. Make a mock schedule from your interview and explain how the cross training helps with the overall schedule.
2. Telephone or interview in person a foodservice manager about his of her insight about having high productivity when scheduling foodservice employees. Make a mock schedule from your interview and explain how the productivity is addressed with the overall schedule.
3. Telephone or interview in person a chief clinical dietitian about how he or she cross trains dietitians to cover a schedule. Make a mock schedule from your interview and explain how the cross training helps with the overall schedule.
4. Telephone or interview in person a chief clinical dietitian about how he or she measures the productivity of the dietitians. Make a mock tracking form from your interview.
5. Call three hospitals and ask how many patient beds are available. Also, contact the foodservice department and ask how many FTEs there are for both foodservice and clinical dietitian staff. Explain how you can account for the difference between each hospital.

CASE STUDY #1: ABLE KITCHEN

Employee Information: Week of June 11, 2006

Employee Name	Title — FT/PT	Skills	Hourly Rate	Worked Hours	Total Paid Hours
Eric	Cook, full-time	8 years experience	$15.00 per hour	44 hrs	44 hrs
Debbie	Cook, full-time	6 years experience	$12.50 per hour	34 hrs	42 hrs
Juanita	Cook, full-time	1 year experience food prep worker for 15 years	$13.25 per hour	41 hrs	41 hrs
Wesley	Cook, full-time	5 months experience	$11.45 per hour	39 hrs	43 hrs
Linda	Prep, full-time, has trained for cook position	22 years experience	$13.00 per hour	40 hrs	40 hrs
Vanessa	Prep, part time, has	8 years experience	$10.50 per hour	42 hrs	46 hrs
Ralph	Prep, part time, has trained for cook position	3 years experience	$10.00 per hour	16 hrs	16 hrs
Carey	Prep, part time	2 months experience, college student	$9.50 per hour	24 hrs	24 hrs

---

Other information:

Budgeted positions: 7 worked FTEs; 7.75 paid FTEs
UOS: Total meals produced: 6,300 meals/week
Target worked hour standard: .041 worked hour/meal
Overtime: 1.5 times hourly rate for worked hours greater than 40

1. Calculate the total worked and paid hours.
2. Calculate the worked FTEs and total paid FTEs.
3. Calculate employee wages. How many hours of overtime were paid?
4. Calculate flexible target FTEs.
5. Calculate two different productivity percentages.
6. Describe productivity for the operation.
7. What is the labor cost per UOS?

References

1. Thompson, G. (1999). Labor scheduling, part 4: Controlling workforce schedules in real time. *Cornell Hotel and Restaurant Administration Quarterly, 40*(3), 85-96. Retrieved August 3, 2006, from http://www.hotelschool.cornell.edu/chr/research/inbrief/laborsched.html.
2. National Restaurant Association. (2005). State of the restaurant industry workforce: An overview. Retrieved August 3, 2006, from http://www.restaurant.org/pdfs/research/workforce_overview.pdf.
3. Biesemeier, C. (2004). *Achieving excellence: Clinical staffing for today and tomorrow.* Chicago, IL: American Dietetic Association.
4. Bertagnoli, L. (2004). *The 10-minute manager's guide to cross-training staff.* Retrieved August 3, 2006, from http://www.rimag.com/archives/2004/08b/10-minute-manager.asp.
5. Minimum wage laws in the states. (2006). Retrieved August 3, 2006, from http://www.dol.gov./esa/whd/flsa/.
6. Restaurant employer assessment tool. Retrieved August 3, 2006, from http://www.youthrules.dol.gov/selfassess_restaurant.htm.
7. HFM express. Retrieved August 3, 2006, from http://www.hfm.org/benchmarking.html.
8. Kelson, A. (2002). Cost-cutting technology: Beating back labor expenses with equipment upgrades. Retrieved August 3, 2006, from http://www.rimag.com/archives/2002/05a/bus5.asp.
9. Sherer, M. (2004). *The cook-chill factor.* Retrieved August 3, 2006, from http://www.fermag.com/sr/v8i7_sr_cookchill.htm.

10. Sheehan-Smith, L. (2006*).* Key facilitators and best practices of hotel-style room service in hospitals. *Journal of the American Dietetic Association, 106,* 581–586.

11. McCaffree, J. (2006). Clinical staffing: Determining the right size. *Journal of the American Dietetic Association, 106*(1), 25–26.

12. Kieselhorst, K., Skates, J. & Pritchett, E. (2005) American dietetic association: Standards of practice in nutrition care and updated standards of professional performance. *Journal of the American Dietetic Association, 105*(4), 641–645.

13. CDR certifications and state licensure. Retrieved August 3, 2006, from http://www.cdrnet.org/certifications/index.htm.

14. *Comprehensive accreditation manual for hospitals: The official handbook.* (2006). Oakbrook Terrace, IL: Joint Commission on the Accreditation of Healthcare Organizations.

Web Sites

Action O-I Benchmarking Tool: http://www.solucient.com/.
Premier Clinical Nutrition Benchmarking Tool: http://www.premierinc.com/.

PART III

DAILY MANAGEMENT OF OPERATIONS

## CHAPTER 9

FISCAL MANAGEMENT IN FOODSERVICE

Esther C. Okeiyi, PhD, RD, LDN, CHA

Reader Objectives

At the end of studying this chapter and reflecting on the contents, the student will be able to perform the financial functions found in the foodservice operation from these areas:

1. **Menu**
   Percent popularity (menu mix)
   Percent food cost, food cost, and selling price
   Menu engineering

2. **Food Purchasing**
   Amount to purchase based on percent yield
   Reorder point
   Determining unit cost and extended cost

3. **Inventory**
   Computation in physical and perpetual inventory
   Percent food cost
   Average inventory and inventory turnover rate
   Determining percent food cost using adjusted inventory data
   Valuing product in inventory

4. **Production**
   Adjusting or modifying the menu
   Costing the menu to determine portion cost and total cost
   Cooking and trimming

5. **Cost and Profit Determination**
   Sales mix, break even point, and fixed/variable cost
   Calculating total sales

6. **Labor**
   Meals per hour
   Labor costs
   Full-time equivalents (FTE) calculation
   Employee turnover rate

7. **Profit and Loss Statement**
   Income statement
   Balance sheet

Key Terms

AP: as purchased, the actual price paid for food.

Contribution margin (CM): is the same as gross profit and CM is equal to sale price minus the variable cost.

Cost plus method: prices are calculated for menu items based on the entire actual cost to produce the item—per portion costs for food, direct labor, operating expenses, fixed expenses, and profit.

Covers per labor hour: determined by dividing the total number of customers served by total number of hours worked.

D'hote: table d'hote is when several food items are sold together for one unit price.

EP: edible portion, the portion of the food that can be eaten or yielding portion.

Factor method: the raw food cost is multiplied by a predetermined factor that takes into account labor, supplies, and any projected profit margin.

Labor cost per cover: calculated by dividing total payroll by number of covers (customers or meals) during the period of the payroll.

Labor cost per labor hour: calculated by dividing total payroll by total labor hours.

Menu engineering: an evaluating tool used to determine how well a menu item is doing in foodservice business. It determines the menu mix and contribution margin for each product and compares them with an average menu mix or average contribution margin.

Menu mix: the percent popularity of a menu item in comparison to other items sold with it.

Par stock level: the maximum amount of food item that should be in inventory at a time. It is the same as maximum inventory level.

Percent food cost method: figure reached by dividing the cost of a particular food by the cost of the total food bill.

Percent popularity: measures how popular a menu item is in comparison with other menu items sold with it.

Physical inventory: an actual count of the inventory items and a paper record of them to determine the total cost of inventory. The inventory data can be used to determine the amount of food available for sale for that month, average inventory, inventory turnover rate, cost of food sold, and percent food cost.

Prime cost method: the sum of food and labor costs is multiplied by a predetermined pricing factor that accounts for food and labor through separate percentages.

Reorder point: computation relating to the reorder point or economic order quantity is a concept that balances ordering cost and inventory holding cost. It is used to determine size and ordering frequencies of orders.

Safety level: an additional amount of food allowed in inventory to safeguard against running out in the middle of the week or before the ordered food is received. Every operation can determine its safety level for its foods based on experience.

Sales per labor hour: determined by dividing the total sale by the number of total labor hours.

Variable cost: the cost (for example food cost) that goes up and down depending on the volume of sales.

Variable rate (VR): the ratio (expressed in decimal form) of variable cost to a dollar.

Contribution rate (CR): the ratio (expressed in decimal form) of the sum of fixed cost and profit to sales or the difference between one and variable rate.

Introduction

This chapter serves as an introductory gateway to restaurant math, emphasizing the financial impact of food and production costs and labor. The menu, food production, and labor are the center of every foodservice operation. While planning the menu, the foodservice manager must be aware of food costs, availability, and the production cost to bring the prepared food item to the customer's table. Food costs, along with production costs in terms of labor, all impact the net profit a foodservice operation reaps from its menu.

The recipe is the backbone of the menu. A poorly used recipe can make or break a foodservice because of the cost of poor quality. Important aspects of properly using recipes to the foodservice operation advantage would be:

1. Adjusting menu (recipe modification)
2. Costing menu to determine portion cost and total menu cost
3. Determining food cost based on cooking and trimming loss
4. Determining meal per hour, meal per meal period, meals per labor hour, meals per full-time equivalent (FTE), and labor minutes per hour

Foodservice budgets are affected by inventory control. Inventory data can be used to determine the amount of food available for sale in a given month, average inventory, inventory turnover rate, cost of food sold, and percent food cost. It will be important for foodservice managers to be familiar with:

- The use of physical and perpetual inventory data to determine food cost
- Costing the inventory
- Determining average inventory
- Calculating inventory turnover rate
- Determining percent food cost using information on inventory
- Valuing the inventory using various methods, such as First In First Out (FIFO), weighted average, latest purchase price, and Last In First Out (LIFO)

The third component of financial mastery involves the ability to utilize staff in a productive and efficient manner. As a part of this chapter, many of the formulas intrinsic to labor will be learned, such as:

- Sales per labor hour
- Covers per labor hour
- Labor cost per labor hour
- Labor cost per cover

The Menu

In this section, several fiscal concepts about planning a menu will be introduced to the reader. These include the percent of popularity of each menu item within the **menu mix**, the food cost of each menu item to determine the selling price, and menu engineering, which is based on the financial information discovered about food costs and selling prices.

Percent Popularity

Percent popularity (% of the menu mix) measures how popular a menu item is in comparison with other menu items sold with it. The formula to make this determination is shown below:

$$\text{Percent popularity index} \ = \ \frac{\text{Portion sales for Item A}}{\text{Total portion sales for all items}} \times 100$$

Example:

Item	Portion sold	% of total sale (Popularity index)
A	23	14.2
B	60	37.0
C	34	21.0
D	45	27.8
Total	162	100%

Example:

1. Twenty portions of chicken, 45 portions of beef, 60 portions of fish, 80 portions of scallions, and 16 portions of beef patties were sold on Monday in a King restaurant. What is the popularity index for fish?

   Chicken   = 20
   Beef   = 45
   Fish   = 60
   Scallions   = 80
   Beef patties = 16
   Total   20 + 45 + 60 + 80 + 16 = 221
   Menu mix for fish: 60/221 = 27.15%

2. Mahi restaurant is expecting a 40% increase in sales on the second Monday of the month due to several events occurring in the city where the restaurant is located. Using the example figures given in the first example, how many portions of item "C" should be prepared on Monday?

Total portions sold   = 162
A 40% increase   = .40 × 162 = 64.80
Total expected   = 162 + 64.8 = 226.8
Portion of "C" to be made   = .21 × 226.8 = 48 portions

Food Cost

Food cost is one of the prime costs in foodservice. Percent food cost determines the dollar cost of food to generate a $100 sale. The selling price of the food can also be determined using the same formula. Actually, when two of the factors are known, the third unknown factor can be calculated using this formula. Cost percents are useful for comparing cost relative to sales for two or more periods of time, and they also provide a means of comparing two or more similar operations or making a comparison with industry averages. The formula for computing relationship between cost of food, volume of sales, and percent food cost is shown below.

Computing percent food cost:

$$\% \text{ food cost (\%FC)} = \frac{\text{Cost of food}}{\text{Sales (sale price)}} \times 100$$

Example:

Given the following information, calculate the percent food cost.

A. Cost $30; Sales $500.00

$$\frac{\text{Cost}}{\text{Sales}} \times 100 = \% \text{ FC (food cost)}$$

$$\frac{300}{500} \times 100 = 60\%$$

What does this 60% food cost mean?

It means that for every $100 sale, $60 is used to purchase food.

Example:

Given the following information, calculate cost percentages. Round your answers to the nearest tenth of a percent.

a. Cost $150; Sales $500   Answer: 30.0%
b. Cost $127.80; Sales $450   Answer: 28.4%
c. Cost $610; Sales $2,000   Answer: 30.5%

Example:

Calculate cost, given the following figures for cost percent and sales.

a. Cost % 28.0%; Sales $500   Answer: 140 cost/500 = .28
                                  Cost = .28 × 500
b. Cost % 34.5%; Sales $2,400   Answer: 828
c. Cost % 24.8%; Sales $225   Answer: 55.8
d. Cost % 31.6%; Sales $1,065   Answer: 336.54

Example:

Calculate sales, given the following figures for cost percent and cost.

a. Cost % 30%; Cost $90   Answer: $300 90/sale = .30
                                  Sale = 90/.30
b. Cost % 25%; Cost $500   Answer: $2000
c. Cost % 33.3%; Cost $1,000   Answer: $3003
d. Cost % 34.8%; Cost $1,113.60   Answer: $3200

Example:

a. How much would you sell an a la carte item for if it cost .85 and the desired percent food cost is 35%?

Answer: .85/sale = .35%
          Sale = .85/.35 = $2.43

b. For how much would a table **d'hote** menu with a 40% food cost and $2.25 (edible portion) EP cost of the menu sell?

Answer: $2.25/sale = .40
          Sale = 2.25/.40=$5.62

Example:

If the sales factor is 4, and the raw food cost is $1.75, what is the selling price of the food item? See formula in Table 9.1.

Answer: $7

Example:

What is the food cost percent if the cost of food is $325 and the income is $865?

Answer: $325/$865 = 37.5%

Example:

A foodservice operates with a 35% food cost. If a menu item has a raw cost of $1.25, and it takes an employee 45 minutes at $6 an hour to prepare, what is the traditional selling price?

Answer: There are different ways of determining the selling price of a menu item or a meal. The methods are:

1. Percent food cost method
2. Factor method
3. Prime cost method
4. Cost plus method

The last three methods are presented in Table 9.1.

Food Purchasing

Amount to Purchase Based on Yield

There are several basic concepts in food purchasing the food manager will need to know. These include the **As Purchased (AP)** price and the **Edible Portion (EP)** price. AP represents the actual price paid for food at market, while the dollar made on the food is the EP or yield. The higher the yield, the more portions there are to sell. Therefore, the actual cost is based on yield and is used to determine the actual food cost. These figures help to determine what price the

Table 9.1 Determining Selling Price of Menu Item

Method	Concept	Formula	Example
Factor (also referred to as fixed factor and markup)	The raw food cost is multiplied by a predetermined factor that takes into account labor, supplies and any projected profit margin.	Selling price = food cost × pricing factor Pricing factor = 100% ÷ desired food cost objective (stated as percentage of the selling price)	Desired food cost % = 40 100 ÷ 40 = 2.5 If menu item food cost is $.90. then selling price = .90 × 2.5 = $2.25
Prime Cost	The sum of food and labor costs is multiplied by a predetermined pricing factor that accounts for food and labor through separate percentages.	Selling price = prime cost × pricing factor Prime cost = food cost + direct labor cost (.90 + .24 = 1.28) Pricing factor = 100% ÷ (food cost % + labor cost %)	Food cost % = 40 Labor cost % = 38 Food cost for roast beef = $.90 Labor cost for roast beef = $.24 Pricing factor = 100 ÷ (40 + 38 = 1.28) Selling price = ($.90 + $.24) × 1.28 = 1.46
Cost Plus Profit (also referred to as recovery plus profit and actual cost)	Prices are calculated for menu items based on the entire actual cost to produce the item. Based on per portion costs for food, direct labor, operating expenses, fixed expenses, and profit.	Selling price = food cost ($) + direct labor ($) ÷ 100 – operating expenses (% of sales) + fixed expenses (% of sales) + profit (%)	Roast beef: If: Food Cost = $.90 Labor Cost = $.24 Op. exp. = 10% Fixed exp. = 7% Profit = 5% Selling Price = ($0.90 + $0.24) ÷ (100 – 22) = $1.46

food should be sold at, as well as evaluate purchasing sources. Examples of how EP prices are determined are presented below.

Computation Relating to Food Purchasing:

Amount to purchase based on % yield

$$\text{Quantity} = \frac{\text{Number of portions} \times \text{portions size}}{\text{Yield percentage}}$$

Example:

Mr. Wang is catering for 500 people this evening. Each person will be served 3 oz. of beef. The beef has a yield of 70%. How much meat should be purchased to adequately serve the 500 people?

$$500 \times 3 = 1,500 \text{ oz. meat}$$

$$\frac{1,500}{.70} = 2,142 \text{ oz.} = 2,142/16 = 134 \text{ lbs. approximately}$$

Example:

An 8 lb. roast beef cost $2.79 per pound. The EP is 65%. What is the EP price per pound of the roast?

Answer: $2.79 per lb./.65 = $4.29

Example:

Desiring to lower the food cost, should you buy the beef that cost $2/lb. with a yield of 75% or one that cost $3.25/lb. with a yield of 95% if 4 oz. is the portion size and you need to serve 200 guests?

Answer: $2.00/.75 = $2.67 per lb. EP cost
$3.25/.95 = $3.42 per lb. EP cost

Example:

Chicken breast with skin and bones has 34% waste. What size per pieces of chicken do you need to serve 3 oz. of meat?

Answer: Yield = 100 − 34 = 66%.
          Therefore to get 3 oz. EP = 3 oz./.66 = 4.55 oz.

Example:

If the chicken in the previous question is purchased for $1.25 per pound. What is the cost per pound and cost per serving EP?

Answer: 1 lb. (16 oz.) = $1.25. Therefore, 3 oz. = .23
          (AP cost)
          4.55 oz. = .36 (EP cost)

Example:

A can of number 10 peaches serves 60 people. How many cans do need to serve 300 guests if the portion size is 4 ounces?

Answer: There are 10–12 cups (12 cups × 8 oz. = 96 oz.) in one
          10 lb. can
          96 oz. serves 60 people = 1 can
          If 60 people use 96 oz.
          Therefore, 300 will use 96/60 × 300 = 480 oz.
          480 oz./96 oz. = 5 cans

Distinguish AP and EP in food purchasing and preparation.

Trimming, cutting, peeling, cleaning, de-boning, and cooking result in cooking or preparation loss and therefore the yield, which is the EP (edible Portion) of the food item sold. The loss increases the actual AP price.

Reorder Point

Computation relating to the **reorder point,** or economic order quantity, is a concept that balances ordering cost and inventory holding cost. It is used to determine size and ordering frequencies of orders. Readers should be familiar with the following terminologies: minimum and maximum stock level, par stock inventory levels, lead time, and safety level. Reorder point is an inventory managing strategy that is used to determine at what level or point an item in the inventory will be ordered to avoid dollars being tied up in the inventory. Other bench marks that management will set to control cost of inventory and waste are **par stock level, safety level,** and minimum and maximum inventory level for each food item. Par stock level is the maximum amount of food item that should be in inventory at a time. It is the same as maximum inventory level. And, safety level is an additional amount of food allowed in inventory to safeguard against running out in the middle of the week or before the ordered food is received. Every operation should determine its safety level for its foods based on experience.

Example:

For each of the following three items, calculate the quantity of each item to be ordered given the following information in Table 9.2.

With this example, use items 2 and 3 of Table 9.2 and practice with 1, 2, and 3 below.

Table 9.2   Figuring Reorder Points

	Item 1	Item 2	Item 3
Consumption rate	14 a week	7 a week	10 cases a month
Ordering frequency	every 2 weeks	weekly	monthly
Safety level	3	1	1 case
Present stock	6	1	3 cases
Delivery time	2 days	1 day	1 week

Note that Item 3 can be only ordered in full cases.

Solution to Item 1:
   Usage = 2 per day (uses 14 per 7 days)
   Available now = 6
   In 2 days = 2 × 2 = 4 (would be used) and 2 will be left
   Amount needed for safety level is 3.
   But for the safety level, only 2 will be available, making safety level
      short of 1.

Amount needed to order will be the amount needed for 2 weeks (2 × 14 days) + 1 short in safety level = 28 + 1 = 29

Item 2

Answer: Consumption rate = 1 per day
Order every week = will need 7 for the week
Safety level is 1. Therefore, add 1 to 7 = 8.
Present stock is 1. Therefore, need only 7.
Delivery will take one day. Need additional (1) for that
day. Therefore will need (1 + 7) = 8 to order.

Item 2

Answer: Consumption rate = 10 cases per month
Order monthly = will need 10 cases for the month
Safety level is 1 case. Therefore add 1 case to 10 cases
= 11 cases.
Present stock is 3. Therefore, need only 11 − 3 = 8.
Delivery will take 1 week. Need additional 10/4= 2.5
(approximately 3 cases for that week). Therefore, will
need (8 + 3) = 11 to order.

Example:

Determine the proper order quantity for each item below if the periodic order method is used.

Item	Par Stock	Usage	Quantity on Hand	Amount to Order
Smirnoff	72	48	24	Answer: 48 (72-24)
Gordon's Gins	36	24	3	Answer: 33
Jack Daniels	5	3	4	Answer: 1
Canadian Club	36	24	10	Answer: 26

Hint to solution (Par Stock − Quantity at hand = Amount to Purchase

Example:

Nestor's Restaurant uses the periodic order method, placing orders every 2 weeks.

Determine the quantity of canned peaches to order today given the following:

1. Normal usage is one case of 24 cans per week.
2. Quantity on hand is 10 cans.
3. Desired ending inventory is 16 cans.

Answer: 48 cans used for 2 weeks
          – 10 cans on hand
          + 16 ending inventory
          _____
          54 cans = 9 cases if 10 lb. can @ 6 per case to order

Example:

Harvey's Restaurant uses the periodic order method, ordering once a month.

Determine the proper quantity of tomato juice to order today given the following.

1. Normal usage is one case of 12 cans per week.
2. Quantity on hand is 6 cans.
3. Desired ending inventory is 18 cans.

Answer: 48 cans used for 4 weeks (orders once a month)
          – 6 cans on hand
          + 18 ending inventory
          _____
          60 cans

Determining Unit Cost and Extended Cost

It is important that managers and employees who are involved in any foodservice-related mathematical calculations be able to determine the total cost of an item given the number of units and cost per unit. Employees working with inventory, pantry, and recipes must be confident with these calculation where units and extended costs are computed.

An example of determining unit cost and extended cost is below:

If 12 legs of lamb were purchased at $8.99 per leg, what is the extended cost?

Answer: $12 \times 8.99 = \$107.88$

Example:

Twelve cases of apple juice containing six bottles of 128 oz. juice cost $35.25 per case.

What is the cost of a bottle of apple juice?

> Answer: Twelve cases (each with six bottles = 72 bottles) cost
> $35.25. Therefore, one bottle will cost $35.25/72
> = .49.

Example:

If one bottle serves about 10 people, how many would one case of apple juice serve?

> Answer: One bottle serves 10 people. Therefore, one case of six
> bottles will serve 6 × 10 = 60 people.

Inventory

This section deals with calculation relating to inventory control. **Physical inventory** is an actual count of the inventory items and a paper record of them in order to determine the total cost of inventory. The inventory data can be used to determine the amount of food available for sale for that month, average inventory, inventory turnover rate, cost of food sold, and percent food cost. Determining the physical inventory involves mathematical problem solving. For example:

- The use of physical and perpetual inventory data to determine food cost
- Costing the inventory
- Determining average inventory
- Calculating inventory turnover rate and what it means
- Determining percent food cost using information on inventory
- Valuing the inventory using various methods, such as FIFO, weighted average, latest purchase price, and LIFO

Note: Inventory costing can be used to determine the following: percent food cost (% FC); inventory turnover; and average inventory.

Computation in Physical and Perpetual Inventory

Physical inventory is the actual count of items on hand at any given time. This differs from perpetual inventory; physical represents the knowledge of what is in inventory at all times because items are continually tracked as they enter and leave the storage area. Keeping these definitions in mind, the following formula can be used to figure several factors related to inventory:

Costing the Inventory

Food cost = Beginning inventory
+ Purchase
– Ending inventory
_____
= Gross food cost

Gross food cost
+ Transfer from other area like bar
– Employees meal
– Complimentary meals
– Food to other departments
_____
= Net food cost

$$\% \text{ food cost} = \frac{\text{Cost of food}}{\text{Food sales}} \times 100$$

$$\text{Average inventory} = \frac{\text{Beginning inventory} + \text{Ending inventory}}{2}$$

$$\text{Inventory turnover rate} = \frac{\text{Cost of food}}{\text{Average inventory}}$$

Determining food cost using adjusted inventory data =
Opening inventory
+ Purchases
– Closing inventory
_____
Total available for sale

= Total cost of food issued
+ Cooking liquor
+ Transfer from other units
− Foods to the bar
− Transfer to other units
− Grease sale
− Steward sale
− Gratis to the bar
− Promotion expenses
───────────────────────
= Cost of food consumed

$$\frac{\text{Cost of food consumed}}{\text{Total sale}} \times 100 = \% \text{ food cost}$$

Example:

The following figures for November 2006 have been taken from the financial records of three units in the Pasta Pit chain. Determine total food issued for each.

1. Opening inventory $1,500.00
   Purchases $4,600.00
   Closing inventory $1,722.00   Answer: $4,378.00

2. Closing inventory $12,083.00
   Opening inventory $10,371.00
   Purchases $28,468.00   Answer: $26,756.00

3. Purchases $65,851.08
   Closing inventory $18,335.10
   Opening inventory $19,874.77   Answer: $67,390.75

Example:

Opening inventory   = $1,500.00
Purchases   =   +4,600.00
Closing inventory   =   −1,722.00
Cost of food issued   = $4378.00
Average Inventory   =

$$\frac{\text{Beginning inventory (\$1,500) + ending inventory (\$1,722)}}{2} = \$1,611.00$$

Inventory turnover rate =

$$\frac{\text{Food cost}}{\text{Average inventory}} = \frac{\$4,378.00}{\$1,611.00} = 2.7$$

Approximately = 3

Example:

For three units in a chain of restaurants operating under the name Grandma's Kitchen, calculate the cost of food issued and cost of food consumed for each restaurant given the figures below.

1. Purchases $8,300.00
   Opening inventory   2,688.00
   Closing inventory   2,540.00

   Answer: Cost of food issued = Opening + purchases – ending inventory
   $2,688 + $8,300 – $2,540 = $8,448

   Cost of food consumed =
   Cost of food issued + cooking liquor – grease sale – gratis to the bar

   $8448 + $94 -$76 – $119 = $8,347

2. Food to bar (directs) $189.00
   Closing inventory   6,647.00
   Transfers to other units   19,472.00
   Purchases   25,000.00
   Steward sales   53.00
   Transfers from other units   223.00
   Opening inventory   6,531.00

   Answer: Cost of food issued = $6,531 + $25,000 – $6,647 = $24,884
   Cost of food consumed = $24,884 + $223 – $189 – $19,472 – $53 = $5,393

3. Opening inventory $ 6,622.40
   Transfers from other units   47.35
   Cooking liquor   253.65
   Purchases   24,182.55

Closing inventory	6,719.30
Transfers to other units	347.60
Food to bar (directs)	337.40
Grease sales	91.85
Gratis to bar	177.35

Answer: Cost of food issued = $6,622 + $24,182 − $6,719.30 =
$24,084.70
Cost of food consumed = $24,084.70 + $253.65 +
47.35 − $347.60 − $337.40 − $91.85 = $23,608.85

Average Inventory and Inventory Turnover

The following figures for November 2006 have been taken from the financial records of three units in the Pasta Pit chain. The sale for the month is $20,000 for the first unit, $1,000 for the second unit, and $2,500 for the third unit. Determine the average inventory and inventory turnover. Explain what the value obtained in inventory turnover rate means. Calculate the percent food cost. Should a manager aim for a higher or lower turnover rate?

1. Opening inventory $1,500.00
   Purchases   4,600.00
   Closing inventory   1,722.00

Answer: Food cost = $1,500 + $4,600 − $1,722 = $4,378
Average inventory = $1,500 + $1,722/2 = $1,611
Inventory turnover rate = $4378/$1611 = 2.7 =
approximately 3
The higher the turnover may mean more sales

$$\text{Percent food cost} = \frac{4{,}378}{10{,}000} \times 100 = 43.78\%$$

2. Closing inventory $12,083.00
   Opening inventory   10,371.00
   Purchases   28,468.00

Answer: Food cost = $10,371 + $28,468 − $12,083 =
$26,756
Average inventory = $11,227
Inventory turnover rate = 2
Percent food cost = 26.75%

3. Purchases $65,851.08
   Closing inventory   18,335.10
   Opening inventory   19,874.77

   Answer: Food cost = $19,874.77 + $65,851.08 –
            $18,335.10 = $67,390.75
            Average inventory = $19,104
            Inventory turnover rate = 3.5
            Percent food cost = 26.96%

Example:

Opening inventory is $2,000; closing inventory is $3,000, and food cost is $4,600.

Calculate the average inventory and inventory turnover.

   Answer: Average inventory = $2,000 + $3,000/2 = 2,500
            Turnover rate = 4,600/2,500 =1.8 approximately = 2

What is an acceptable difference when the record shows a difference between physical and book or perpetual inventory?

An acceptable difference between book and physical inventory is what that particular operation has established and what is acceptable and not acceptable. It varies from facility to facility. Typically, a 3–5% difference is the norm.

Valuing Inventory Method

The valuing inventory method is the designation of any of the following terms when deciding what items to utilize in the inventory:

1. Actual Purchase Price Method
2. FIFO
3. Weighted Average
4. LIFO
5. Latest Purchase Price Method

Examples:

Open inventory on May 1, 10 cans at $2.35 = $23.50
Purchased on May 7,   24 cans at $2.50 = $60.00

Purchased on May 15,   24 cans at $2.60 = $62.40
Purchased on May 26,   12 cans at $2.30 = $27.60

       70 cans   = $173.50

At the end of May, inventory shows 20 cans remaining (so 50 cans were used).

The actual price for the 20 remaining cans was found to be 4 @ $2.35, 12 @ $2.30, and another 4 @ $2.60.

Calculating cost of inventory using various methods of inventory costing:

1. Actual Method
   4 @ $2.35 = $9.40
   12 @ $2.30 = $27.60
   4 @ $2.60 = $10.40
   Total = 20 cans at $47.40

Prices have to be marked on cans to use this method or use other method.

2. FIFO—of the 20 cans left, the remaining will come from:
   Latest   12 × $2.30 = $27.60
   8 from May 15   8 × $2.60 = $20.80
   Total   20 (12+8) = $48.40

3. Weighted—used when one is unsure of proper rotating or when large amount of inventory is involved:
   From actual cost—there were 70 cans at $173.50
   (1 can = 173.50/70) 1 can = 2.48
   For 20 cans = It will be $2.48 × 20 = $49.60

4. LIFO—means the last purchased is used first;
   20 cans will come from:
   On ending inventory 10 at $2.35 = $23.50
   next   10 at $2.50 = $25.00
   Total   20 = $ 48.50

5. Latest Purchase Price Method—is most recent price. So use the latest purchase price, which is $2.30:
   20 × $2.30 = $46.00

Compare Cost

Actual = $47.40
FIFO = $48.40
Weighted = $49.60
LIFO = $48.50
Latest Purchase = 46.00

Valuing the Inventory

FIFO: Inventory value will be the highest.

LIFO: Inventory value will be the lowest. For tax purposes you want to be as low as possible (minimize inventory).

FIFO—Inventory value is based on the price if purchases on today's price of goods is good.

LIFO—Ending inventory is valued at the cost of the oldest stock.

Example:

The following information about one of the items carried in the food inventory of the Yellow Dog Restaurant is taken from inventory records for the month of January.

January 1	Opening inventory	12 units @ $1.05 each
January 5	Purchased	18 units @ $1.15
January 12	Purchased	18 units @ $1.20
January 19	Purchased	12 units @ $1.30
January 26	Purchased	6 units @ $1.40

On January 31, the physical inventory indicated nine units remaining on the shelf. Determine both the value of the closing inventory and the cost of units issued, using each of the five methods identified above.

Answers:

Open Inventory on January 1	12 units @ $1.05	= $12.60
Purchased on January 5	18 units @ $1.15	= $20.70
Purchased on January 12	18 units @ $1.20	= $21.60
Purchased on January 19	12 units @ $1.30	= $15.60
Purchase on January 26	6 units @ $1.40	= $ 8.40
	66 units	= $78.90

At the end of January inventory show 9 units remaining (so 57 were used and 9 remained).

The actual prices for the 9 remaining units as marked on the cans were 6 @ $1.40 = $8.40; 3 @ $1.30 = $13.90

Calculating cost of inventory using various methods of inventory costing.

1. Actual Method
   6 @ $1.40 = $8.40
   3 @ $1.30 = $3.90
   Total 9 units = $12.30

Prices have to be marked on cans to use this method or use other method.

   Therefore, total available in the inventory = $78.90
   Ending inventory   = $12.30
   Cost of Units issued   = $66.60

2. FIFO—of the 20 cans left, the remaining will come from:
   Latest   6 × $1.40 = $8.40
   3 from January 19   3 × $1.30 = $3.90
   Total   20 (12 + 8) = $12.30

   Total available in the inventory = $78.90
       Ending inventory   = $12.30
       Cost of units issued   = $66.60

3. Weighted—used when one is unsure of proper rotating or when large amount of inventory is involved:
   From actual cost—there were 66 units at $78.90
   (1 unit = $78.90/66); 1 unit = $1.20
   For 9 units = $1.20 × 9 = $10.80

   Total available in the inventory = $78.90
       Ending inventory   = $10.80
       Cost of units issued   = $68.10

4. LIFO—means the last purchase is used first;
   9 units will come from:
   On ending inventory 9 at $1.05 = $9.45

   Total available in the inventory = $78.90

Ending inventory   = $9.45
Cost of units issued   = $69.45

5. Latest Purchase Price Method—is most recent price. So use the
   latest purchase price, which is $1.40:
   Therefore, 9 × $1.40 = $12.60
   Total available in the inventory = $78.90
   Ending inventory   = 12.60
   Cost of units issued   = $66.30

Food Production

Food production and the menu are the center of every foodservice.
The recipe is the backbone of the menu, and a poorly used recipe
can make or break a foodservice because quality of food is greatly
affected by the recipe. Therefore, it is important that everyone who
works in the kitchen be familiar with how to develop and modify a
recipe. Recipes may be obtained from friends, books, magazines,
food labels, etc., but usually require modification for the number of
people being served. Formulas and examples of how to convert
recipes are shown below.

1. Adjusting menu (recipe modification)
2. Costing menu in order to determine portion cost and total
   menu cost
3. Determining food cost based on cooking and trimming loss
   (butcher test and cooking loss test)
4. Determining meal per hour, meal per meal period, meals per
   labor hour, meals per FTE, and labor minutes per hour

Adjusting or Modifying the Recipe

The recipe below, curried black-eyed pea potash, is for 25 portions,
and the recipe is to be modified to serve 75 guests. This is figured by
computing a conversion factor that is obtained by the following
method.
Formula for recipe modification or adjustment is:

$$\frac{New}{Old} = Factor$$

Then multiply all ingredients in the recipe with the factor 3. For example, for the new recipe, the amount of black-eyed peas will be: 2 lbs. × 3 = 6 lbs.

Costing the Menu

Cost control is paramount to successful foodservice management. Portion cost determination is important for establishing the food selling price. The correct selling price will result in achieving the desired percent food cost and, therefore, the desired profit. The portion cost is obtained by determining the total cost of the recipe and dividing it by the number of portion sizes the recipe will yield. The total cost is determined by adding the cost of each item in the recipe. The recipe usually indicates the number of yields or portions to be obtained in that recipe. Examples of how to determine the portion cost is as follows:

Curried Black-Eyed Pea Potash (yield = 25)

Black-eyed peas (beans)	2 lbs. @ $1.50	$3.00
Onions	3 medium @ .59 a piece	$1.77
Vegetable oil	1 cup (8 oz.) @ $.45/8 oz.	$.45
Crayfish (dry)	8 oz. @ $6.50/8 oz.	$6.50
Maggie cubes	4 pieces @ $5.00/100	$.20
Curry	1 tablespoon @ $5.50/8 oz.	$1.38
Water or beef	2 quarts	
Chicken stock	1 quart @ 4.50/qt.	$4.50
Salt	2 tablespoons	$.20
Total cost		$18.00

If 25 portions made from the recipe cost $18.00, one portion will cost:

$$\frac{\$18.00}{25} = \$.72$$

Example:

If one portion of black-eyed pea potash costs $.72 and the desired percent food cost is 33%, how much should a portion size be sold to maintain that percent food cost?

$$\frac{.72}{X} = .33 \qquad .33X = .72 \qquad \text{Therefore, } X = \frac{.72}{.33} = \$2.18$$

Cost and Profit Determination

Costs in foodservice include all expenses incurred to generate sales. They consist of all costs found in income statements. Income from sales minus total cost yields the net profit. Gross profit is obtained by subtracting the prime cost, that is, the cost of food and beverage and plus labor cost from total sale income. Foodservice managers calculate costs in dollars and compare those costs to sales dollars.

Any money made after variable or controllable costs have been accounted for is gross profit. The net profit is made after all costs (controllable and noncontrollable) costs have been taken care of. Controllable costs include variable cost consisting of prime costs: the food, beverage, and part of the labor costs. Noncontrollable cost can be changed in a short term, while the long term cannot be changed in a short term. Examples of controllable costs that are usually variable cost include food cost. These costs can be controlled by reducing portion size, changing the ingredients, reducing employees' work hours, controlling the payroll clock in, and overtime. Noncontrollable are such costs as rent, interest on mortgage, salaried employees, real estate taxes, depreciation, license fees, and insurance.

Calculating Total Sales

How well sales are progressing can be determined by calculating total sales generated, total sales by category of food items, sales per server, sales per seat, average sale per customer, and check average. Total sales expressed in dollars can be computed for any given period such as a week, a month, or a year. Sales by category can be tallied by category, such as steak sales, seafood sales, entree sales, or beverage sales, etc. When sales are calculated by server, the number of sales for the meal period is divided by the number served and used to determine employee service performance and productivity. Sales per seat are obtained by dividing total sales in dollars by the number of seats in the restaurant for a given period. Average sale per customer is calculated by dividing the total sale by the number of customers served. Seat turnover rate calculation determines the number of times that a given seat in a dining room area is occupied during a meal period. This is obtained by dividing the number of guests by the number of available seats.

$$\text{Cover per hour} = \frac{\text{Total covers}}{\text{Number of hours worked}}$$

$$\text{Cover per day} = \frac{\text{Total covers}}{\text{Number of days of operation}}$$

$$\text{Cover per server} = \frac{\text{Total covers}}{\text{Number of servers}}$$

$$\text{Seat turnover} = \frac{\text{Number served during meal period}}{\text{Number of seats in restaurant}}$$

$$\text{Check average} = \frac{\text{Total sale (\$)}}{\text{Number of guests served}}$$

Cover is a term used to describe one diner regardless of amount of food and number of foods consumed.

Total covers refers to the total number of guests served. Covers per meal, covers per day, and covers per server can be calculated.

Seat turnover is the number of seats occupied during a given period, or number of customers served during that period, divided by the number of seats available.

These ratios are used to determine or evaluate efficiency of service in a dining room, the effectiveness of a particular promotional campaign, or effectiveness of a particular server.

Labor

Labor productivity is the measure of output in relation to the labor hours (input) used. There are different indices used to measure labor productivity, such as total labor hours, **sales per labor hour, covers per labor hour, labor cost per labor hour,** and **labor cost per cover.** Each time payroll is processed, total labor hours worked is tallied. If there is a variance in the total actual hours worked compared to those scheduled, management must investigate to determine the reasons for the difference. This calculation should be done for each job category.

Sales per labor hour are determined by dividing the total sales by the number of total labor hours worked. If the sales per labor hour worked is equal or exceeds the standard labor hour, the manager is said to be scheduling his labor hours productively. The only disadvantage of this indicator is that an increase in sales may affect the ratio, therefore skewing the accuracy of the employee productivity. Covers per labor hour are determined by dividing the total number of customers served by the total number of hours worked. This calculation can be done for each job category. This method of evaluating employee productivity is preferred and more effective than sales per labor hour.

The labor cost per labor hour is calculated by dividing total payroll by total labor hours. The information can be used to see the wage differences between employee job classifications. Management can use this information to establish wage ranges for the various job categories. The labor cost per cover can be calculated by dividing total payroll by number of covers (customers or meals) during the period the payroll spans. This can provide information on the group of employees with the highest and lowest cost per cover. Other productivity indices that can be calculated are percent efficiency, cover per day, cover per server, and sales per hour.

Meals Per Hour

Percent Efficiency is used to calculate work efficiency of employees. The formula used is:

$$\text{Efficiency \%} = \frac{\text{Earned (standard) hours}}{\text{Actual (worked) hours}} \times 100$$

Results are compared with the standard or national average, which is usually between 40% and 55%.

Formula for determining how long it takes to accomplish a given task:

$$\text{Probable time required} = \frac{a + 4m + b}{6}$$

Where:

    a = is the least time to do the task
    b = the most time to do a given task
    m = the most likely time to do the given task

Example:

How long would it take to prepare salad for 500 customers if the fastest worker will take 100 minutes and the extremely slow, efficient, thorough operator will take 30 minutes? If done effectively and adequately, it will take 60 minutes?

A = 30 minutes, b = 100 minutes, m = 60 minutes

$$\frac{30 + (4 \times 60) + 100}{6} = \frac{370}{6} = 61.66 \text{ minutes}$$

Meals per hour and meals per meal period are used to determine employees' labor productivity.

$$\text{Meals per hour} = \frac{\text{Total number of meals}}{\text{Total hours of labor to produce the meal}}$$

$$\text{Meals per full-time equivalent (FTE)} = \frac{\text{Total number of meals served}}{\text{Total FTE to produce the meal}}$$

$$\text{Labor minutes per minute} = \frac{\text{Total minutes of labor to produce the meals}}{\text{Total number of meals served}}$$

Labor Costs

Labor cost percent is calculated by dividing the total number of hours worked (payroll dollar) to produce the sale by total sale. Traditionally, only hourly wages are used, and an operation may include benefits such as employees' meals as part of payroll cost. Usually, management salaries are not included.

$$\text{Percent labor cost} = \frac{\text{Labor cost} \times 100}{\text{Total sale}}$$

Assume you have 7 full-time cooks paid $15 per hour with 20% of wage benefit.

Labor cost can be determined by computing how much per hour is paid each employee × hours worked + benefit for the employees.

Example:

Wages 7 cooks × 35 hours × $15 per hour = $3,675

Benefits $3,675 × 20%   = $735
Total labor cost   = $4,410

Example:

Given the following:

Sales total		$16,946

Cost of goods sold (COGS):
1. Beginning inventory $9,087
   [+] Purchases $4,067
   [=] Cost of goods available $13,154

2. Cost of goods available $13,154
   [–] Ending inventory $7,211
   [=] COGS $5,943   (–)$5,943

Labor Expenses

1. Works 160 hrs @ $9.00/hrs   = $1,440
2. Works 160 hrs @ $8.75/hrs   = $1,400
3. Works 120 hrs @ $7.35/hrs   = $882
4. Works 120 hrs @ $7.00/hrs   = $840
5. Works 80 hrs @ $6.15/hrs   = $492
6. Works 60 hrs @ $5.50/hrs   = $330

Fringe benefits $1,250
Taxes $682
Administrative expenses [$300] $300
                                    ———————
Subtotal $7,616
Operating expenses $385
                                    ———————
Total expenses   = $8,001   (–)$8,001
Net profit [loss] $3,000

Hourly wages for employees:

1 = $9.00/hr	3 = $7.35/hr	5 = $6.15/hr
2 = $8.75/hr	4 = $7.00/hr	6 = $5.50/hr

Determine how the following data were obtained from the information above.

Labor cost %	= 45		Food cost %	= 35
Labor cost/meal	= 3.11		Food cost/meal	= 2.43
Minutes/meal	= 17		FTEs needed	= 17.5
Meals/labor hour	= 3.5			

Please note that there were 2,450 meals produced in February. The operating expenses = $385, Sales = $16,946, BI = $9,089, EI = $7,211, and Purchases = $4,067.

Note: How these figures were obtained is shown here.

$$\% \text{ Labor cost} = \frac{\text{Labor cost}}{\text{Sale}} \times 100 = 18001/16946 \times 100 = 44.94 = 45\%$$

$$\text{Labor cost per meal} = \frac{\text{Labor cost}}{\# \text{ of meals}} = \frac{7,616}{2,450} = 3.108 = 3.11$$

Minutes per meal

Minutes = 160 + 160 + 12 + 12 + 80 + 60 = 700 hours × 60 = 42,000 minutes

Number of meals = 2,450

$$\text{Minute per meal} = \frac{42,000}{2,450} = 17$$

$$\text{Meals per labor hour} = \frac{2,450}{700} = 3.5$$

$$\text{Food cost percent} = \frac{\text{Cost}}{\text{Sale}} \times 100 = \frac{5,943}{16,946} \times 100 = 35.07\%$$

$$\text{Food cost per meal} = \frac{5,943}{2,450} = 2.426 = 2.43$$

FTE needed = 700 = 17.5

Full-Time Equivalents (FTE) Calculations

Full-time equivalent is obtained by dividing the total number of labor hours worked by all employees by 40. It is the minimum number of employees needed to staff the establishment. If, for example, a restaurant requires 200 hours of labor per day, and the normal working period is 8 hours per day, it needs 25 FTE (that is 200 divided by 8). Many times management may reduce the number of FTEs while adding part-time or relief employees in an attempt to reduce the labor cost. Food cost, beverage cost and labor cost are the prime costs in foodservice and may account for up to 65% of the total sale. FTE information is important for staffing and determining productivity.

$$\text{Cost per meal} = \frac{\text{Total cost}}{\text{Number of meals prepared}}$$

$$\text{Meals per labor hour} = \frac{\text{Total number of meals served}}{\text{Total labor hours to produce the meals}}$$

$$\text{Meals per labor minutes} = \frac{\text{Total labor minutes to produce meals}}{\text{Total number of meals served}}$$

Full-time equivalent (FTE)

25 employees × 40 hours = 1,000 hours
12 employees × 20 hours = 240 hours
6 employees × 10 hours   = 60 hours

Total hours   = 1,300 hours per week

$$\frac{1,300 \text{ hours}}{40} = 32.5 \text{ FTE}$$

Although the department has 43 employees, it has only 32.5 FTEs.

Note: A relief employee can cover 2.5 FTEs.

Each FTE works 5 days per week and has 2 days off. A full-time relief employee works 5 days a week and has 2 days off. Therefore, the relief worker can work 2 days for 2 employees plus 1 day for another employee, giving her a 5-day-a-week (40 hours per week) workweek.

Employee Turnover Rate

Employee turnover rate is the number of departing employees divided by total number of staff. Employee turnover rate in foodservice is usually very high. The higher the employee turnover, the higher the tax levied by the government to cover unemployment compensation and therefore increased labor cost. Managerial effectiveness is the key to a lower employee turnover rate.

$$\text{Labor/employee turnover rate (\%)} = \frac{\text{Number of employees departed}}{\text{Number of employees on the staff}} \times 100$$

It is important to compare turnover rate with industry average and with the establishment's previous year.

XYZ restaurant had 150 employees on its staff for 2005. Of this number, 45 resigned or quit their job in that year. What is the employee turnover rate for XYZ restaurant for 2005?

Answer:

$$\frac{45}{150} \times 100 = 30\%$$

Profit and Loss Statements

Income Statement

Income statement, also known as a profit and loss statement, is a managerial tool used to evaluate the financial status with a given time period, usually for 12 months. It lists revenues, expenses, and gains and losses for a given period. The net income (or loss) for a given period is the bottom line. Variable costs are the costs that change as volume sales change such costs as food, beverage, and wages part of the payroll. Fixed cost does not change even when volume of sales increases, for example, insurance cost, mortgage, taxes etc. Overhead costs are costs for running the business and will include such costs as utilities and maintenance. Gross profit is the profit before subtracting the overhead or operating costs.

Balance Sheet

Balance sheet is a statement of financial condition that shows the financial position of the enterprise at a particular time, including the economic resources (assets, economic obligation [liabilities], and the residual claims made by the owners [owners' equity]).

Total Assets = Total Liabilities + Owner's Equity

There are two types of assets—current assets and fixed assets. Current assets include cash, account receivables, marketable securities, and inventory to be converted into cash, sold or exchanged within 1 year. Fixed assets are the monetary value of equipment, land, buildings, patents, and other items used to produce goods and services.

Liabilities are the amount of debt owed by the business to an outside entity, payable money such as a bank loan, outstanding bills, and payroll. Long-term liabilities include such items as mortgages, bonds, and other debts that are being paid off gradually.

Owner's equity or capital is the owner's share of the assets or the amount the owner has invested in the business. It may include the shareholders equity or stockholders equity.

Example:

Problems relating to financial records

Income Statement in Foodservice
The Graduate Restaurant
Operating Budget

			Percentage (%)
Sales			
Food	$303,875		
Beverage	53,625		
Total Sales		$357,500	

Cost of Sales			
Food	$106,356		29.75
Beverage	13,406		3.75
Total		$119,762	
Gross Profit		$237,738	66.50
Controllable Expenses			
Fixed Salaries and Wages	$ 42,120		11.78
Variable Salaries and Wages	28,600		8.00
Employee Benefits	17,680		4.95
Other Controllable Expenses	55,250		15.45
Total		$143,650	
Income Before Occupancy Costs		$ 94,088	26.31
Occupancy Costs		29,500	8.25
Income Before Int. & Dep.		$ 64,588	
Interest		5,000	
Depreciation		16,250	4.55
Restaurant Profit		$ 43,338	12.12

Discussion Questions

1. What is the percent food cost? How was that obtained?

   Answer:

   $$\frac{106,356}{303,875} \times 100 = \$34.99 = 35\%$$

2. What is the beverage percent cost?

   Answer:

   $$\frac{13,406}{53,625} \times 100 = \$24.99 = 25\%$$

3. What is the total labor cost? What is the percent labor cost? How was it obtained?

Answer:

$$\frac{88,400}{357,500} \times 100 = 24.72\%$$

4. What makes some costs controllable?

   Answer: Cost you can control such as wages, utilities, and food costs, etc.

5. List other controllable costs that may exist in foodservice.

   Answer: Payroll cost
   Utility cost
   Operational cost

6. How does gross profit differ from net profit?

   Answer: Gross profit is obtained by subtracting food and beverage cost from total sales, while net profit is obtained after costs have been subtracted.

7. How does this restaurant's net profit, percent food cost, and labor cost compare with industry averages?

   Answer: Restaurant food costs range from 30% to 65%, depending on the type of food served. Those serving seafood and steak may have higher costs, and institutional foodservice may have costs ranging between 30% and 33%. In terms of labor costs, industry average ranges from 20% to 25%, while the net profit may range from 5% to 10%.

Summary

The menu, food production, and labor are the center of every foodservice operation. While planning the menu, the foodservice manager must be aware of food costs, availability, and the production cost to bring the prepared food item to the customer's table. Food costs, along with production costs in terms of labor, all impact the net profit a foodservice operation reaps from its menu. This chapter has served as a review for managing these costs.

Suggested Reading

Dittmer, P.R. & Griffin, G.G. (1994). *Principles of food, beverage, and labor cost controls.* New York: Von Nostrand Reinhold.
Creamer and Breeding & Associate (19th ed.) R.D. Exam Review Guide.
Palacio-Payne, J. & Theis, M. (2005). *Introduction to foodservice.* Upper Saddle River, NJ: Pearson Prentice Hall.
Pavesic, D.V. & Magnant, P.E. (2005). *Fundamental principles of restaurant control.* Upper Saddle River, NJ: Pearson Prentice Hall.

CHAPTER 10

SCHOOL FOODSERVICE

Raymond Papa, EdD, RD, LD/N, Darlene Moppert, MS, RD, LD/N, and Sari Edelstein, PhD, RD

Reader Objectives

After reading this chapter and reflecting on its contents, the student will be able to:

1. Articulate the history of the National School Lunch Program (NSLP).
2. Explain the concepts of the meal plans.
3. Acknowledge the importance of good nutrition for children.
4. Understand the school foodservice food procurement process.
5. Conceptualize the school foodservice commodity program.
6. Explain why Hazard Analysis Critical Control Point (HACCP) is important in the school foodservice programs.

Key Terms

Commodity foods: foods that the federal government has the legal authority to purchase and distribute in order to support farm prices.

Dietary Guidelines for Americans: published jointly every 5 years by the Department of Health and Human Services and the Department of Agriculture (USDA). The *Guidelines* provide authoritative advice for people 2 years old and older about how good dietary habits can promote health and reduce risk for major chronic diseases.

Entitlement foods: foods available through a government program providing benefits to members of a specified group.

Federal subsidies: funding by the government to an individual or organization to assist in an enterprise deemed advantageous to the public.

Hazard Analysis and Critical Control Point (HACCP): refers to a systematic approach to food safety that focuses on each step in the preparation of food from receiving to serving the product.

Nonprofit program: a program that is exempt from income tax under section 501 (C) (3) of the Internal Revenue Code.

Nutrient Standard Menu Planning or the Assisted Nutrient Standard Menu Planning: meal planning that utilizes USDA-approved nutrient analysis software to plan school meals that meet the nutrient standards for the appropriate age/grade group.

Offer Versus Serve (OVS): a serving method that may be used in schools participating in the National School Lunch Program or School Breakfast Program. It allows the students the opportunity to select foods that they plan to eat and reject foods that they do not want.

Recommended Dietary Allowances (RDA)/Daily Reference Intakes (DRI): RDAs are nutritional intake values that meet the needs of most Americans to stay healthy. DRIs are nutrient reference values.

Reimbursable meal: a meal that meets the requirements of the National School Lunch Program for lunch and of the School Breakfast Program for breakfast.

Traditional/Enhanced Food Based Menus: meal planning that requires specific food components in specific amounts for specific age/grade groups.

Introduction

Almost 29 million U.S. children receive lunch each day through the NSLP.[1] With an annual cost of 7.1 billion dollars in 2003, the NSLP is the largest federally subsidized food program in the United States.[2] Approximately 88% of public schools participate in the NSLP and 67% in the School Breakfast Program (SBP). These meal programs are regarded as a safety net for ensuring that children and adolescents at risk for poor nutritional intake have access to safe, adequate, and nutritious foods that promote optimal physical, cognitive, and social growth and development.[3]

Both public and nonprofit private schools, high schools, and elementary schools may participate in the NSLP and the SBP. School districts and independent schools that participate in these school lunch and breakfast programs receive cash subsidies, and the USDA donates **commodity foods** for providing meals that meet federal requirements. Additionally, participating schools are required to offer free and reduced price meals to eligible students.[4]

President Harry S. Truman signed the National School Lunch Act into law in 1946 in response to claims that many U.S. men had been rejected for World War II military service because of diet-related health problems.[5] The NSLP was established as a "measure of national security, to safeguard the health and well-being of the nation's children and encourage the consumption of nutritious domestic agriculture commodities and other foods."[6]

In 1966, President Lyndon B. Johnson signed the Child Nutrition Act, which established the SBP. Like the NSLP, this federally subsidized program provides nutritionally balanced, low-cost, or free breakfasts for children in public and nonprofit private schools and non-profit childcare institutions. This act also authorized the Special Milk Program. The Special Milk Program reimburses schools and other programs that do not participate in the NSLP for milk that they serve. The Summer Foodservice Program provides federal resources to local sponsors to combine a feeding program with summer activities programs.[7]

Over the years, research has documented the benefits of these school-related child nutrition programs. Good nutrition has been linked to learning readiness, academic achievement, decreased discipline problems, and decreased emotional problems.[8] Studies have shown that children who eat school lunch consume more fruit, vegetables, and dairy foods than children who bring meals from home. School lunch meals also were shown to provide more protein, fiber, vitamins A, D, B_6, folate, niacin, riboflavin, calcium, iron, and zinc.[9]

In an essay in 1971, Gordon W. Gunderson, the first head of the NSLP, reviewed the benefits of the NSLP. These benefits still hold true today.[10] See Table 10.1.

Table 10.1   Benefits of Participating in the National School Lunch
                 Program

a. The nutrient content of school lunch meals must meet one-third of the
    child's daily nutrient requirement.
b. Through federal, state and local support, the price of a meal is likely
    to be within most children's ability to pay.
c. Federal regulations provide free and reduced price meals for children
    who are unable to pay for school lunch whose families meet
    established income requirements.
d. The USDA required meals platter gives latitude to local districts in
    menu planning while providing that child nutrition requirements are
    met when a wide variety of foods are used.
e. The program provides the opportunity to introduce foods that the
    student may not be familiar with at home, thus broadening their
    selections, helping to ensure an adequate and balanced diet.
f. Daily participation in the School Lunch Program develops good food
    habits that will carry on into adult years and the community.
g. Coordinated with classroom work, the cafeteria becomes a learning
    laboratory for experience in the principles of nutrition, sanitation,
    safety, personal hygiene, food service management, courtesies and
    social graces, budgeting, accountability, food storage and handling,
    food preservation, delivery systems and other subjects important to
    society.

Compiled by the authors from Gordon Gunderson, 1971.

Funding for School Lunch Programs

Through the NSLP and the SBP, the School Food Authority (SFA)
receives **federal subsidies** in the form of cash and USDA commodity foods based on the number of **reimbursable meals** served. The
SFA is the governing body that is responsible for the administration
of one or more schools and has the authority to operate the NSLP.
To qualify for reimbursement, meals must meet federal quality
requirements. Additionally the SFA must offer free and reduced
price meals to eligible children.[2] The SFA must submit an application annually to the state authority to operate under the NSLP.

The SFA receives money for each reimbursable meal based on the eligibility status of a child participating in the NSLP. Student eligibility is divided into three categories: free, reduced price, and paid. The eligibility for free or reduced price meals is based on the student's family financial status. Students whose family income is within 130% of the poverty level are eligible for free meals. Those with family incomes between 130% and 185% of the poverty level are eligible for reduced price meals. The remainder of the students pay prices set by the SFA. The SFA must operate the program as a non-profit program.[11]

A reimbursable meal is one that meets the requirements for lunch of the NSLP and for the SBP for breakfast. The requirements include specifications that ensure schools provide nutritious, well-balanced meals to all the children served. Lunch must provide one-third of the **Recommended Dietary Allowances (RDA)** set by the **Daily Reference Intakes (DRI)** for protein, calcium, iron, vitamin A, vitamin C, and energy appropriate for the different age levels. School breakfast is required to provide one-fourth of the RDA for these nutrients. Meal planning must adhere to the *Dietary Guidelines for Americans*[1]:

1. Offering a variety of foods
2. Limiting fat to 30% of the total calories and saturated fat to less than 10% of total calories
3. Providing a diet low in cholesterol
4. Providing a diet with plenty of grains, vegetables, and fruit

Meal Planning

The USDA through Food and Nutrition Service implemented the School Meals Initiative for Healthy Children (SMI) in 1995. The SMI includes all of the NSLP and the SBP regulations and policies that pertain to the nutrition standards for school meals. The SMI rule, along with federal legislation, allows School Food Authorities to select from a variety of menu planning options. SMI is an ongoing process to provide nutritious school meals to children and motivate children to make healthy choices.[1] Menu planning options fall into two categories: food based and nutrient based.

Traditional Food Based Menu Planning

Traditional or Enhanced Food Based Menu Planning utilizes meal patterns to establish nutritional adequacy of the menu. Schools using these options must offer specific food components in at least the minimum quantities required for specific age groups. The four meal components are milk, meat or meat alternate, vegetable or fruit, and grains-breads. The student must select at least three components. Tables 10.2 and 10.3 show the required meal pattern for Traditional Food Based Menu Planning and the Enhanced Food Based Menu Planning.[12] The USDA provides sample meal patterns for all menu-planning options used at breakfast and lunch. Under the SBP, participating SFAs must adhere to similar USDA meal-planning guidelines.

Nutrient Standard Menu Planning or Assisted Nutrient Standard Menu Planning

Nutrient Standard Menu Planning or the Assisted Nutrient Standard Menu Planning is used to develop the breakfast or lunch menu based on nutrient analysis to ensure meals meet the nutrient standards for the appropriate age/grade group. A reimbursable lunch must offer three menu items that include an entrée, fluid milk, and a side dish. Students must select the entrée and one other item. Table 10.4 outlines the Nutrient Standard Menu Planning or the Assisted Nutrient Standard Menu Planning requirements.[12]

Offer versus Serve

Offer Versus Serve (OVS) is a term used in school menu planning and is the basis for determining if the school meal is reimbursable. OVS allows the student to decline some of the foods offered in the breakfast and lunch program. There are a variety of methods that may be used in school menu planning, but OVS is applicable no matter what method is selected, OVS is applicable. OVS was incorporated into the NSLP in 1975 and

> **Learning Point:** School food-service managers will have to research the area for the appropriate menu planning format for their district, county, or school.

Table 10.2 Traditional Food-Based Menu Planning

Food Components and Food Items	Minimum Quantities				Recommended Quantities
	Group I Ages 1–2 Preschool	Group II Ages 3–4 Preschool	Group III Ages 5–8 Grades K–3	Group IV Ages 9 and Older Grades 4–12	Group V Ages 12 and Older Grades 7–12
Milk (as a beverage)	6 fluid ounces	6 fluid ounces	8 fluid ounces	8 fluid ounces	8 fluid ounces
Meat or meat alternate (quantity of the edible portion as served):					
Lean meat, poultry, or fish	1 ounce	1½ ounces	1½ ounces	2 ounces	3 ounces
Alternate protein products[1]	1 ounce	1½ ounces	1½ ounces	2 ounces	3 ounces
Cheese	1 ounce	1½ ounces	1½ ounces	2 ounces	3 ounces
Large egg	½	¾	¾	1	1½
Cooked dry beans or peas	¼ cup	⅜ cup	⅜ cup	½ cup	¾ cup
Peanut butter or other nut or seed butters	2 tablespoons	3 tablespoons	3 tablespoons	4 tablespoons	6 tablespoons
Yogurt, plain or flavored, unsweetened or sweetened	4 ounces or ½ cup	6 ounces or ¾ cup	6 ounces or ¾ cup	8 ounces or 1 cup	12 ounces or 1½ cups
The following may be used to meet no more than 50% of the requirement and must be used in combination with any of the above:					

continues

Table 10.2 (continued)

Food Components and Food Items	Minimum Quantities				Recommended Quantities
	Group I Ages 1–2 Preschool	Group II Ages 3–4 Preschool	Group III Ages 5–8 Grades K–3	Group IV Ages 9 and Older Grades 4–12	Group V Ages 12 and Older Grades 7–12
Peanuts, soy nuts, tree nuts, or seeds, as listed in program guidance, or an equivalent quantity of any combination of the above meat/meat alternate (1 ounce of nuts/seeds = 1 ounce of cooked lean meat, poultry, or fish)	½ ounce = 50%	¾ ounce = 50%	¾ ounce = 50%	1 ounce = 50%	1½ ounces = 50%
Vegetable or fruit: 2 or more servings of vegetables, fruits or both	½ cup	½ cup	½ cup	¾ cup	¾ cup
Grains/breads: (servings per week): Must be enriched or whole grain. A serving is a slice of bread or an equivalent serving of biscuits, rolls, etc., or ½ cup of cooked rice, macaroni, noodles, other pasta products or cereal grain	5 servings per week[2] — minimum of ½ serving per day	8 servings per week[2] — minimum of 1 serving per day	8 servings per week[2] — minimum of 1 serving per day	2 servings per week[2] — minimum of 1 serving per day	10 servings per week[2] — minimum of 1 serving per day

Source: www.fns.usda.gov/
[1] Must meet the requirements in Appendix A of 7 CRF 210.
[2] For the purposes of this table, a week equals five days.

Table 10.3 Enhanced Food-Based Menu Planning

Lunch

The Enhanced Food-Based Menu Planning Approach
The Enhanced Food-Based Menu Planning Approach is a variation of the Traditional Menu Planning approach. it is designed to increase calories from low-fat food sources in order to meet the Dietary Guidelines. The five food components are retained, but the component quantities for the weekly servings of vegetables and fruits and grains/breads are increased.

Food Components and Food Items	Minimum Quantities				Option for Grades K–3
	Ages 1–2	Preschool	Grades K–6	Grades 7–12	
Milk (as a beverage):	6 fluid ounces	6 fluid ounces	8 fluid ounces	8 fluid ounces	8 fluid ounces
Meat or meat alternate:	1 ounce	1½ ounces	1½ ounces	2 ounces	1½ ounces
Lean meat, poultry, or fish	1 ounce	1½ ounces	2 ounces	2 ounces	1½ ounces
Alternate protein products[1]	1 ounce	1½ ounces	2 ounces	2 ounces	3 ounces
Cheese	1 ounce	1½ ounces	2 ounces	2 ounces	1½ ounces
Large egg	½	¾	1	1	¾
Cooked dry beans or peas	¼ cup	⅜ cup	½ cup	½ cup	⅜ cup
Peanut butter or other nut or seed butters	2 tablespoons	3 tablespoons	4 tablespoons	4 tablespoons	3 tablespoons
Yogurt, plain or flavored, unsweetened or sweetened	4 ounces or ½ cup	6 ounces or ¾ cup	8 ounces or 1 cup	8 ounces or 1 cup	6 ounces or ¾ cup
The following may be used to meet no more than 50% of the requirement and					

continues

Table 10.3 (continued)

Food Components and Food Items	Minimum Quantities						
	Ages 1–2	Preschool	Grades K–6	Grades 7–12	Option for Grades K–3		
must be used in combination with any of the above: Peanuts, soy nuts, tree nuts, or seeds, as listed in program guidance, or an equivalent quantity of any combination of the above meat/meat alternate (1 ounce of nuts/seeds = 1 ounce of cooked lean meat, poultry, or fish)	½ ounce = 50%	¾ ounce = 50%	1 ounce = 50%	1 ounce = 50%	¾ ounce = 50%		
Vegetable or fruit: 2 or more servings of vegetables, fruits or both	½ cup	½ cup	¾ cup plus an extra ½ cup over a week[2]	1 cup	¾ cup		
Grains/breads: (servings per week): Must be enriched or whole grain. A serving is a slice of bread or an equivalent serving of biscuits, rolls, etc., or ½ cup of cooked rice, macaroni, noodles, other pasta products or cereal grain	5 servings per week[2] — minimum of ½ serving per day	8 servings per week[2] — minimum of 1 serving per day	12 servings per week[2] — minimum of 1 serving per day[3]	15 servings per week[2] — minimum of 1 serving per day[3]	10 servings per week[2] — minimum of 1 serving per day[3]		

[1] Must meet the requirements in Appendix A of 7 CRF 210.
[2] For the purposes of this table, a week equals five days.
[3] Up to one grains/breads serving per day may be a dessert.

Source: District of Columbia State Education Office. Accessed 8/1/2006. Available at: http://seo.dc.gov/seo/frames.asp?doc=/seo/lib/services/food_nutrition/nslp_mea_pattern_requirement.pdf.

Table 10.4 The Nutrient Standard Menu Planning Approach

The Nutrient Standard Menu Planning Approach
Nutrient Standard Menu Planning (sometimes called "NuMenus") is a computer based menu planning system that uses approved computer software to analyze the specific nutrient content of menu items automatically while menus are being planned. It is designed to assist menu planners in choosing food items that create nutritious meals and meet the nutrient standards.

Here are the required minimums for nutrients and calories for these nutrient standard menu planning approaches:

Minimum Nutrient and Calorie Levels for School Lunches
Nutrient Standard Menu Planning Approaches (School Week Averages)

Nutrients and Energy Allowances	Minimum Requirements			Optional Grades K–3
	Preschool	Grades K–6	Grades 7–12	
Energy allowances (calories)	517	664	825	635
Total fat (as a percentage of actual total food energy)	1	1, 2	2	1, 3
Saturated fat (as a percentage of actual total food energy)	1	1, 3	3	1, 3
RDA for protein (g)	7	10	16	9
RDA for calcium (mg)	267	286	400	267
RDA for iron (mg)	3.3	3.5	4.5	3.3
RDA for Vitamin A (RE)	150	224	300	200
RDA for Vitamin C (mg)	14	15	18	15

[1]The Dietary Guidelines recommend that after 2 years of age ". . . children should gradually adopt a diet that, by about 5 years or age, contains no more than 30% of calories from fat."
[2]Not to exceed 30% over a school week.
[3]Less than 10% over a school week.
Source: www.fns.usda.gov/.

applied only to students in senior high school. Based on its success in high school, OVS was later expanded to include all grade levels, elementary through high school lunch and breakfast. The goals of OVS are to reduce food waste in the school meal program and to allow students choices in selecting the foods they prefer.

The NSLP mandates that OVS be implemented in senior high schools; it is optional in all other grade levels. The SFA has the discretion to implement OVS for the SBP at any or all grade levels. The alternative to OVS is that the student must take all food offered as part of the meal. Providing students a choice in selecting food items enhances the opportunity to learn good nutrition.

Procurement

Federal, state, and local authorities have established the procurement requirements for the SFA. School districts' procurement practices must meet the requirements of the regulatory authorities. The SFA is no different than any other foodservice operation in that it needs to purchase food, paper goods, small kitchen supplies, and large equipment. What makes the SFA somewhat unique from other foodservice operations are the restrictions on what may or may not be purchased, as well as the process that will be used to purchase the items.

Detailed information regarding specific regulations and procedures as they relate to procurement for the NSLP can be found in the Federal Procurement Standards. These requirements ensure that materials and services are obtained for the NSLP efficiently, economically, and in compliance with applicable laws and executive orders.

Learning Point: Diversity Issues

The USDA requires that the cultural background of the students be given consideration in meal planning. School meals provide the opportunity to celebrate the diversity in the school community. By learning about and trying foods from different cultures, children increase their knowledge of the world around them. This increases the likelihood that they will choose a more varied diet when they grow up. [13] Many ethnic recipes provide the opportunity to introduce students to healthy fruit, vegetables, and grain dishes.

The items to be purchased are based on a variety of factors including the menu, the facility, production method, skill level of personnel, food cost, labor cost, USDA-donated commodity foods, and federal regulations.

Commodity Foods

When the commodity distribution program was instituted, it had two major objectives: assist farmers and support the variety of government-sponsored feeding programs, with schools being the largest participant. Participants are entitled by law to receive these commodity foods called **entitlement foods,** based on a dollar amount for each reimbursable meal served. USDA provides SFAs information as to what foods are available and when they can be ordered.[4]

Commodity foods are available as canned, frozen, or fresh products. There are hundreds of foods available directly from USDA commodity distribution. Another option available to the SFA is to have commodity foods further processed. This is when the SFA has a commodity food item sent to a food manufacturer to have that item made into something more useable. An example is when the SFA orders commodity whole chickens but does not want to receive the whole chickens in that form. The SFA may select from a wide range of approved manufacturers that will produce chicken products such as chicken nuggets, chicken patties, or ready-to-cook frozen chicken pieces. Processing commodities increases the variety of foods available to the SFA.

Careers, Staff Development, and Quality Improvement

The USDA does not mandate the requirements for school nutrition program directors and managers.[14] Nutrition services administrators fill diverse roles including spokesperson, manager of the budget, and partner in comprehensive school health programs. In small districts, one person may directly fulfill all of the roles, while larger districts allow for delegation of these duties to a professional leadership support staff. School nutrition directors should have a minimum of a bachelor's degree in a nutrition/foodservice related field. Larger districts often mandate that the school nutrition

administrator have at least a master's degree. The School Nutrition
Association provides credentialing that includes minimum education requirements and the passing of a rigorous exam specific to
school foodservice administration. Individuals who complete these
requirements are awarded the designation of School Food and
Nutrition Specialist.[15]

Management and staffing at individual schools varies based on
the number of students and programs at a school. School districts
typically implement their own recruitment program, with parents of
the school's students often applying to fill vacancies. Food and
Nutrition Services Departments must implement training programs
that provide employees with needed job skills to meet federal regulations and department objectives.

School nutrition managers often come from the ranks of already
employed school foodservice employees. Often managers take on an
active role in educating students about nutrition, marketing the
food and nutrition service program, as well as managing a quality
foodservice operation that meets USDA guidelines and customer
satisfaction.

Meeting these goals necessitates an ongoing professional development program to ensure the highest standards.

The School Nutrition Association established a certification program for all levels of foodservice staff. Requirements include education in sanitation, nutrition, and foodservice operations. Individuals
must also complete required continuing education to maintain certification.[15] The School Nutrition Association provides the Keys to
Excellence, a self-assessment tool that school foodservice operations
can use a part of a continuous quality improvement program.[16]

Hazard Analysis and Critical Control Point (HACCP)

As of July 1, 2006, school food authorities are required to have a
food safety program for the preparation and service of school meals
served to children. This can be referenced in Section III of the Child
Nutrition and WIC Reauthorization Act of 2004.[17] The program
must be based on **Hazard Analysis and Critical Control Point
(HACCP)** principles and conform to guidelines issued by the USDA.
HACCP is designed to reduce the risk of foodborne hazards by following a systematic approach in constructing a food safety pro-

gram. The focus is on identifying each step in the preparation of food from receiving the product to serving the product. The three major components in developing the food safety program are: sanitation, temperature control, and standard operating procedures (SOPs). See chapter 7 for more information and an HACCP manual.

Learning Point: HACCP Steps

1. Develop, document in writing, and implement SOPs.
2. Identify and document in writing all menu items according to the process approach to HACCP.
3. Identify and document control measures and critical limits.
4. Establish monitoring procedures.
5. Establish corrective actions.
6. Keep records.
7. Review and revise your overall food safety program periodically.

Coordinated Review Effort

The USDA requires school districts participating in the NSLP to periodically undergo an administrative review. This review is required by Regulation 7 CFR 210.18 in the *Federal Register* and is known as the Coordinated Review Effort (CRE).[18] State agencies shall conduct administrative reviews of all school food authorities at least once during each 5-year review cycle and provide that each school food authority is reviewed at least once every 6 years. The purpose of the CRE is to ensure compliance with regulations for child nutrition programs.

The primary goals of the CRE are to determine if free and reduced price meal benefits are provided in accordance with regulations, if proper meal counts are taken at the point of service, and if complete, reimbursable meals are offered for the review period.

The critical review areas include two performance standards:

- Certification/ counting/claiming: All free, reduced price, and paid lunches claimed for reimbursement are served only to children eligible for free, reduced price, and paid lunches, respectively, and are counted, recorded, consolidated, and reported through a system that consistently yields correct claims.

- Lunches claimed for reimbursement within the SFA contain food items/components as required by NSLP regulations.

The general review areas include, but are not limited to, the following:

- A review of the free and reduced price policy statement to ensure it is implemented as approved.
- Review the verification of free and reduced price meal eligibility process to ensure that the process is complete.
- Ensure that overt identification of students receiving free and reduced price meals does not occur.
- Through observation and review of records, ensure food quantities are sufficient to provide food components in the quantities required.
- Ensure the SFA is in compliance with civil rights provisions.
- Confirm that SFA submits and retains records as required.
- Review and confirm that the SFA conducts on-site reviews annually as required.
- Review and confirm that the SFA performs edit checks monthly prior to submitting claims for reimbursement.
- Ensure safe food handling/serving/storage practices have been implemented.
- Observe serving/dining areas for compliance with competitive food regulations.[19]

Emergency Plan

The SFA should have an emergency plan in place that will allow it to function under abnormal operating conditions without compromising food safety. Emergencies may affect one school for a short period of time or the entire district for an extended period of time. While it is difficult to plan for every type of emergency, the plan should include emergencies common to foodservice as well as disasters that may be prevalent to school districts in certain regions of the country. Emergencies typical to foodservice operations include kitchen fires, loss of electricity or gas, equipment breakdowns, and water main breaks. Disasters that might be more regional in nature include hurricanes, tornados, blizzards, wildfires, and floods. When natural disasters affect the community, schools may be used as shelters to house and feed those persons in need.

While it would not be realistic to have a separate plan for every conceivable emergency, think about having a plan that different types of emergencies could fit into. For example, one plan could address short-term emergencies affecting one school, several schools, and many schools. Another plan would cover longer-term emergencies for one school, several schools, and many schools. Each variation will have some unique features, but a number of the actions to be taken will be common to many emergencies.

> **Learning Point:** School foodservice managers should have a disaster/emergency plan that is realistic and ready for action at any time.

An effective emergency readiness plan provides a foundation for what actions to take in the event of a disruption. When developing the plan, take one step at a time. A well-conceived plan will help reduce confusion and ensure the health, safety, and satisfaction of customers and employees.

The six steps of a successful emergency readiness plan include:

1. Determine who will do what in the event of an emergency and develop a contact directory.
2. Identify disruptions that may hinder a foodservice operation and determine alternate procedures.
3. Develop the foodservice emergency readiness plan.
4. Teach components of the emergency readiness plan to foodservice staff.
5. Practice emergency readiness drills.
6. Evaluate the emergency readiness plan's effectiveness and update as needed.

Chapter 15 gives more detailed information on planning for a disaster.

Nutrition Education and Promotions

A healthy school environment integrates school nutrition services with a coordinated, comprehensive school health program. This would link comprehensive sequential education access to child nutrition programs, which provide nutritious meals with family, and community health service partnerships that support positive health and education outcomes for all children.[14] School foodservice employees often provide classroom education to students. The cafeteria is a learning laboratory where nutrition education concepts are promoted and practiced.

Marketing the school food and nutrition program ensures a successful business while providing nutrition education. A school food and nutrition services marketing plan involves the following: definition of the business, identification of the target audience, needs of the target audience, services offered that meet the needs of the target audience, knowledge of the competition, and a budget for marketing and promotional objectives.[11] Marketing can convey to the target audiences many important aspects about school food and nutrition services. For example, these can include:

- School meals are convenient, inexpensive, and meet the children's nutrition requirements.
- Free and reduced price meals are available for students who qualify.
- Children who eat breakfast do better in school.
- Lucky tray promotions can entice children to buy school breakfast or lunch or try a new item.

National School Lunch Week™, National Breakfast Week™, and National Nutrition Month™ are annual programs that provide economic ideas for celebrating the value of school nutrition services many times per year.[11,20] Poster contests, games, nutrition quizzes, lucky trays, celebrity guests, coloring sheets, and theme meals provide the opportunity to highlight the food and nutrition services programs.

Inviting parents, teachers, and local dignitaries to enjoy a school meal shows them firsthand the quality foodservice that is provided. It also provides them with a memorable opportunity to enjoy time with the children. Utilizing celebrity servers such as politicians, sports heroes, media persons, and principals at special events also promote the program. Often these individuals are willing to come in and have a meal with the students.

Valuable school foodservice marketing requires efficient mechanisms to effectively communicate to the parents and students about a special event or service. Promotions build awareness of the school foodservice product line. Flyers and banners are one way to deliver the message. School newsletters that are regularly sent home to parents provide additional opportunities to advertise the program and teach nutrition. Daily nutrition messages through the school intercom or school radio stations remind students about service and promotions. Public service announcements can be sent to local radio and television stations creating community interest. Press releases can also be sent to the media. The menu provides terrific marketing opportunities. Local newspapers often print the weekly menu without charge. A department Web site can also underscore the foodservices that are available as well as provide nutrition education for students and families. Chapter 4 gives the reader more information about social marketing.

School Wellness Policy

The Child Nutrition Reauthorization Act of 2004 mandated that each local school agency establish a local wellness policy. This policy must provide assurance that schools meet nutritional standards established by federal law. It must address all foods served on campus. This includes school meals, a la carte cafeteria sales, vending sales, concession stands, classroom celebrations, and fundraising.[6] The plan must include goals for nutrition education and physical activity. School administrators, parents, students, food and nutrition service employees, and the public must have been involved in the development of the policy. The policy must also include a mechanism for monitoring and ensuring that the school district meets the objectives of the policy.

This federal mandate was adopted in response to the obesity crisis facing our nation. The prevalence of overweight children has doubled between 1980 and 2000, and during that same time period the prevalence of overweight adolescents has tripled.[14]

Overweight children and adolescents are more likely to remain overweight or become obese adults. This will lead to development of chronic diseases. One in three children will develop diabetes. Overweight children are less likely to achieve academic success.

The issue of competitive foods from school stores, vending machines, and a la carte cafeteria sales challenges school districts to provide a balance between revenue generation and student health needs. The availability of unhealthy competitive foods undermines the Healthy Schools Meals for America Act, which requires that school meals must meet the *Dietary Guidelines for Americans.* Schools are a critical part of the environment that shapes children's eating behaviors. Other issues that must be addressed are nutritional quality, variety, and acceptability of school meals, mealtime scheduling, physical activity, and foods served outside the classroom. Children receive a mixed message when the value of healthy food choices is taught in the classroom but school vending machines and other venues provide an assortment of snacks and beverages that are not based on nutrition standards.[8]

> **Learning Point:** Because of the obesity crisis among U.S. youth, school foodservice managers should be engaged in doing their part to provide nutritious meals for students.

Summary

The NSLP was designed to nourish U.S. youth, such that they could flourish physically and in the classroom. In order for this to occur, guidelines for procuring foods and providing menus that meet the nutritional needs of children of all ages have been developed. The SFA may select food or nutrient based menu planning options. Those professionals working in the school foodservice industry must know and follow federal guidelines and understand their mission of providing nutritious foods to their students.

Student Activities

1. Using one of the school lunch meal plans, plan a 1-day menu. If possible, use nutrient analysis software to get nutrient information from your planned menu.
2. Obtain one or more of the monitoring sheets from the HACCP manual in the appendix, and record the information from your school cafeteria.
3. Call a foodservice operation or school lunch program office and ask how HACCP is enforced there. Report their examples to the class.

4. Investigate software programs that are used for school foodservice.
5. Write an objective for a school wellness policy that relates to foods served during the school day.
6. Plan a social marketing campaign for an element of school foodservice.
7. Plan possible food storage ideas for a disaster.
8. Plan vending machine items for a school.
9. Visit a school cafeteria and perform a sanitation check (see the HACCP manual in the Appendix for the form).
10. Investigate what other meal plans can be used in the school system and present them to the class.

Web Resources

Food Distribution Program (Commodity Foods)
http://www.fns.usda.gov/fdd/facts/biubguidance.htm

Food Safety, U.S. Department of Agriculture Food Distribution Program http://www.fns.usda.gov/fdd/foodsafety/sda-safety.htm

HACCP
HACCP-based Standard Operating Procedures
http://sop.nfsmi.org/HACCPBasedSOPs.php

HACCP Manager's Self-Inspection Checklist, U.S. Department of Agriculture, 1999
http://schoolmeals.nal.usda.gov/FoodSafety/ManagersChecklist.pdf

Regulations and Guidelines
Food Code, Food and Drug Administration
http://www.cfsan.fda.gov/~dms/fc01-toc.html

National School Lunch Program Facts
http://www.fns.usda.gov/cnd/Lunch/AboutLunch/NSLPFact Sheet.pdf

National School Lunch Program History
http://www.fns.usda.gov/cnd/Lunch/AboutLunch/ProgramHistory .htm

Nutrition Guidelines (Dietary Guidelines, MyPyramid)
Center for Nutrition Policy and Promotion, U.S. Department of
Agriculture
http://www.usda.gov/cnpp/

Dietary Guidelines for Americans 2005, U.S. Department of Agriculture and U.S. Department of Health and Human Services, 2005
http://www.usda.gov/cnpp/dietary_guidelines.html

Dietary Reference Intakes (DRI) and Recommended Dietary
Allowances (RDAhttp://www.nal.usda.gov/fnic/etext/000105.html
MyPyramid: http://www.mypyramid.gov/

School Breakfast Program
Child Nutrition Fact Sheet: School Breakfast Program, Food
Research and Action Center, 2004
http://http://www.frac.org/pdf/cnsbp.PDF

Discover School Breakfast Toolkit, U.S. Department of Agriculture,
2004.
http://www.fns.usda.gov/cnd/breakfast/toolkit/Default.htm

School Breakfast Program, U.S. Department of Agriculture
http://www.fns.usda.gov/cnd/Breakfast/Default.htm

School Breakfast Program Menu Planning, U.S. Department of
Agriculture
http://www.fns.usda.gov/cnd/Breakfast/Menu/sbp-menu-planning.htm

USDA Regulations for the School Breakfast Program
http://www.fns.usda.gov/cnd/Governance/regulations.htm

School Lunch Program
A Menu Planner for Healthy School Meal, U.S. Department of
Agriculture, 1998
http://www.fns.usda.gov/tn/Resources/menuplanner.html

School Nutrition Association: www.schoolnutrition.org
School Nutrition Practice Group, ADA
http://www.eatright.org/cps/rde/xchg/ada/hs.xsl/career_dpg42_
ENU_HTML.htm

National School Lunch Week
http://www.schoolnutrition.org/nslw/

Protocols: How to Analyze Menus for USDA's School Meals Programs, U.S. Department of Agriculture, 2005
http://www.fns.usda.gov/tn/Resources/nutrientanalysis.html

Offer Versus Serve Handout, Minnesota Department of Children and Families
https://fns.state.mn.us/FNSProg/NSLP/PDF/Resources/OVSHANDOUT.pdf#

USDA Regulations for the National School Lunch Program
http://www.fns.usda.gov/cnd/Governance/regulations.htm

Special Milk Program
Special Milk Program, U.S. Department of Agriculture
http://www.fns.usda.gov/cnd/Milk/Default.htm

USDA Regulations for the Special Milk Program
http://www.fns.usda.gov/cnd/Governance/regulations.htm

References

1. U.S. Department of Agriculture. (2006). School meals–regulations. Retrieved September 24, 2006, from http://www.schoolnutrition .org/Index.aspx?id=1078.
2. U.S. Department of Agriculture. (2006). National school lunch program: Program facts. Retrieved September 24, 2006, from http://www.fns.usda .gov/cnd/lunch/.
3. American Dietetic Association. (2006). Position of the American Dietetic Association: Child and adolescent food and nutrition programs. *Journal of the American Dietetic Association, 106*(9), 1467–1475.
4. U.S. Department of Agriculture. (2006). Schools/child nutrition commodity programs: Food distribution fact sheets. Retrieved September 24, 2006, from http://www.fns.usda.gov/fdd/programs/schcnp/.
5. School Nutrition Association. (2006). Program history and data. Retrieved September 24, 2006, from http://www.schoolnutrition .org/Index.aspx?id=71.
6. Russell, Richard B. National school lunch act. (2004). Retrieved September 24, 2006, from http://www.schoolnutrition.org/Index.aspx?id=71.
7. School Nutrition Association. (2006). National school lunch week. National school breakfast week. Retrieved September 24, 2006, from http://www.schoolnutrition.org/Index.aspx?id=31.
8. American Dietetic Association. (2006). Position of the American Dietetic Association: Local support for nutrition integrity in schools. *Journal of the American Dietetic Association, 106*(1), 122–133.

9. Rainville, A.J. (2001). Nutrition quality of reimbursable school lunches compared to lunches brought from home in two southeastern Michigan school districts. *Journal of Child Nutrition and Management, 25*(1).

10. Gunderson, G.W. (1971). The national school lunch program: Background and development. Retrieved September 24, 2006, from http://www.fns .usda.gov/cnd/Lunch/AboutLunch/ProgramHistory.htm.

11. U.S. Department of Agriculture. National school breakfast program: Marketing efforts. Retrieved September 24, 2006, from http://www.fns.usda.gov/cnd/breakfast/toolkit/Default.htm.

12. District of Columbia State Education Office. Retrieved August 1, 2006, from http://seo.dc.gov/seo/frames.asp?doc=/seo/lib/seo/services/food _nutrition/nslp_meal_pattern_requirement.pdf.

13. American Dietetic Association. (2005). An essential component of comprehensive school health programs. *Journal of the American Dietetic Association, 103*(4), 505–513.

15. School Nutrition Association. (2006). Become nationally certified with SNA certification program. Retrieved September 24, 2006, from http://www.schoolnutrition.org/Credentialing.aspx?id=1021http://www.schoolnutrition.org/Credentialing.aspx?id=1021.

16. School Nutrition Association. (2006). Keys to excellence. Retrieved September 24, 2006, from http://www.schoolnutrition.org/KEYS.aspx?ID=1158.

17. School Nutrition Association. (2005). USDA issues HACCP guidance for schools. RetrievedSeptember 24, 2006, from http://www.school nutrition.org/Index.aspx?id=1300.

18. Code of Federal Regulations. (2003). Administrative review 7 CRF 210.18. Retrieved September 24, 2006, from http://www.gpoaccess.gov/cfr/ index.html.

19. Indiana Department of Education. (2005*)*. CRE-coordinated review effort. Retrieved September 24, 2006, from www.doe.state.in.us/food/ pdf/cre_review_explanation.pdf.

20. American Dietetic Association. (2006). National nutrition month-March 2007. Retrieved September 24, 2006, from http://www.eatright.org/cps/ rde/xchg/ada/hs.xsl/shop_4920_ENU_HTML.htm.

## CHAPTER 11

COMPUTERIZED INFORMATION SYSTEMS FOR MANAGING FOOD AND NUTRITION SERVICES

Neeta Singh, PhD

Reader Objectives

After reading this chapter and reflecting on the contents, the student will be able to:

1. Identify the trends in information technology (IT) as they relate to the management of food and nutrition service.
2. Describe the field of database management as an essential component in understanding computerized information systems.
3. Discuss the field of management information systems (MIS) as an essential component in understanding computerized information systems.
4. Explain the applications of computerized information systems for managing various subsystems of nutrition and foodservice.
5. Translate the need for computerized IT as it could be applied to selected subsystems of nutrition and foodservice.

Key Terms

Data modeling: process of structuring and organizing data; used for database management.

Database: organized collection of data.

Direct-reading tables: method used for adjusting yield of recipes with ingredients amount given in weights and measurements.

Excel: a popular spreadsheet program, originally released in 1985 by Microsoft® for Macintosh®, and later adapted by Microsoft Windows®.

Factor method: formula for adjusting yield of recipes.

Hardware: a physical element of a computer system; the computer equipment as opposed to the program or information stored in the machine.

Nonproprietary programming: an open software that uses openly available tools and technologies, allowing add-ons and the ability to connect readily with other technologies.

Proprietary programming: a design or technique that is owned by a company.

Query: form of questioning used for computer software.

Schema: description of the structure of a database.

Software: program that directs computer on what to do. Software is classified as system software and/or application software.

Introduction

Today's rapidly changing healthcare environment demands the efficient use of resources, whether material or nonmaterial. That means that foodservice professionals need to be familiar both with technological trends in their field and the terminology of the technological applications that will positively impact their organizational productivity and quality. More and more, depending on the size and scope of a foodservice organization, professionals should realize that business terms, such as productivity, profitability, strategic planning, multitasking, globalizing, rightsizing, downsizing, and optimizing, carry a significant relevance in their field. Accordingly, the degree to which dietitians and foodservice managers use this terminology depends on the size of the organization, whether it be a "mom and pop" restaurant or a larger, more complex integrated healthcare foodservice. As the structure of the organization becomes more intricate, the complexities of the environment necessitate the application or redesign of technological contents and their application, so that the organization's operation will be more effective and efficient. One might think that application of computerized technology does not affect our immediate environment, but it does. As part of the workforce, and as consumers, we breathe and live within these environments, so we need a better understanding of the application and benefits of computerized information systems for managing food and nutrition services.

Since technology evolves, it seems, at the speed of light, the emphasis of this chapter is on understanding and exploring the functions and application of technology in food and nutrition services systems and subsystems, rather than suggesting specific computer **hardware** and **software** as they may be applied. It is quite possible that many food and nutrition service organizations will have a technology support technician, but it is still necessary that dietetic professionals clearly and proficiently express their departmental technology needs. It is important to understand the basics of information systems and their application of computerized technology for various processes. Merely unpacking computers' fragile components, plugging and starting the right sequence or step-by-step guide to setting up your computer is not enough. Foodservice professionals now need a deeper understanding of the subsystems, with a view to a seamless integration of technology into their system.

Trends

Any profitable business and its strategy is driven by trends. Analyzing business trends helps you to see how information systems have been used in the areas of food and nutrition services so that you may then help shape the strategic efforts of your organization. Since application of technology is not easy on the pockets of the organization, careful planning is critical. Trends can steer this effort.

So far, information systems in healthcare organizations have been used preliminarily in the areas of human resource management and financial functions. One of the main reasons behind slow growth in the application of technology, specifically to foodservice systems, is that foodservice is a labor-intensive business. This does not mean that information systems cannot be used by foodservice. It does mean, however, that a system's application should be carefully selected and designed so that it will not interfere with patient care and customer satisfaction and will increase the organization's productivity through better, efficient management of resources.

As nutrition and foodservice grows as a field, so too does its complexity and, thus, the need to explore the application of computer technology beyond processes. More and more, management needs to refine its computer assistance, especially in the areas of **database** management, data-based decision making, and reporting specific information. The new requirements by regulatory agencies such as the Joint Commission on Accreditation of Healthcare Organizations (JCAHO) will necessitate the application of information systems for the purposes of data collection, data management, and data reporting. Information systems will continue to dominate the technological front in the coming years in foodservice organizations.

The other prominent trend in the application of computerized technology involves the design and implementation of a universal electronic data interchange system for processing healthcare claims. Health care claims have received much criticism because they have always involved a complicated process requiring multiple data entry at each level. Repetitive data entry steers the monetary resources of the organization, which can be used otherwise. This tedious system necessitates the development of a common language for hospitals, regulatory agencies, the federal government, and insurers, along with the standardization of core financial information. A retooled system will not only bring uniformity but will make the process effective and efficient, decreasing the costs associated with the process. Most hospital billing departments do not find it easy to accommodate a common language or method because of the lack of integration of computer systems and the large volume of services billed. The constant changes in healthcare management and claim processing will make it increasingly necessary for hospitals to improve their current computer information systems.

Another trend in health care is that medical professionals are including clinical information systems in their office practices. Much of this technology provides for more accurate diagnosis, improved customer care, and improved patient medical records. These systems will typically be used by patient care teams accessing uniform information at all levels. As the technology becomes more commonplace, future professionals will have greater access and comfort levels with it. Clinical information systems tie diagnostic testing results directly to nurses' stations or physicians' offices; this linkage allows quick review and action on the test results and facilitates improved patient care. This linkage will also aid the transferability and accessibility of patient records by appropriate and authorized personnel. Besides compiling vital data regarding patients' care, computerized medical record information can expedite the reimbursement process.

Information systems also are important in foodservice departments where management control systems are numerous and their applications vary considerably. Systems may include software packages designed to manage information for clinical management and meal service; menu planning; forecasting and purchasing; production; catering; inventory management; food safety; payroll; financial management; and material data sheets. With computerized technology, menu vendors and distributors can offer foodservice operators a direct link to their warehouse for the purpose of placing orders and accessing information regarding inventory, prices, and purchase history. Foodservice inventory systems range from department-specific personal computer and software to mainframe systems designed specifically for the organization.

Other software programs include nutrition analysis and additional clinical applications. As it becomes increasingly important to evaluate past and current information to make the best decisions for tomorrow, advanced information systems will become more significant. The use of computer systems may not decrease staff needs, but in today's environment, these systems are necessary to manage the increasing amount of information needed by managers to run their department effectively. Computer software should be purchased based on individual needs, because one size doesn't fit all. What works for a hospital department may not work for school foodservice, and what works for a conventional production system may not work for a cook-chill production system.

Another trend in the last decade is found in vendors increasingly providing customized business solutions. Once the food and nutrition services information systems needs are assessed by the vendor, it is easier to translate those needs into appropriate information systems for the organization. That is one of the reasons that the organization needs to be able to effectively communicate system needs to the vendor, thus synchronizing the need with the solution.

Understanding Information Systems Applications

In the foodservice field, computer applications tend to be used for database management, which includes data entry, data processing, data management, and data reporting. The auxiliary applications of

Learning Point

1. The new requirements by regulatory agencies such as JCAHCO will necessitate the application of information systems for the purposes of data collection, data management, and data reporting.
2. The application of computerized technology now involves a universal electronic data interchange system for processing healthcare claims.
3. Computerized technology has brought about the electronic medical record where clinical information systems have evolved.
4. Information systems have enabled management control systems, such as software packages that are designed to manage information for clinical management and meal service; menu planning; forecasting and purchasing; production; catering; inventory management; food safety; payroll; financial management; and material data sheets.
5. Software programs continue to get more and more sophisticated in providing nutrition analysis and additional clinical applications.
6. Foodservice vendor orders can now be synchronized to cut down on phone calls and paperwork.

computer systems include integration with other computer systems, education (presentation and graphic applications), and communication (word processing, Intranet and Internet). Often, the boundaries of these applications blur.

As computer technology continues to emerge, food and nutrition services professionals are faced with new possibilities of exploring applications of information systems. Any more, depending on the size of the organization, the issue is not which applications to computerize, or whether to computerize recipes, nutritional analysis, accounting, inventory, purchasing, and diet office or clinic functions. Today, the industry recognizes the benefits of all. *Now, the issue is how to weave a seamless integration of various applications, improve usability, and adapt technological tools to achieve business objectives.*

Traditionally, food and nutrition services management software systems have been based on **proprietary programming**. Proprietary software programs are "as is" programs. Typically, if someone buys a software program from a store, the buyer cannot then alter that program. For modifications, a user might work through a users group to persuade a software vendor to release enhancements to achieve desired functions or customizations. At times, if different software is produced by the same vendor, those programs may share compatibility and have the capacity to transfer data. And, if a software vendor should go out of business, the user might be left holding expensive software that can no longer be updated or integrated with other applications.

In addition, traditional proprietary software offers little means for connecting information systems. A case in point is the foodservice director who wants to plug sales data from a point-of-sale (POS) system and data from inventory records into a spreadsheet for budget planning. With a proprietary software program, the director would have to perform the cumbersome task of transferring data from one program into another because the formats for handling data do not match. More typically, though, a foodservice director or secretary enters numbers from a printout into another program. Or, the director simply has to forgo the benefits of pulling all the information together for informed decision making.

A typical computerized foodservice operation uses several proprietary software systems. One may be for kitchen management, another for POS, another for nutritional analysis. Perhaps the operation also uses separate packages for desktop publishing, word processing, spreadsheets, employee scheduling, meeting room scheduling, and more. In case-by-case instances, vendors of proprietary foodservice software have developed custom interfaces (links) from one program to another to attempt to open communications among applications. These interfaces are expensive to develop and of limited availability. For example, one package may offer a link to one prime vendor's ordering system but not to another's system. Or, it may link to one nutritional analysis tool but not to another. One may offer no link whatsoever to an accounting package or a catered event room scheduling package. These situations leave individual foodservice directors in the lurch with few choices and no easy solution to achieve a highly integrated MIS.

In contrast to proprietary programming, industry leaders may choose **nonproprietary programming** (open architecture software), which uses openly available tools and technologies. With open architecture software, customizing and connecting systems becomes possible and allow a system to connect readily with other technologies. This can make for a less expensive software solution as integration can become an option rather than buying several different software applications that may or may not interface with one another. For example, an open system from one developer may easily accommodate a bar coding or radio frequency device developed by another. Open architect systems are more like LEGO® pieces, where a person can interlock the various pieces to create a desired structure. Open systems provide flexibility to advance with the technology regardless of which developer has the technology in demand. A choice for open systems also arms the foodservice operator with shopping power with the ability to shop among vendors for the best product fit and the most competitive price. Furthermore, nonproprietary, open systems permit users to keep pace with advancing technology because the software can be updated or added on to.

With the advent of the Microsoft Windows® operating platform, which supports standard data transfer protocols, the basic operation of personal computers has been modified to allow simple integration of a variety of functions. Programs written specifically for Windows® may support object linking and embedding, a feature in which data readily pass from one program to another. Windows® allows computer users to multitask (let the computer and the user work on more than one task at a time), and it offers a graphical user interface (use of icons or pictures and an input device such as a mouse to allow users to direct the computer). Because it is becoming increasingly easier and less cost-prohibitive, foodservice professionals are using computer technology systems in the areas of purchasing, receiving, inventory, menu planning, POS integration, and enhancing overall seamless systems integration.

> **Learning Point:** More useable software programs will have the ability to provide object linking and embedding, a feature in which data readily pass from one program, which will allow seamless systems integration. Managers should evaluate hardware and software products on this basis.

Database Management Systems (DBMS)

Since the earliest days of electronic computing, databases have been used, but the vast majority of these were custom programs written to access custom data. These systems were tightly linked to the data to gain speed at the expense of flexibility, unlike modern systems which are compatible with different data and computing needs. The term database refers to the collection of related records, and the application used to access those records is referred to as the "database management system" or DBMS. Many professionals would consider a collection of data to be a database only if it meets certain criteria; for example, if the data are managed to ensure integrity and quality, if they allow shared access by a community of users, if they have a **schema**, or if they support a **query** language. However, there is no standardized definition of these properties.

Generally speaking, DBMS are computer applications designed to manage a database. A database is a large set of structured data, saved to view the operational, historical, tactical, or strategic operation of a company, individual, or a business. Examples of typical customers using DBMS to perform daily operational business functions include groups like accounting, human resources, and customer support systems. Historically only supported by large organizations with the computer hardware and resources needed to support large data sets, DBMSs have more recently emerged as a fairly standard part of any company's technical infrastructure. There are many different types of DBMSs, ranging from small systems that run on personal computers to huge systems that run on mainframes. Examples of popular commercial DBMS, are Oracle®, DB2®, Informix®, and Microsoft SQL®.

A database is a collection of records stored in a computer in a systematic way so that a computer program can consult it to answer questions. Each record is usually organized as a set of data elements, for better retrieval and sorting. The data retrieved by queries become information that can be used in decision-making processes.

Structural grouping of related information held in a database is known as a schema. The schema describes the information objects that are represented in the database and the relationships among them. An example of a schema used in a company would be a Sales Schema, containing all the tables that store information regarding the sales data of a company, or a Customer Schema, which would likewise contain a grouping of the tables containing customer information of the organization and their relationships.

Different ways of organizing a collection of information objects or schema is known as **data modeling**. Data modeling is a logical representation of the information objects or schema. The most commonly used data model is a relational model, which, in laymen's terms, represents all the information in the form of multiple related tables, each consisting of rows and columns. Other widely used data models are the hierarchical model and the network model.

DBMSs are usually categorized according to the data model that they support: relational, object relational, network, and so on. The data model tends to determine the query languages that are available to access the database. A great deal of the internal engineering of a DBMS, however, is independent of the data model and is concerned with managing factors such as performance, concurrency, integrity, and recovery from hardware failures.

Use of databases in every industry is anticipated to grow exponentially. Commercial products like Microsoft Acess®, which are designed to be used by individual users or groups of small users, are on the rise. These products are being designed to be managed by nontechnical users and can be stored on a personel computer or a removable disk, thus making them highly flexible, manageable, and scalable.

Use of highly structured and complex databases used by large organizations is also on the rise. Companies are spending more and more resources to efficiently manage different business processes with the help of these databases. These databases are helping organizations to manage customer information more easily by providing

Learning Points: An example of how to retrieve dietary information:

a. Search the database for the patient record.
b. Receive a structural grouping of related information held in the database (the schema).
c. Schema shows up on the screen in a predesigned format (data modeling) from which useful dietary information can be extracted.

information regarding differerent aspects of business and customer behavior. Some companies are applying highly sophisticated business metrics to historical data stored in the databases to predict future performances of those companies. Customer spending trends are profiled, thereby enhancing profitability.

Management Information Systems (MIS)

IT management is the study of information systems with a focus on the integration of computer systems with business operations and processes. In business, MIS support decision making and competitive strategies. This area of study differs from computer sciences because computer science is more theoretical in nature and deals mainly with software creation, while computer engineering focuses more on the design of computer hardware. Apart from supporting business processes and operational needs of an organization, MIS use extends to every function of an organization. Those functions can be broadly classified into three roles: functional support, decision support, and performance monitoring.

Functional support roles aid the maximum use of an organization's potential by analyzing, processing, and referencing organizational data stored in a company's databases. Business processes and operations support functions are carried out by collecting, recording, storing, and basic processing of data. For example, the data stored in an accounting department of an organization might include sales data, purchase data, investment data, and payroll data.

Decision support systems help an organization's competitive positioning by providing access to timely and current information critical in a dynamic, competitive environment. This information helps decision makers and managers by providing a holistic view of the company, revealing to an organization its weaknesses and strengths, and helping devise strategies accordingly.

The performance monitoring role helps organizations establish relevant and measurable objectives and monitor results and performances accordingly. Use of technology enables functionality to preestablish objectives and budgets at each level of the organization and send alerts in case there are deviations between them, thus helping managers to realize their established deliverables and perceive how their functional objectives fit and contribute to the overall success of the organization.

Investing in information systems, especially investment in core operations of the company (supply chain networks or logistics), can potentially pay off for a company in many ways such as faster delivery times, problem-free delivery, and an assured supply. Investment in business and production processes can produce economies of scale in promotion, purchasing, and production. It can also produce economies of scope by streamlining distribution by reducing overhead, resulting in absolute cost advantage and greater profits and revenue for most organizations. For most companies, IT investment has helped the organization to expand their business

---

How Some of the Software Programs Work

What-if Analysis

Various software programs used by food and nutrition services use what-if analysis. What-if analysis is a process of changing the values in a spreadsheet cell to see how those changes affect the outcomes. For example, for nutrient analysis, when you know the caloric content of one gram of brown sugar, using the same data and formula (a sequence of values, cell reference, name, functions, or operations in the cell that together produces new value), you can determine the nutrient content of any amount of brown sugar. When you use any nutrient analysis software, the program already has a nutrient database (developed by professionals) on the nutrient content of a variety of foods. You are entering the amount of a specific food you consumed; then as an output, it gives you a calculation of your nutrient intake.

Goal-Seek

Another command commonly used for forecasting is called Goal-Seek. Goal-Seeking is a method used to find a specific value for a cell by adjusting the value of one other cell. For example, Goal-Seek can determine the unknown value that produces a desired result, such as number of $6 entrées a foodservice must sell to break even with food costs or to reach its goal of daily revenues of $5,000.

and has provided round-the-clock business availability, thus adding to bottom-line profitability.

Food and Nutrition Services Applications

The next section of this chapter will discuss the information systems applications for various functions of food and nutrition services. The potential of the application of information systems is broader than the scope of this chapter, so for the ease of understanding, the functions of foodservice are divided into five areas:

1. Menu-planning
2. Procurement
3. Production
4. Managing food and nutrition services
5. Clinical functions and overall systems integration

Menu-Planning

Menu-planning is one of the primary functions of any foodservice subsystem. Planning menus is a multifaceted process because it encompasses several variables, including food preferences, nutritional adequacy, budget, equipment, purchasing systems, production system, and meal patterns, to name a few. When the tasks are repetitive, encompass several variables, and require processing, using computer systems can maximize efficiency and reduce duplication of effort. From a menu-planning perspective, what-if analysis is commonly used. In this analysis, a user can experiment with various menu offerings and recipe ingredients to find the most cost-effective choice that meets nutritional, aesthetic, and quality requirements. As food prices change, a user can experiment with alternatives, immediately viewing the impact on the per-serving cost, menu cost, forecasted revenue, or other user-defined financial criteria. Queries (special question form) may help the user identify possible inventory items that meet specified criteria, such as a tomato-based product that costs less than $.15 per serving or the salad green with the lowest price that particular week. As alternatives are selected, they may be plugged in on a menu screen, with real-time updates carrying through to published menu descriptions, inventory requirements, ingredient pull lists, production instructions, scaled recipes, nutritional analysis totals, and so forth.

Recipe Modification

In an integrated health foodservice, often the menu for modified diets is based on the regular menu, and the primary difference is in modification of calories, nutrients, seasoning, and method of preparation. Generally, software using what-if analysis can help modify regular menus regarding calories, nutrients, seasoning, and method of preparations for various therapeutic diets, such as purée diet, diabetic diet, low-fat diet, and low sodium diet. A very simple application such as MS **Excel®**, which is generally used for storing the menus, can be set up with formulas for what-if analysis to help modify the menu items.

Recipe Standardization

Information systems may also be applied to foodservice in the area of recipe standardization, which is mandated for use in medical foodservice operations by outside accrediting agencies. A standardized recipe refers to one that has been tested and adopted for use in a particular facility. The purpose of standardization is to ensure that all meals served meet quality and quantity standards. The auxiliary benefit of recipe standardization is mainly that it reduces waste, thereby increasing profits. There are several relatively inexpensive stand-alone software programs available in the market that may be used for recipe standardization or the integrated menu management software may have recipe standardization as one of its functions.

Recipe Adjustment

Adjusting the recipes for volumes and weights is generally considered a time-consuming and expensive task. Frequently used methods to perform this task are **direct-reading tables** and the **factor method**. These methods are relatively easy to use but may require training the foodservice workers and are considered expensive in terms of labor and food cost. This task can also be easily computerized on a simple spreadsheet, which increases the efficiency of the process while reducing labor costs and the possibility of errors.

Preparatory programs are available for the recipe adjustment faction of the market and can be used for regular production, catering, or similar activities in any foodservice.

Recipe Costing

Recipe costing is another crucial function for any foodservice. Foodservice professionals use several calculations to find out food cost, portion cost, labor cost, food cost percentage, As Purchased, Edible Portion, prime cost method, mark-up method, etc., to determine the cost of a recipe. These processes can be easily designed, formulated on a spreadsheet, or purchased from the market. For bigger operations, it is always advisable to purchase this function as part of integrated software so the costing function can seamlessly integrate into other functions, like purchasing for real-time price codes by venders.

Several software programs in the market today will perform the functions relevant to recipe cost analysis, such as calculating the suggested selling price of cafeteria items based on actual food cost in conjunction with user selected formulae and variables, comparing projected costs with anticipated revenue, and showing the expected gross profit and the percentage of profit to sales. This software can be used like an electronic spreadsheet to determine the best menu item mix and pricing methodology to obtain the desired profit objectives in the retail areas of the department.

Menu Marketing

Marketing a menu is like marketing any product or service. There has been tremendous progress in the area of marketing because there are numerous texts, research, and software available on the use of information and data for marketing. Most colleges and universities offer courses in various aspects of marketing. Since menus can be considered a product and service, IT can utilize various tactics to lure customers into purchasing. Since data are considered a powerful tool that can be used to steer business efforts, use of information systems can create a reservoir of data, thereby providing a great marketing tool for a foodservice. The simplest example, the POS system, can create a database and further reports to analyze data, which can be used to improve the sales. Some of the information that may be synthesized from those data includes: menu items not selling well, the relationship of a physical location of various stations and sales, sales by days, employee versus visitor purchases, and so on. Foodservice managers can use this information to improve their operation's productivity, profitability, sales, quality, and issues of such nature.

Integrated Menu-Planning Applications

A foodservice operation can purchase separate proprietary software based on the size, needs, and typical functions performed in the operation, or the operation can approach a vendor to design integrated software. One example of such integrated software application deals with menu management at a hospital, which includes all the functions of menu-planning. Typically, menu management software allows patient menus to be printed by a computer. The menu is headed with the patient's name, room number, diet order, etc. Menu selections are printed according to menu day and individual dietary restrictions, and they consider the specific requirements of the patient, including allergies, dislikes, preferences, food/drug interactions, etc. Other functions of such software will typically include printing of patient menus, patient nourishment labels, and reports on patient status in total or as exceptions occur.

With contemporary and emerging technologies, it is also possible to provide paperless menu alternatives that reduce menu-related costs even further and can support a just-in-time meal service. Technologies currently in use with relational database and client/server systems include interactive voice technology (a patient orders meals through a bedside telephone), wireless networking using notebook personal computers at the patient's bedside, and bedside workstations permanently located in patients' rooms. These devices, connected to a client/server system, can later retrieve menu selections, which can then be used to calculate personalized nutritional analysis.

A menu management system compares a patient's choices with that patient's exchange pattern and makes corrections to the selections, based on preestablished criteria developed by the facility. Concurrence with specific nutrient amounts can also be identified. Tray cards can be printed for each patient, based on his or her selections, modified selections, or computer-generated selections. Production tally information is available at any time. Nourishment, supplement, and tube-feeding labels can be printed for all patients for each delivery time or for the entire day. Nourishment, supplement, and tube-feeding tally information is also available. Charges for nutritional supplement products can be maintained in the patient records for future billings. Billing reports can be generated at any time. The menu management system can be integrated in a nutrient analysis system, which can accurately perform calorie counts and detailed nutrient-intake analysis. The benefits of integrated menu management systems are mainly:

- Increasing productivity
- Recordkeeping
- Adhering to diet restrictions
- Interfacing with real-time data
- Using information for analysis and reporting

Procurement

Procurement refers to the process of acquiring goods for production. Procurement is based on the planned menu. The basic goal of procurement is acquisition of the desired product at the right time, right quality, and right quantity. Depending on the size of the foodservice facility, orchestrating procurement can be a very complex process because it encompasses several factors/variables (purchasing systems, vendors, specifications, and quality control). Furthermore, multi-unit operations (a school district foodservice) will perform cooperative functions like group purchasing and use computer technology more extensively as they require integration among various systems.

Because procurement is a process used by practically all businesses and consumers, tremendous advances have been made in the area of purchasing at the organizational as well as consumer level, which, in turn, improves the operational efficiency of a company. Bar codes, cashier-free checkout, direct payment methods, to name a few, are technologies that benefit the consumer end of the purchasing process.

Purchasing

Purchasing for the foodservice industry is based on the specific menus and needs of the operation. The goal of this function is to obtain desired product(s) at the right time, right amount, right price, and at the specified level of quality. Purchasing can be performed in several ways, including group purchasing, one-stop buying (buying from one vendor), or competitive bidding. In any type of purchasing, a computerized information system can both improve the process and save time and labor.

To manage food costs effectively, managers are employing several strategies. One is just-in-time purchasing, which requires finely-tuned product forecasting as well as the ability to place and process orders with a short turnaround time. Technologies such as electronic data interchange, singular user interfaces for placing electronic purchase orders through a variety of distributors' computer systems, and fax modem transmission are all replacing traditional telephone ordering. Two-way communications supported by computers means that purchasers can receive feedback and troubleshoot order fulfillment problems more efficiently. Today, food-service purchasers have the ability to generate an ingredient list from a menu management system, automatically consolidate the ingredient list, check its specifications, set the inventory par-level, and give vendor access to the information so they can supply the materials if the inventory par-level goes down. Again, the procurement process is not only used by foodservice but by practically every business, necessitating the constant demand to implement better IT solutions.

Managers who use bid analysis as a basis for purchasing decisions can obtain price information electronically and automate the process. What about the single bid involving multiple vendors? Complex variations of the bid system can be accommodated through relational database systems. Purchasing flexibility based on price poses additional issues. The manager who does not wish to be locked into a single distributor for any one product needs a robust information system to support flexibility. To make cost-effective decisions as prices fluctuate, the manager needs to know current prices and which purveyor offers the lowest price on any given day. An information system built to accommodate electronic price updates can provide real-time price information and identify the lowest price for each item, if desired.

If the system is designed using a relational database, it can also permit queries and user-defined reports to identify products with significant price swings. For example, a user might choose to query a relational database to find out which items have changed in price by more than 10% since the last order or which five items contribute the highest cost to tomorrow's menu. A query is a tool that permits users to "mine" their own databases for useful information in a self-directed, dynamic fashion. Today's software tools even allow users to word their queries in plain English, rather than having to understand data fields and database design. Based on information received through queries and customized reports, a manager can make up-to-the-minute decisions to control food costs.

To track and control product flow, many operators use bar coding technology or pen-based computing for data entry. Radio frequency devices may be used to transmit information from a bar code scan to a computerized inventory system wirelessly and in real-time. As among consumers, voice recognition technology is also gaining popularity. Voice recognition technology allows navigations through prompts using voice and provides the customer with hands-free access. Each of these technologies is broadly available on an open platform.

Inventory Management

Another aspect of procurement is inventory management. Today's information systems offer several functions to manage inventory. A user can switch vendors and/or products frequently to reap cost advantages. Maintaining product information in a relational database system makes it easier for users to specify multiple sets of data related to a single item, multiple vendors, prices, and packaging. Inventory changes sometimes require changes to recipes, too. These are accomplished easily through real-time, global data inventory updates.

Foodservice operators who use POS equipment are increasingly seeking connectivity with back-of-the house systems. By establishing communications between POS systems and foodservice management systems, operators can capture sales data to plug into forecasting formulas, profitability analyses, menu-planning, and pricing activities. They can make POS records flow into routine financial reports, such as cash reporting and profit/loss statements. Finally, sales records can provide information that assists managers in making cost-effective staffing decisions.

Steps of procurement include ordering, receiving, storing, and issuing. IT is best suited to the complex processes of ordering, whereas use of technology in other processes is somewhat limited to bar code systems for receiving, storing, issuing, and maintaining databases for computation and reporting. Another emerging use of IT in procurement is in the area of food safety. Systems such as Hazard Analysis and Critical Control Point (HACCP) are used as a model for implementing food safety systems. Information systems are frequently used at various steps of HACCP. For example, a cook-chill system uses software to record temperature while cooked food is being blast-chilled. The software can also alert the manager to improper temperatures according to the set default values.

Again, the complexity of any process necessitates the application of IT. Some of the benefits of the stand-alone procurement software or integrated procurement software systems include improved efficiency, control of processes (inventory and purchasing), cost control, tracking, access to data for reporting, and constant price updates for an efficient procurement process.

Production

After a menu is planned and the materials are procured, the next stage is production. Production varies according to the production system. The use of IT will vary according to production systems such as cook-serve, assembly-serve, cook-chill, cook-serve, or cook-freeze. Besides the differences in the various food production systems, there are some similarities in the processes of production (forecasting, storeroom requisition, processing sheet, thaw schedule, etc).

Foodservice production-related software will perform the task of expanding the stored ingredients in each recipe to the amount needed for production of the forecasted number of portions; also, the system can round ingredient amounts to preparation sizes (the number of portions in a specific cooking pan, major ingredient pack size, or batch cooking size). Such software is also able to print labels showing the recipe description and each ingredient.

Storeroom Requisitions

Storeroom requisitions (pick lists) combine the ingredients needed for all recipes to be produced and give a cumulative listing of these ingredients sorted by storage location. The software will list items in issue units and/or order units and will consider ingredient waste. The form can be used to retrieve items from the storage locations.

Processing Sheets

A processing sheet can be generated, detailing the amount of each ingredient that must be pre-processed in any variation. For example, the listing will show the total amount of onion that must be chopped for the day's production, the amount that must be minced, sliced, etc. A thaw schedule details all of the items and the required amounts of each that must be transferred from a frozen location to a tempering location for proper thawing prior to production. Freezer pull labels can also be generated for identification of the items placed in the tempering location.

Production System Management

Production system software is more useful in big foodservice operations with several storerooms, or is more beneficial for the cook-chill or cook-freeze production systems that requires constant monitoring. Some of the other benefits of production-related software include standardization of the processes, reduction in food waste, control of production, and overall effectiveness of the production process.

Managing Food and Nutrition Services

Management functions are variable, depending on the type and size of the organization. In bigger organizations such as health care facilities, the managerial functions become more complex. Typical management processes include planning, directing, integrating, and coordinating.

Human Resource Management

Human Resource Management (HRM) is the crux of management, because employees of any organization carry on the management processes. The HRM function is still, to a large degree, administrative and common to all organizations. To varying degrees, most organizations have formalized selection, evaluation, and payroll processes. Since the management functions are typical for any organization, applications in IT have advanced greatly. Several integrated and well-designed HRM systems are available on the market, enabling managers and administrators to access and update all types of employee-related information.

The HR function consists of tracking innumerable data points on each employee from personal histories, data, skills, capabilities, and experiences to payroll records. To reduce the manual workload of these administrative activities, organizations began to electronically automate many of these processes. The benefits of automation of these processes include (but are not limited to) accessibility of personnel data to management, scheduling, reporting, and tracking of vacation time. Automation of these factors increases efficiency.

Other standard modules that integrate HR and IT and are available in the marketplace today are known as Enterprise Resource Planning (ERP). Metaphorically speaking, ERP is the autoimmunization of business practices associated with the operations or production and distribution aspects of a company engaged in manufacturing products or services. ERP systems are back office systems dealing with business activities like billing, shipping, sales, inventory management, HR, distribution, and so on. One example of the users of ERP in foodservice is the national foodservice suppliers/distributors who deal with issues of logistics/shipping.

During the 1980s, the HR automation process was limited to large organizations because they required high-capital investment. Today some types of proprietary software and nonproprietary software are available even for small businesses that effectively address the four principal areas of HRM: payroll, scheduling, benefits administration, and HR management. The payroll module automates the pay process by gathering data on employee time and attendance, calculating various deductions and taxes, and generating periodic paychecks and employee tax reports. Data are generally fed from the HR and time-keeping modules to calculate automatic deposit and manual check writing capabilities. The scheduling module applies new technology and methods (time collection devices) to cost-effectively gather and evaluate employee time/work information. The most advanced modules provide broad flexibility in data collection methods, as well as labor distribution capabilities and data analysis features. The benefit administration module permits HR professionals to easily administer and track employee participation in benefits programs ranging from healthcare provider, insurance policy, and pension plan to profit sharing or stock option plans. The HR management module is a component covering all other HR aspects from application to retirement. The system records basic demographic and address data; selection, training, and development; capabilities and skills management; compensation planning records; and other related activities. Leading-edge systems provide the ability to "read" applications and enter relevant data to applicable database fields, notify employers, and provide position management and position control.

Web deployment of HRM applications is becoming common–software systems (in-service training) that can be Web deployed for remote access by employee and administrators. Web deployment and access reduce time spent to do repetitive and tedious activities, and managers can direct more of their time toward customer care, arguably the most important aspect of any business.

Clinical Functions and Overall Systems Integration

In health care, systems integration takes on special significance for clinical nutritional care applications. Traditionally, the major expenses in managing patient menus have been recording and updating patient information, whether manually or through data entry into a computer. Ease of integration means ease of electronically updating data such as a patient's name, location, and diet order. In addition, integration is consistent with current JCAHO standards, which require eliminating duplicate data entry. Full integration translates into labor efficiency and cost savings. If integration is also used to connect clinical data (laboratory results and prescribed medications) with clinical nutrition records, additional benefits ensue from improved nutrition screening, effective nutrition intervention, and thorough diagnosis-related groups assignment/billing.

Nutrition Risk Screening Modules

Other IT modules and clinical systems used by nutrition professionals who assist in clinical functions are nutrition risk screening modules that accept data from the existing hospital A/D/T, order entry, lab, and pharmacy systems and then share and compare those data with a selected facility that screens criteria and generates specific screening reports. These screening reports show all patients currently in the hospital who meet the risk criteria established by the facility. The data generated by such systems can be further integrated into menu-planning modules and also be used for patient education upon discharge.

Nutrition Assessment

IT can also be integrated into a nutrition assessment function. The input for such software includes general patient information, laboratory data, physical parameters, etc. The software is then able to analyze these data and generate information to assist in assessing a patient's nutritional status (calculating values of transferrin, arm muscle circumference, energy expenditure, required kilocalories/kilojoules, body mass index (BMI), protein requirements, etc.). The individual patient's values can then be compared to age and gender matched standards and deficiencies.

Drug-Nutrient Interaction

Other clinical software programs are designed to assist in identifying patients with whom a potential drug-nutrient interaction may occur. The system will assist in specifying those drugs that have a possibility of affecting the patient's nutritional status and where a drug's interaction with nutrients will alter absorption and distribution. Lists of drugs meeting specific nutrient-related criteria (reduced or delayed absorption, decreased appetite, alcohol affected, etc.) are accessible by the clinical staff. Most of these software models generate reports for staff and patients. Some of the benefits of using the clinical systems include increased staff productivity, accuracy of analysis, and more time for patient care.

Overall Systems Integration

Traditional foodservice information systems planning has focused on stand-alone operations. This type of planning finds scheduling and nutritional analysis software useful. Since the size and complexity of the healthcare processes are increasing, however, the software systems are leaning more toward interfacing and integration. Integrated systems may use a data warehousing approach. A data warehouse may use one, massive database system for all of an organization's information. As designated, users can access the information they need. As users enter data, the information immediately becomes part of the single, enterprise-wide database. This approach is being adopted in major materials management systems as well as in healthcare organizations.

To share information over distances is a strategic goal of any organization with multiple sites, and information systems professionals are taking advantage of other new technologies to facilitate that communication. For example, remote access may be used to link a facility to a corporate office. Payroll time sheets, invoices, and other time-sensitive electronic documents may be transmitted this way. A manager, for example, may also use remote access while telecommuting to check on the day's sales, print reports, and/or place orders.

MS Windows® has many built-in capabilities that support communications. Built-in to MS Windows® is connectivity to the Internet. The Internet and Intranets (internal networks operating under browser software and supporting Internet connections) can improve communications by e-mail, and make common applications and data available to a multitude of users. At the same time, the technologies allow users to tap into selected resources on the Web.

Summary

While the state of technology changes daily, it is important for a professional in any field, especially health care and foodservice, to know and understand the concepts of technology so that he or she may translate those needs clearly, effectively, and efficiently. There has always been resistance toward changing to the processes with information systems. This resistance has been especially felt in the area of foodservice. Even though foodservice is a labor intensive field, several processes can use IT and potentially free up more valuable time for quality improvement and patient care. It is advisable for the food and nutrient services professional to stay connected with the trends and potential applications of IT to be part of planning and the decision-making process. In today's world it is nearly impossible to isolate IT from any process, so it's quite sensible to become part of it.

Student Activities

1. Briefly discuss the trends in information technology that you have observed and have felt affected your food supply chain during the last 5 years.
2. At your place of work or by phone interview, determine what software programs are being used for various processes.
3. List all the software you have used in the past. Briefly describe how that software has improved your work.
4. Select a type of foodservice (correctional facilities, school foodservice, retirement home, or healthcare foodservice). Plan a 10-minute class presentation about the potential use of information systems for the various subsystems (menu, procurement, production, distribution, and management) of the selected foodservice.
5. Discuss in a small group each person's example of experiences with information systems in their work and home environments.
6. Examine the forces that drive organizations/companies to adopt information systems. Are they related to productivity and profitability or are they related to customer/patient care?

Suggested Reading

Database. (2006). Wikipedia, the free encyclopedia. Retrieved May 30, 2006, from http://en.wikipedia.org/wiki/Database.

Grossbauer, Sue. (1999). *Computer technology in foodservice and hospitality.* Goodlettsville, TN: Vision Software Technologies, Inc.

Puckett, Ruby P. & Green, Carlton. (2004). *Foodservice manual for healthcare institutions* (3rd ed.). San Francisco: Jossey-Bass.

Sullivan, Catherine F. & Atlas, Courtney. (1998). *Healthcare foodservice systems management* (3rd ed.). Gaithersburg, MD: Aspen Publishers, Inc.

CHAPTER 12

NATURAL RESOURCE MANAGEMENT

Bonnie Gerald, PhD, DTR

Reader Objectives

After reading this chapter and reflecting on the contents, the student will be able to:

1. Manage energy, water, and air resources to preserve quality of life for future generations.
2. Use conservation practices that also control operating costs.
3. Include natural resource management as part of a facility's food procurement, food production, and sanitation and maintenance procedures.

Key Terms

Biological Oxygen Demand (BOD): the amount of dissolved oxygen consumed by microorganisms as they decompose organic material in polluted water.

Demand charge: a charge for electricity based on the maximum amount of a system's electricity a customer uses.

Energy audit: systematic examination of a home's energy performance provided by trained personnel.

Indoor Air Quality: indoor environmental quality of a site.

Kilowatt-hour (kWh): a unit of energy equivalent to one kilowatt (1 kW) of power expended for 1 hour of time.

Production waste: defined as drilling wastes, salt water, and other wastes associated with exploration, development, and production.

Service waste: those solid waste materials that are potentially capable of causing disease or injury.

Solid waste: any solid, semi-solid, liquid, or contained gaseous materials discarded from industrial, commercial, mining, or agricultural operations or community activities.

Solid waste audit: the proper identification of all solid waste that a particular organization generates.

Water audit: accurately determines the amount of unaccounted-for water in a water distribution system.

Introduction

When thinking of sustainability of the food system, some basic principles may come to mind: balancing a growing economy, protecting the environment, and social responsibility. When combined, these principles lead to a better life for us and future generations.[1] As a food and nutrition professional, it is important to look at your everyday life and work routine to determine how you can make improvements by conserving natural resources. Water, energy, and air are integral to foodservice management; without them work would not be as efficient or as cost-effective. In this chapter, you will learn more about the importance of this subject and how it affects on-site foodservice management.

Role of Natural Resources in Food Production

The natural resources of water, energy, and air have a role in nearly every aspect of foodservice systems. They are essential inputs for food production. The procurement process is influenced by quality and availability of water and energy. Distribution and service of food are determined by the form of energy used in the facility. The quality of the system's output (food) is affected by the quality of water used to produce it and how effectively energy for heating and cooling food was used in the process.

Consideration of natural resources when allocating resources within a facility has several benefits. Utilities typically consume 30% of the operational budget; therefore any savings will flow to the bottom line. The Environmental Protection Agency (EPA) estimates that every dollar a nonprofit healthcare operation saves on energy is equivalent to generating $20 in new revenues. For-profit healthcare operations can increase earnings per share by one penny if energy costs are reduced by 5%.[2] Wise use of natural resources will minimize environmental impact, thus preserving the quality of life for future generations. Natural resource management can generate goodwill in the community and has the potential to increase staff commitment to the organization.

Environmental Considerations When Allocating Resources

Every foodservice director must consider social, legal, technological, and natural environments when making resource allocation decisions. For example, some municipalities have had recycling programs for years, which increase public awareness and acceptance of resource conservation issues. A facility in a community with no history of recycling will confront different issues, such as convincing the public of cost savings from recycling when managing natural resources. The federal government has established minimum quality standards for water, air, and solid waste disposal guidelines through the Safe Drinking Water Act, the Clean Air Act, and the Resource Conservation and Recovery Act (RCRA). Each state is responsible for promulgating the standards or developing its own standards that are at least as stringent as federal guidelines. The Occupational Safety and Health Administration (OSHA) is responsible for workplace safety, including **indoor air quality** and hazardous materials. Foodservice directors must comply with all state and federal regulations regarding waste disposal and air quality.

The federal government has encouraged manufacturers to make efficient food production and sanitation equipment since 1992, the year Energy Star was established. The Energy Star program set energy efficiency goals for gas and electricity-using equipment. Advances in computer chip technology and materials science have made possible equipment that uses less energy and is self-regulating. Equipment purchased in the mid-1990s may be less efficient than similar models available today. The decision to repair or replace existing equipment should include energy efficiency as one of the decision factors.[3]

The cost and availability of electricity and natural gas in a specific region also will influence natural resource allocation decisions. Regional climatic conditions may impact resource decisions as well.

For example, child nutrition programs in rural northern Alaska must use disposable service ware and transport solid waste by air because the permafrost makes dish machine use and landfill waste disposal prohibitive. Lightweight, non-bulky products with minimal packaging would be major considerations for a foodservice director in this environment. Heating oil for buildings is widely used in the northeastern United States but is unavailable in other regions of the country. Access to metropolitan areas may influence natural resource allocation. A facility located in a rural area may only receive weekly deliveries. Adequate cold storage space, including the energy required to maintain the space, would be factors to consider when making resource decisions due to geographic location.

> **Learning Point:** It is important to consider your external environment when making natural resource decisions. Conservation practices that are successful in other regions of the United States may not be feasible in your area.

Facilities in rural locations may have limited energy choices; for example, natural gas pipelines may be unavailable, necessitating use of propane for food production. Propane historically has been a more costly energy source than natural gas. Solid waste disposal may be more costly in rural areas because of the lack of recycling outlets and increased distance to landfills, which increases tipping (disposal) fees.

Energy Management

Energy's Role in Food Production

Foodservice operations are intensive users of energy. Food processing and production consumes approximately 10% of the energy produced in the United States. Energy is essential for production of safe, quality food. Several forms of energy may be used for food production. Delivery vehicles transporting food to satellite dining centers may use either gasoline or diesel fuel. All forms of energy convert their basic unit of measurement to BTU, or British Thermal Unit. One BTU is the amount of energy required to increase the temperature of one gallon of water one degree Fahrenheit. Nearly 100 quadrillion BTUs were consumed in the United States in 2005, of which 10% were used by the food system.[4] In general, gas equipment requires fewer input BTUs to generate heat energy than electricity, but the gas equipment will require more BTUs to maintain the equipment's heat energy level compared to similar electric equipment.

Natural gas is considered a better option than oil or gas to generate electricity. Natural gas burns cleaner than gas and coal, which has the added benefit of reducing greenhouse gas emissions. World energy consumption is expected to increase by 59% between 1999 and 2020.[5] However, natural gas and electricity costs will vary by region; energy consumption, energy costs, equipment maintenance costs, payback period, and desired outputs will be factors in energy management.

Energy Audits

Energy consumption can be monitored by reading the electric meter and gas meter located in the kitchen on the same date every month. The resulting data can be used to establish an energy management plan. A team of staff members responsible for the energy management plan surveys equipment and practices used in the kitchen and measures energy consumption and identifies areas where energy may be conserved.[6] Many kitchens do not have separate gas and electric meters, so an **energy audit** is needed prior to developing an energy management plan. The energy audit is a method to identify all energy-consuming equipment, the amount of energy consumed, and energy consumption patterns. Analysis of the data may indicate areas where energy consumption can be decreased. Energy should be monitored by time period: day, week, and month.

Energy consumption patterns will emerge as a result of the energy audit. Peak energy consumption typically occurs prior to meal service. Peak demand for electricity may occur on certain days of the month, such as Mondays when patient census is highest. Electricity providers must have generating capacity sufficient to

> **Learning Point:** The form of energy your local utility company uses to generate electric power will influence the cost of that energy source for your facility. Generation of electricity can impact local air and water quality.

meet peak demand. Electricity is charged by the amount consumed and the **demand charge,** a fee based on the maximum amount of electricity consumed. Practices that can be shifted to non-peak consumption hours will conserve energy and reduce costs. For example, it may be possible to run the dish machine at times other than during meal service to reduce the demand charge.

Payback and Incentives

Replacing older equipment can save money in addition to conserving energy. There are various tax credits available depending on the type of equipment being replaced. The decision of what to replace older equipment with and when to replace it can be determined by using economy studies and the payback period. An economy study compares the costs of operation based on maintenance, potential savings, depreciation, and payback period. The payback period is the amount of time needed to recoup the cost of purchasing a specific piece of equipment. Generally, the most energy efficient equipment in such comparisons will have the shortest payback period.

General Energy Management Practices

Purchase Specifications

As stated previously, technology development has created more energy efficient equipment. Energy efficiency can be included in equipment purchase specifications. This can be accomplished by stating the desired level of performance and power consumption in the specification bid.

Integrating system controls for food production, sanitation, cold storage, and climate control also may be considered when remodeling or constructing a new facility. Energy conservation systems control all on-and-off equipment by controlling hours of operation. This has the effect of establishing the lowest energy demand and maintaining it for the facility. Dish machine systems will only operate with a dish rack inside the machine. A water reduction system for a dish machine diverts water overflow to disposers or scrappers. Heated overflow water from the dish machine can be routed back to the hot water tank, thus reducing energy needed to heat water. Water-cooled ice makers use less electricity and generate less heat than air-cooled ice makers.[7]

New types of cooking equipment produce food more efficiently. Induction cookers generate a magnetic wave at the cooking surface. The cooker heats more quickly than gas equipment and consumes less energy. Because it generates heat only at the cooking surface, the energy required for air-conditioning is reduced. Super cookers, which combine convection, microwave, and impingement methods, can cook a wide variety of products using less time and energy than conventional equipment.[8] It also is important to match equipment to the appropriate circuit size when making purchasing decisions. Plugging equipment into a circuit that is rated at a lower voltage than the equipment can result in blown fuses and inefficient operation, and could create a fire hazard. Using a higher rated voltage circuit for a lower voltage appliance can shorten equipment life and also create a fire hazard.

Food Production

There are many opportunities for energy conservation using existing equipment. Simple procedural changes can result in significant energy savings. The following recommendations are a starting point for all foodservice managers for developing an energy conservation plan for their facility.

Refrigeration

- Keep doors closed; limit the amount of time the unit's doors are open.
- Organize shelves so that foods are easy to locate, limiting the number of door openings.
- Store all perishable items immediately following delivery.
- Install plastic strip curtains on walk-in refrigerator and freezer doors.
- Cool cooked food appropriately before storage.
- Keep coils and condensers clean.
- Make certain that condensers have air circulation and protection from extreme temperatures so they can function efficiently.
- Check the entire system for coolant and air leaks and obstructions of the air intake and vents.
- Use the correct operating temperature for the unit.

Cooking

Preheat equipment only to the cooking temperature; setting to a higher temperature will not heat any faster.

- Operate equipment only when needed; do not leave ovens and fryers on for the entire shift.
- Operate with full loads when possible.
- Use equipment that is the appropriate size for the food.
- Clean equipment at specified intervals.
- Filter oil and clean fryers at least daily.

Ware Washing and Hot Water

- Clean dish machines daily and regularly de-lime the dish machine.
- Run full loads whenever possible.
- Run the dish machine at slack times whenever possible (refer to energy audit) to reduce demand charge.
- Repair leaking faucets.
- Insulate hot water pipes and refrigerate cold suction lines.

Lighting

- Turn off lights in parts of the kitchen not being used during the shift.
- Upgrade fluorescent lights to T-8 lamps with electronic ballasts.
- Install occupancy sensors in areas not in continuous use.

Ventilation

- Clean air filters and hoods regularly.
- Turn off fans (man coolers) in areas not used during the shift.
- Position fans so they do not blow directly on temperature-sensitive equipment such as fryers.
- Consider air cleaners to reduce the amount of outside air required for adequate turnover of air. Outside air must be filtered, then either heated or cooled before entering the workplace. [9]

Maintenance

Performing routine maintenance on appliances and HVAC (heating, ventilation, and air-conditioning) systems can significantly impact the amount of energy consumed. Regular cleaning of all food production equipment keeps the equipment operating within its optimal energy consumption range. Documenting cleaning and maintenance schedules will help with tracking operating costs, identifying energy consumption patterns, and indicating areas that need intervention.

Water Conservation

Role of Water

Water is essential for food production, sanitation, and climate control. Only 0.3% of the earth's water is fit for human use; the other 99.7% of global water is either unusable or unavailable.[10] Potable water, or water fit for human consumption, is projected to become a scarce resource. Therefore it is important to use this resource wisely. Foodservice operations must have access to water for sanitation and food production.

Foodservice operations are affected by the two standards established in the Clean Water Act of 1970. These standards include: receiving (incoming) water and waste (effluent) water. It is important to know your source of water, whether it is a private well or an approved public water system. If water is provided by a public well, it must meet 40 CFR (Code of Federal Regulations) standards. If water is distributed by a private well, it must meet state and local regulations linked to the Safe Drinking Water Act and standards of quality.[11] The National Water Quality Inventory reports that the majority of domestic water sources are rated as "good." However, waterborne disease outbreaks have been reported in public water systems. Foodservice operations should monitor the annual required local water quality reports from municipal systems to determine if filtration is needed.[12]

Water is often considered a free good; this is because the true cost of water treatment and delivery is not borne directly by consumers. Delivery of water to consumers includes water disinfection,

Learning Point: Water quality can affect the quality of beverages and food. Water with a high mineral content can cause dish machines to operate inefficiently. Bottled water is popular with consumers but can have higher levels of organic and mineral substances than tap water. Several brands of bottled water actually come from the municipal water sources!

filtration, energy for transport, construction of waterways, and wastewater treatment. Because of its low cost to consumers, water is often wasted. Wasted water ultimately is wasted energy. [6,13]

Water Audits

Climatic conditions, expanding populations in arid areas, and growing food place demands for clean water, which are likely to shift more of the cost of water to consumers in the near future. Some communities in the southwestern United States already have restrictions on domestic water use.

Foodservice directors can manage their water costs by establishing a water management plan similar to an energy management plan. The amount of water consumed can be monitored by reading the water meter at the same time every month. However, some facilities may not have a separate water meter for the kitchen. A **water audit** should then be conducted to identify all equipment consuming water and the amount of water consumed per time period. Equipment manuals may provide consumption by time period or operation cycle. For example, dish machine and disposal service manuals will have water consumption data. The average single tank dish machine uses 1.2 gallons of water per rack. A typical garbage disposal consumes 8 gallons of water per minute.

A reasonable estimate of water use can be obtained by determining the hours of operation or number of cycles used per day. For equipment with no consumption information, the amount of water used can be determined by operating the equipment for a specific time and then measuring water in the equipment. For example, the amount of water produced by faucets can be determined by placing a bucket under the faucet and measuring the amount of water generated in one minute with the faucet completely open. A form similar to an energy audit form can be developed. Careful monitoring of water should reveal usage patterns and potential areas for conservation.

General Water Management

Purchase Specifications

Producing water efficient equipment has not yet had the widespread attention similar to energy conservation. In order to conserve resources and control costs, foodservice directors should be aware of the energy-water connection when making equipment purchasing decisions. Several options already exist for water-consuming equipment. For example, dish machines that recycle rinse water for use in the prewash cycle conserve water and energy. Dish machines with sensors that shut down after a specified idle time also conserve resources. Water use can be minimized by purchasing a dish machine the correct size to handle the number of meals served. For example, a single-tank door-style dish machine is adequate for 50 to 250 meals produced per hour. Facilities producing 1,500 or more meals per hour should use a flight-type conveyor dish machine for efficient operation. Pulpers are similar to garbage disposals except that wastes are collected in a container for disposal as solid waste. Excess water is removed from the waste. The water from a pulper may be routed to a prewash tank of a dish machine.

Hands-free sinks conserve water while increasing the frequency of employee hand washing.[14] Technology development and the foodservice industry's drive to control costs will generate more choices for energy and water efficient equipment in the future.

Food Production, Sanitation, and Wastewater

Just as with energy conservation, there are many opportunities to conserve water using existing resources. Several of the bulleted points in the food production section also will conserve water. Foodservice directors can conserve water by implementing the following practices:

Food Preparation

Install flow restrictors on faucets. However, some equipment may not operate efficiently with flow restrictors. Check the equipment manual before installing flow restrictors.

- Turn off all faucets when not in use.
- Do not allow water to run while cleaning produce or other foods.
- Follow recipes when using water for cooking. Using more than the recipe amount will waste water and increase cooking time.
- Defrost frozen foods in refrigerator instead of under running water.

Sanitation

- Install sensors in hand sinks.
- Install flow restrictors in toilets and showers.
- Use dish machines and pot and pan washers only for full loads.
- Use garbage disposals only when needed; do not allow disposals to run the entire time service ware is washed.
- Do not dispose of large amounts of starchy foods, such as leftover pans of pasta, rice, or potatoes in the garbage disposal. Starches require extra water to flush through the lines without clogging the drain pipes.
- Scrap instead of rinsing dishes before washing.

Wastewater

City and/or state regulations determine the type and amount of wastewater that may enter a sewer system. Generally, dish machines, garbage disposals, grease traps, and oil and grease disposal are affected by these regulations. Oil and grease can clog sewer lines; therefore grease traps are installed on drain lines from a production kitchen. Food particles can decrease water quality after the water is discharged into the sewer system by increasing the water's **Biological Oxygen Demand** (BOD). BOD is a method of measuring the amount of dissolved oxygen required to decompose the organic matter in the water. Excessive organic matter content in streams, lakes, and rivers causes algae blooms and fish kills. Poor water quality is indicated by a high BOD. High BOD levels increase water treatment costs because more chemicals are needed to treat the water. Numerous municipalities monitor facilities that generate wastewater with high BOD levels and assess them higher treatment costs. Wastewater practices that minimize BOD include:

- Cleaning grease traps on a regular basis.
- Installing pulpers in place of garbage disposals.
- Removing grease and oil from pans before washing.
- Collecting used fryer oil and grease and disposeing of in a grease container. The containers may be picked up for recycling into other products.
- Collecting leftover food for composting, animal feed, or food bank donations instead of flushing it down the sewer.

Types of Waste

Solid Waste

Solid waste, sometimes labeled "trash" or "garbage," includes any solid, semi-solid, or liquid that is discarded. There are many categories of solid waste, but for the purposes of this chapter the focus will be on municipal solid waste (MSW). MSW encompasses all non-hazardous waste from domestic, commercial, and institutional sources. MSW generated from foodservice operations can be further divided into two categories: production waste (food preparation) and service waste (from plates or trays served to customers). Which inputs generate the most waste in foodservice? It depends on whether the waste is measured by weight or by volume. Food waste is the largest category by weight. Packaging waste generates the largest volume of waste. MSW removal is charged by volume; any practice that reduces the volume of solid waste also will reduce costs. Solid waste removal is charged by the cubic yard.

On average for food prepared outside the home, 0.32 to 1.47 pounds of food and packaging wastes are discarded per meal served.[15] Americans generate an average 4.6 pounds of solid waste per day. Of the total MSW generated in 2001, more than 11% by weight or 96 billion pounds of food were discarded.

Solid waste management will depend on several environmental and internal factors. The type of food system will influence the

Learning Point: Are we running out of landfill space? Older landfills that did not meet EPA guidelines were closed. Modern landfills are similar to manufacturing facilities in that greater capacity is not built until needed. The trend of fewer but larger landfill sites will impact a facility's solid waste management practices.

types of waste generated. A ready-prepared system may generate significant volumes of **production waste** from packaging. A conventional from-scratch system may generate the most production waste from raw ingredients. Service waste may be affected by the number of prepackaged menu items served and whether disposable or permanent service ware is used. The presence of recycling centers in the community will impact decisions initiating a recycling program in the facility. The distance to the nearest landfill will impact frequency of waste pickup. The trend for landfills is for fewer but larger regional landfills. This means waste may be transported to an intermediate site before removal to the landfill. The intermediate site incurs a "transfer fee" before final disposal, which is a "tipping fee" for tipping or dumping the waste from the truck.

Solid Waste Audits

The EPA has the long range goal of reducing by 50% the amount of solid waste going to landfills. The hierarchy of solid waste management is a strategy to prevent pollution before it occurs. The management hierarchy, from most to least preferred methods, is: source reduction, recycling, landfilling, and incineration.

To realize cost savings and reduce pollution, foodservice directors must first understand the types of waste generated within their facility. Solid waste can be measured by a **solid waste audit** or solid waste analysis. A solid waste audit measures the volume of one category of waste for a period of 3 to 5 days. The category may be a specific item such as cardboard or it may include all production waste. The volume of waste is converted from gallons to cubic yards and averaged for the time period.

A solid waste analysis is a comprehensive measurement of waste generated. All categories of waste are measured for a period of 7 days. Waste is sorted into categories such as cardboard, plastic, paper, aluminum, steel, food, and glass. The volume of each category and the total volume of waste are converted to cubic yards and averaged to give a picture of the daily waste stream.[16]

Solid Waste Management

Information from a waste stream audit or analysis is the first step for managing waste. There are several approaches for reducing the volume of waste generated. The most common ones for foodservice are source reduction and recycling.

Source Reduction

Source reduction limits potential waste-generating inputs to the system before they can become waste. It is part of forecasting, purchasing functions, and reusing items within the facility. Accurate forecasting reduces overproduction so there is less food and associated packaging waste. Purchasing can "close the loop" by specifying recycled content where possible. Paper products such as napkins with a percentage of post-consumer waste are available. Paperboard and cardboard packaging may be made from recycled materials. Some vendors may reuse their cardboard boxes. The boxes are folded flat when empty and picked up by the vendor at the next delivery. Vendors use these cardboard boxes for snack foods such as potato chips. Alternative packaging materials such as Mylar™ bags for bulk ketchup reduce the volume of waste compared to rigid plastic containers.

Some facilities may reuse food packaging such as plastic sour cream containers for storage or cleaning. Any containers used for these purposes must be clearly labeled and dated. A reusable cup/mug program in cafeterias can reduce the need for disposable cups. Purchasing pre-processed fruits and vegetables can reduce the volume of food production waste. Directors should conduct a yield study to determine whether the cost of the processing and reduced waste volume offsets the labor cost and edible portion cost of processing your own produce.

The decision to use permanent service ware can reduce the volume of plastic and paper waste generated from disposable service ware. However, there is no one "correct" decision. Foodservice directors must evaluate factors including:

- Adequate ware washing equipment
- Adequate labor for cleaning
- Cost of chemicals, water, and energy
- Adequate storage space for disposables
- Adequate dumpster space
- Cost of disposal to the landfill
- Replacement costs for permanent service ware compared to cost of disposables

Recycling

Recycling is the next level of the waste hierarchy. Instituting a recycling program requires support from administration and willingness of staff to perform the recycling tasks. Using data from the waste stream audit or analysis, the foodservice director must decide whether sufficient recyclable material is available on a regular basis to justify allocating resources for a program. The most frequently recycled materials are cardboard, aluminum, and paper.

Assuming the facility generates sufficient quantities of recyclable materials and then locating a market for the items at a reasonable distance from the facility would be the next step. The materials must be cleaned and stored before they are transported to the recycling site. The labor and storage space required would be factors to consider. Decisions about transporting items to the pick-up site would include labor and energy considerations. Some vendors are willing to pick up items and transport them to the recycling center as part of their delivery schedule.

Food waste represents another opportunity for recycling. In 2003, food waste accounted for 2.7% of the U.S. total recycled MSW. Leftover food may be donated to local food banks. Composting food waste is another recycling option. The food waste may be

Learning Point: Food and nutrition departments can practice source reduction through the purchasing function. Specify products with less packaging material or purchase products in bulk and store in reusable containers. Purchasing precut fruits and vegetables also reduces production waste.

used as part of a community composting program or composted by schools. The composted material can be used for school gardens as a soil amendment or as mulch. Other facilities may collect food waste, such as vegetable trimmings for use as animal feed. EPA has created WasteWise, a voluntary source reduction program that is open to all organizations.[11]

Hazardous Waste

RCRA defines hazardous waste as a material that exhibits ignitability, corrosiveness, reactivity, or toxicity. Foodservice staff may be exposed to hazardous chemicals such as solvents, cleaners, and pesticides. The Hazard Communication Standard of 1987 ("Hazcom"), or the "Employee's right to know" is promulgated by OSHA.

The facility is required to maintain a list of all hazardous chemicals, have Material Safety Data Sheets (MSDS) for the chemicals, proper labels on all chemical containers, and provide staff training in the safe use of the hazardous chemicals. MSDS are generally provided by the chemical manufacturer. They describe potential hazards of the specific chemical and list the chemical's ingredients. Multiple copies of the MSDS should be on file in the kitchen. In the event of an accident, an MSDS will be given to emergency medical personnel so the victim receives appropriate treatment.

The Agency for Toxic Substances and Disease Registry (ATSDR), part of the Centers for Disease Control and Prevention, sponsors a Hazardous Substances Emergency Events Surveillance (HSEES) system to monitor uncontrolled or illegal release of hazardous substances or by-products. Operator error, equipment failure, or improper mixing are the most frequently reported causes of events.[17] Hazardous chemicals must be disposed of in a manner described by the manufacturer. Products such as paints or solvents may require special disposal to prevent pollution. Communities often have "hazardous chemical days" where the hazardous material is collected by a community agency for proper disposal.

A written Hazcom plan is required for all employers using hazardous materials. The plan must include a list of all hazardous chemicals, MSDS storage location, employee training procedures, and how the plan is evaluated. The state environmental health agency can be contacted for more information regarding storage and disposal of hazardous waste. Foodservice directors may want to investigate alternative cleaning agents that are not harmful to the environment.[18]

Indoor Air Quality

Most people spend between 80% and 90% of their day indoors;therefore the quality of indoor air is important for good health. The quality of indoor air is affected by humidity levels, airflow, particulates, and volatile organic compounds (VOCs). High humidity levels can foster growth of harmful molds and bacteria. Legionnaire's Disease was linked to mold growth inside an air conditioning system of a large hotel. Inadequate levels of make-up air or air exchange can lead to upper respiratory distress. Particulates from smoke also can cause reactions. VOC emit fumes that can trigger allergic reactions and respiratory distress. Examples of VOCs include new paint, new carpet, cleaning agents, and radon.[19]

Adequate ventilation is key in controlling exposure to indoor air pollutants. The kitchen and dining areas should be monitored for adequate airflow. The American Society of Heating, Refrigerating and Air-Conditioning Engineers (ASHRAE) recommends levels of CO_2, humidity, temperature, and particulates for optimal comfort and safety. ASHRAE recommends that a production kitchen with a cafeteria should have 13 air changes per hour. Another method to determine air exchange is by the number of people using the space. A kitchen with a staff of 20 would need 1,000 cubic feet per minute of make-up air. Poor air quality has been associated with Sick Building Syndrome (SBS). SBS is characteristic of a facility with inade-

Learning Point: Energy efficiency measures implemented in the 1970s and 1980s may have contributed to poor indoor air quality. Sealing windows and doors to reduce air leaks without ensuring adequate ventilation led to SBS in many buildings. Foodservice directors should work with building engineers to provide adequate air exchange in the kitchen and dining areas.

quate HVAC systems. Staff working in such conditions increase the facility's labor cost due to their absences because of health issues. OSHA has proposed all employers develop an indoor air quality program. The document would record compliance with air quality standards and also record employee complaints and building-related illnesses.

Other Air Quality Issues

Environmental tobacco smoke (secondhand smoke) and asbestos both can affect the health of staff and customers. Numerous state and local governments have imposed "no smoking" in public areas. If employees do have a smoking area outside the building, it should be located away from public view with adequate receptacles for the smoking waste generated. All kitchen staff must wash their hands and wear clean aprons after a smoking break. OSHA has proposed regulations for designated smoking areas indoors. The purpose is to limit employees' exposure to secondhand smoke.

Asbestos was an effective industrial insulating material as well as a fire retardant. It was widely used in buildings until the 1970s. However, it was found to be carcinogenic as well as an air pollutant. Its use was banned, but asbestos is still part of many buildings. OSHA has ruled that all buildings constructed before 1981 are assumed to have high levels of asbestos. Removal of asbestos requires personnel who have completed OSHA and EPA training for asbestos handling. Transportation and disposal of asbestos must follow EPA guidelines because it is considered a hazardous air pollutant. Guidelines for compliance with OSHA standards for asbestos are available in 29 CFR 1910.1001 and 29 CFR 1926.58. Foodservice directors should work with the facility's maintenance staff and building engineers to identify asbestos in the kitchen and dining areas.

Particulates in smoke created from char broilers, fryers, ovens, smokers, and other heat-producing equipment can impact outdoor air quality. Facilities located in areas with high levels of air pollution may be regulated for particulates. Through the Clean Air Act, the EPA has established outdoor air quality guidelines called the National Ambient Air Quality Standards (NAAQS). These standards include levels of particulates from smoke, which can be imposed on foodservice operations. Noncompliance with the NAAQS can result in fines.

Learning Point: Asbestos was used for many products, including ceiling materials, floor tiles, and insulation. Consult with the building engineers before doing any repairs or remodeling. Friable asbestos crumbles easily, releasing harmful asbestos fibers into the air. Nonfriable asbestos does not release fibers unless it is disturbed, for example drilling through a ceiling. Certified asbestos removal professionals must be used to remove any friable or nonfriable asbestos.

Summary

This chapter is meant as an introduction to natural resource management. You can see that many issues are interrelated and include both human and environmental components. Natural resource management can result in cost savings. However, it goes beyond cost control. It is a philosophy of not using more than is necessary so future generations can meet their needs. Foodservice directors practice natural resource management because it is the right thing to do.

Student Activities

1. Pick a resource such as energy, water, or air. Brainstorm to generate a list of other resources and management practices interrelated with the selected resource.

Cultural Diversity Issues: In the past, low-income neighborhoods often were located next to sources of pollution. These pollutants could result in increased disease rates and birth defects in addition to degrading the environment. The concept of Environmental Justice emerged in the 1970s to address problems created by pollution for these neighborhoods. Polluters were mandated to clean up toxic wastes. Residents were relocated to new housing, and medical expenses resulting from the pollution were paid by the polluting organization. Brownfields is a term EPA uses to designate potential areas for rehabilitation, often located in low-income areas, as eligible for rebuilding if certain conditions are met.

2. Develop a strategy for enlisting support from your staff for a resource conservation program (energy, water, recycling). Describe the steps you will take to change your staff's behavior toward this resource.
3. Assume you are the director of food and nutrition services and housekeeping for a hospital. Generate a list of resource management practices that both foodservice and housekeeping staff could perform. Would it be possible to form a resource management "task force" from these two groups to develop a conservation program? Justify your answer.

CASE STUDY: MAGNOLIA MEMORIAL HOSPITAL

Magnolia Memorial Hospital (MMH) is a health care facility located in the southeastern United States. MMH specializes in cardiac health, oncology, orthopedics, rehab, and transplants. Magnolia Memorial has 298 beds and offers a variety of services including outpatient care, a wellness center, and seminars offered to the public on various health issues.

MMH has a conventional foodservice production system with a 7-day patient cycle menu. Patient trays are delivered to the floor by foodservice employees and are distributed by the nursing staff. A nutrition assistant is available to assist patients with menu choices, visiting the patients on a daily basis.

Susan Blanco, RD, is MMH director of food and nutrition services. She is preparing a capital budget request for kitchen renovations. The kitchen was built in 1968. Most of the appliances date from 1968 to 1975. Mrs. Blanco is concerned about increasing utility costs and would like to install energy- and water-saving equipment. Hospital administration has set a goal of reducing operating costs by 3% for the coming fiscal year.

The community where MMH is located receives its water from the local river. Treated wastewater is discharged to the same river. Solid waste is transported to a site within the

---

continues

county about 15 miles away. A community recycling drop-off center collects aluminum cans, newspaper, plastic, and clear glass. The center's board of directors is considering accepting other recyclable material.

Sue Blanco had her staff conduct audits for water, energy, and solid waste. The results are listed below.

Table 12.1　Energy Audit

Electric Equipment	Energy Consumed, kW/hour	# Hours Operated per Day	Estimated Energy Usage per Day
Walk-in, 100 sq ft refrigerator/freezer	7 kW	24 hrs/day	
Deep fat fryer, 18 lb fat capacity, floor model	5.5 kW	2.5 hrs/day	
Ice Machine, 225 lb production/hr, 1/2 HP motor	6.1 kW	24 hrs/day	
Dish machine, 3 tank flight type	15 kW	4.5 hrs/day	
Natural Gas Equipment, BTUs converted to kW			
Combi oven/steamer, 4 shelf	2.4 kW	3 hrs/day	
Steam jacketed kettle, gas-generated steam, 20 gallon tilting, floor mount	3.8 kW	2 hrs/day	
Griddle, 18 × 24″	3.5 kW	3 hrs/day	
4 burner Range, floor mount	14 kW	8 hrs/day	

1. Calculate the estimated energy usage for the equipment and enter data in the empty column. Rank the equipment's energy consumption from the highest (1) to the lowest (8).
2. Current electricity charges are: $0.08/kWh, demand charge $0.02/kWh for usage 7:00 A.M. to 8:00 A.M., 12:00 pm to 1:00 P.M., and 5:00 P.M. to 6:00 P.M. Electricity cost

will increase by 10% for usage and demand charges in the next fiscal year. Starting next year, the utility will reduce the demand charge by 2% if usage during the times listed above is reduced by 25%. Identify the equipment with the largest potential savings.

3. Current natural gas charges are: $1.00/100 cubic feet of gas. The cost of gas will increase to $1.20/100 cubic feet of gas next year. Calculate the current cost of gas usage for the equipment per week and per month (assume 4 weeks – 1 month) and the cost of operating the equipment in the next fiscal year.

4. Conduct a search on the Internet and in trade journals to locate similar-sized equipment using electricity and similar equipment using gas. Determine this for as many pieces of equipment as possible. For example, equipment such as refrigerator/freezers will not use gas as an energy source.

5. Using the specifications from question #4, calculate the cost of energy consumption using the cost data in question #2 and question #3. Identify equipment that could decrease utility costs. Are there other factors to consider when replacing equipment?

6. Make a recommendation to Susan Blanco on the most efficient equipment to purchase, providing at least one reason for each recommendation.

Table 12.2   Water Audit

Equipment Type	Gallons used/ Minute	Average run time (hours/meal) B	L	D	Consumption (gallons/day) B	L	D
Dish machine	5 gallons/min	1 hr	2 hr	1.5 hr			
Food waste disposer	8 gallons/min	.5 hr	1 hr	1 hr			
		Total gallons/meal					

continues

1. Calculate the water consumption for the dish machine and disposer. Enter the data in the blank columns. Which uses the most water per *day*—the dish machine or the disposer?
2. The cost of water is $0.04/gallon, including sewer treatment ($0.03). Calculate the cost of water per day, per week, and per month to operate both of these machines.
3. The sewer-use fee, which is based on a facility's BOD reading, will increase the next fiscal year due to higher wastewater treatment costs. The sewer-use fee will increase the cost of water $0.01/gallon to $0.05/gallon. Describe several potential actions that could be taken to decrease the sewer-use cost for MMH. Calculate any potential savings. Would the proposed actions be a significant contribution to the utility cost reduction goal? Explain your decision.

Table 12.3   Solid Waste Audit

Category	Waste/day gallons	Cubic yards	Cost/cubic yard @ $2.50/cu yd
Paperboard	25		
Plastic[1]	80		
Aluminum	12		
Cardboard	100		
Clear glass	8		
Steel	45		
Paper (not newspaper)	20		
Production waste	30		
Service waste	30		

[1] There are many categories of plastic. Not all plastics are recyclable. For the purposes of the case study, all plastics are assumed to be recyclable.

1. Calculate the volume of waste in cubic yards and the waste removal cost per cubic yard, and enter the data in the columns above.
2. MMH has one 6 cubic yard dumpster for the kitchen. Trash is collected 3 times per week. Calculate the total volume of waste for the day in cubic yards. Assuming the audit represents a typical day, how much waste is generated per week? Per month?
3. Calculate the total cost of waste generated per day and per month. Describe several actions that could be taken to reduce the volume of waste generated. How would these actions affect the frequency of trash pick up?
4. Mrs. Blanco estimates the cost of recycling is $.03/cubic yard, including cleaning, storage, and transport to the redemption center. Assuming all plastic, steel, aluminum, and clear glass waste can be recycled, what is the cost of recycling these materials? Compare the cost of recycling with the cost of trash removal. Would you recommend a recycling program be started? Describe other factors to consider besides financial issues.

(See Table 12.4 Two-Week Meal Production Data for MMH on next page.)

Notes: "Regular" means regular diet and "Modified" means modified diet. All modified diets are combined for the purposes of this case study. The meal counts may be used to calculate costs or consumption per patient, per day or waste generated per patient, per day. Meal counts are from actual production records from a hospital in the southeastern United States.

continues

Table 12.4   Two-Week Meal Production Data for MMH

Day	Breakfast		Lunch		Dinner	
	Regular	Modified	Regular	Modified	Regular	Modified
1	36	101	36	104	33	102
2	35	103	34	105	33	101
3	31	82	32	97	39	120
4	38	98	39	105	45	103
5	36	104	37	105	36	108
6	32	97	36	99	38	98
7	31	90	33	89	33	86
8	29	89	29	94	30	92
9	34	93	34	89	31	93
10	27	94	27	91	34	89
11	37	89	35	91	43	101
12	43	101	42	102	46	106
13	36	118	36	117	38	108
14	36	114	57	114	36	117

Web Sites

Solid Waste
www.epa.gov/epaoswer/non-hw/muncpt/facts.htm

WaterSense Program
www.epa.gov/owm/water-efficiency

Indoor Air Quality
www.epa.gov/iaq

Energy Star Program
www.energystar.gov

Consortium for Energy Efficiency
www.cee1.org

Plastic Recycling
www.plasticresource.com

Energy and Water Efficiency
www.watergy.org

Conservation Practices
www.food-management.com

U.S. Green Building Council
www.usgbc.org

References

1. Environmental Protection Agency. (2006a). Sustainability. Retrieved May 4, 2006, from www.epa.gov/sustainability/basicinfo.htm.
2. Energy Star. (2005). Making the business case for energy management in healthcare. Retrieved July 28, 2006, from www.energystar.gov/index.cfm?c=healthcare.businesscase.
3. Stevens, J. & Scriven, C. (1999). *Food equipment facts.* Weimar, TX: Chips Books.
4. Energy Information Administration. (2005). Energy consumption by source 1949–2004. Retrieved May 4, 2006, from www.eia.doe.gov/emeu/aer/overview.html.
5. Solocomhouse.com. (2006). Energy. Retrieved May 5, 2006, from www.solocomhouse.com/Energy.htm.
6. Shanklin, C.W. & Hackes, B.L. (2001). Position of the American Dietetic Association: Dietetics professionals can implement practices to conserve natural resources and protect the environment. *Journal of the American Dietetic Association, 101,* 1221–1227.
7. Bendall, D. (2005a). Playing it cool. *Food Management, 40,* 88, 93.
8. Bendall, D. (2005b). High speed cooking. *Food Management, 40,* 76, 80.
9. Restaurant-Food Service Industry. (2005). Energy conservation standards. Retrieved May 7, 2006, from www.thimmakka.org/Activities/Energy_guidelines.
10. United States Geological Survey. (2006). Water on and in the earth. Retrieved April 19, 2006, from www.ga.water.usgs.gov/edu/earthwherewater.html/.
11. Environmental Protection Agency. (2006b). EPA wastewise program overview. Retrieved May 5, 2006, from http://www.epa.gov/wastewise/about/overview.htm.

12. Perkin, J.F. & Gerald, B.L. (2003). Position of the American dietetic association: Food and water safety. *Journal of the American Dietetic Association, 103.*

13. Watergy. (2004). The link between energy and water: Watergy efficiency. Retrieved April 19, 2006, from www.watergy.org/activities.

14. Shea, E.J. (2005). Hands-off success. *Restaurants and Institutions, 115,* 32.

15. Environmental Protection Agency. (2006c). Waste not, want not. Retrieved April 23, 2006, from www.epa.gov/epaoswer/non-hw/muncpl/yard.htm.

16. Mason, D.M., Shanklin, C.W., Wie, S.H., & Wolfe, K. (1999). *Environmental issues impacting foodservice and lodging operations* (2nd ed.). Manhattan, KS: Kansas State University Press.

17. Berkowitz, Z., Haugh, G.S., Orr, M.F., & Kaye, W. (2002). Releases of hazardous substances in schools: Data from the hazardous substances emergency events surveillance system 1993–1998. *Journal of Environmental Health, 65*(2), 20–28.

18. Byers, BA, Shanklin, CW, & Hoover, LC. (1994). *Foodservice manual for healthcare institutions.* (4th ed.). Chicago, IL: American Hospital Publishing, Inc.

19. Lawrence Berkley National Laboratory. (1996). Indoor air pollution. Retrieved April 28, 2006, from www.lbl.gov/Education/ELSI/Frames/pollution-indoor-f.html.

The author gratefully acknowledges the work of Elizabeth Mangrum, RD, LDN for her contributions to this chapter.

CHAPTER 13

PEST MANAGEMENT IN THE FOODSERVICE INDUSTRY

Paul B. Baker, PhD and Robert W. Hartley

Reader Objectives

After studying this chapter and reflecting on the contents, the student should be able to:

1. Recognize when a pest problem exists and the treatment options available.
2. Be aware that there are strict state and federal regulations associated with commercial food handling establishments that include pest control.
3. Understand the critical components of any good Integrated Pest Management program are inspection, preventive measures, monitoring, pest identification, and action thresholds.
4. Realize that all control strategies should be focused around the biology of the pest.

Key Terms

Arthropods: the largest phylum of animals that includes the insects, arachnids, crustaceans, and others.

Cyfluthrin: the active ingredient in many insecticide products.

Environmental Protection Agency: sometimes referred to as USEPA, an agency of the federal government of the United States charged with protecting human health and with safeguarding the natural environment, air, water, and land.

Fumigant: a pesticide vaporized to kill pests. Used in buildings and greenhouses.

Integrated Pest Management (IPM): a pest control strategy that uses an array of complementary methods: natural predators and parasites, pest-resistant varieties, cultural practices, biological controls, various physical techniques, and pesticides as a last resort. It is an ecological approach that can significantly reduce or eliminate the use of pesticides.

Muridae: the largest family of mammals. It contains over 600 species found naturally throughout Eurasia, Africa, and Australia.

Oothecae: plural of ootheca, the egg case of some insects and mollusks.

Pest Management Professional (PMP): refers to the regulation or management of another species defined as a pest, usually because it is believed to be detrimental to a person's health, the ecology, or the economy.

Phorid: a small, humpbacked fly of the highly diverse family Phoridae, and resembling a fruit fly in appearance. Phorid flies can often be identified by their escape habit of running rapidly across a surface rather than taking to the wing.

Pyrethroid: a synthetic chemical that kills most insects and is similar to the natural chemical pyrethrin produced by the flowers of a chrysanthemum. Pyrethroids are common in commercial products such as household insecticides and insect repellents.

Introduction

Every foodservice professional will have to deal with a pest problem at some point. As such, he or she should be aware that although "do it yourself" pest control is an option, it is not recommended due to the strict state and federal regulations associated with commercial food handling establishments. The objectives of these regulations are to ensure that the food preparation areas, the equipment used to prepare the food, and serving surfaces are not contaminated with pesticide residues. It is also imperative that procedures be in place to restrict unwanted contaminates such as rodent droppings, insects, and other foreign body parts that could contaminate surrounding areas where food is being prepared, cooked, served, or eaten. However, it is not our intent to prevent a restaurant owner or foodservice manager from performing his own pest control, but instead, to give

this individual a working knowledge of pest control strategies and
programs to make an informed
decision about how he wants to
handle pest control.

> **Learning Point:** Pest control technologies change frequently; the foodservice professional should consult a reputableWeb site, using a good search engine, to keep up with these innovations.

Pest control strategies within a
food handling establishment are
primarily focused on maintaining
very low levels of pests with little
or no pesticides, while at the same
time ensuring a minimum expo-
sure to chemicals in both the work and eating environments. Maintaining pests at low levels takes a plan and requires a commitment
by the management. With a good plan and management's inputs,
the use of pesticides can be kept to a minimum, which results in
reduced chemical exposure in the air, on food surfaces, and in the
food.

Basic Principles of Pest Control

Understanding basic pest control principles are important for all
managers of foodservice facilities. Essentially, the objective of any
pest control program in a foodservice facility is to minimize the
invasion and establishment of
pest species. To meet that
objective, one has to have a
plan or strategy to keep the
facility clean and operational.
The key, then, is sanitation.
However, sometimes despite the
best efforts, pests invade a
facility and get established.
Then the responsible party must
decide whether to attempt to

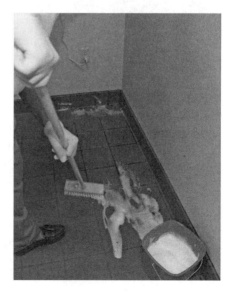

FIGURE 13.1 Cleaning and
Sanitizing Floors
Photo courtesy of Scott Nolen, Truly
Nolen of America, Inc.

remedy the situation himself, or to call a **Pest Management Professional** (PMP). In either case, this foodservice professional must have a working knowledge of the strategies used on pests associated with foodservice establishments.

Integrating pest management principles is critical in any control strategy. The clear objective is to minimize pesticide exposure by employing an integrated approach or an **Integrated Pest Management** (IPM) strategy. IPM principles employ several measures including physical, mechanical, cultural, biological, and educational tactics to maintain pest numbers at extremely low levels. By maintaining pests at low numbers, the need for chemical controls is minimized. However, if a pest is present in sufficient numbers to warrant action, the least-toxic chemical controls are used as a last resort.

Critical components of any good IPM program are inspection, preventive measures, monitoring, pest identification, and "action thresholds." The most successful pest control program starts with thorough inspection of the facilities before any type of control strategies is implemented. A professional level inspection reveals the extent of the infestation, the location of the harborages, the entry points, and the appropriate control tactic to be employed. A detailed written plan is best. As part of the plan, preventive measures should

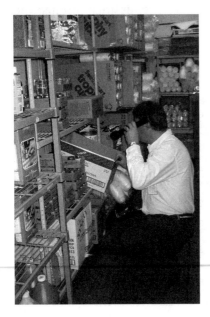

be discussed and implemented. These measures could consist of simple operations such as caulking holes, moving the trash receptacle away from the service entrance, or rotating stock off the floor and away from the walls. In order to keep on top of the potential problem, a monitoring program is encouraged because it enables the facilities manager to keep focused on the issues. Monitoring programs consist of such things as

FIGURE 13.2   Inspection Storage Room in Box
Photo courtesy of Scott Nolen, Truly Nolen of America, Inc.

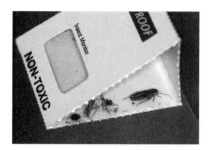

FIGURE 13.3 Insect Monitoring
Photo courtesy of Scott Nolen, Truly
Nolen of America, Inc.

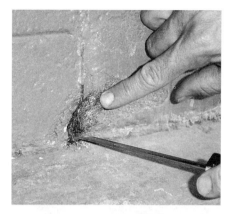

FIGURE 13.4 Exclusion
Photo courtesy of Scott Nolen, Truly
Nolen of America, Inc.

monthly inspections, glue boards, and pheromone traps.

All of these techniques are designed to keep facility management apprised of the pest situation. In the event a pest arrives at the facility, it is critical that a proper identification be made. Without proper identification, wasted effort and resources could lead to larger problems. Several pests look alike but have distinctively different biology and thus, different tactics for control. For example, the red flour beetle and confused flour beetle look identical to the layperson. However, because the former can fly and the latter cannot, proper identification is of primary importance in establishing a control strategy and estimating the potential extent of infestation. Once a pest has been properly identified and has established itself to the point that some response is required, the action threshold has been reached. Usually, once the action threshold is reached, a

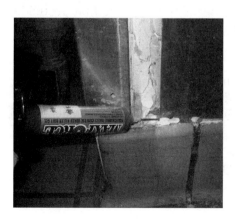

FIGURE 13.5 Gel Bait Applied to Damaged Tile
Photo courtesy of Scott Nolen, Truly Nolen of America, Inc.

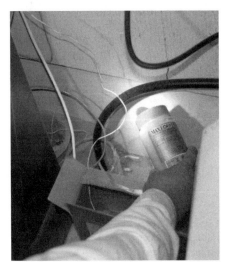

FIGURE 13.6   Granules Bait
Photo courtesy of Scott Nolen, Truly Nolen of America, Inc.

pesticide is applied with the intent of eliminating the pest population. As part of that action, re-evaluation of the current control strategy is important so that the pest problem can be prevented in the future.

Part of the goal in any IPM program is to reduce the risk of pesticides to the applicator, foodservice workers, and the public; the application of pesticides should be target-specific. Pesticides are never applied over a food surface. Instead, they are applied to specific locations such as a spot application or a crack and crevice application. The intent is to control the pest in its harborage area. Pesticides come in various forms (dry and liquid), with different concentrations and target specific requirements. However, pesticides used in the foodservice industry are limited to liquid, dust, or bait applications. Liquid and dust applications are primarily directed at specific targets located in harborages such as cracks and crevices, while baiting is passive in that the pest must come to the food, ingest it, and either die or pass it on to nest mates. In almost all cases, the type of pest and the severity of infestation dictate the treatment methodology. One also needs to be aware that pesticide labels are the law and are enforceable by regulatory agencies such as the **Environmental Protection Agency.** Thus, because the label is the law, any deviation from the label instructions can result in fines and or license suspensions by the applicator. Therefore, it is important that the PMP be licensed by the state and federal governments for those categories under

> **Learning Point:** Keys to good pest control in foodservice establishments: sanitation, monitoring, records and maintenance logs, and PMPs.

which the food establishment is covered. This licensure demonstrates to the public and to the facility manager that the individual
is competent to be applying pesticides in your facility.

One of the most important keys to establishing a good IPM program is proper identification. Listed below are some of the more
common pests encountered in foodservice establishments: **arthropods**
(such as ants), cockroaches, stored product pests, flies, and vertebrate
pests (such as rats and mice). Each pest will be profiled so that relevant information is available. These profiles are not exhaustive, but
they do provide sufficient information to enable a restaurant or foodservice manager to have a basic understanding of the pests.

Pest Profiles

Ants

Ants are social insects that live in colonies with large numbers of
individuals. The colony functions as one despite the division of
labor. Ants vary greatly in their physical characteristics, nesting
habits, food preferences, dispersal methods, health importance, and
distribution. Ants have complex food needs and forage for both
solid and liquid foods and water. Pest ants divide into two primary
groups based on their nesting preferences—either in the ground or in
wall voids. Common wall nesting ants are the carpenter ant, crazy
ants, odorous house ants, Pharaoh ants, and the thief ant. Ground
dwelling ants are the Argentine ant, pavement ant, the little black
ant, and the fire ant.

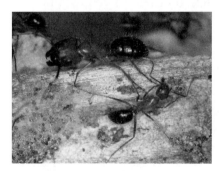

FIGURE 13.7 Carpenter Ants
Photo courtesy of Scott Nolen, Truly
Nolen of America, Inc.

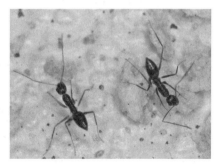

FIGURE 13.8 Crazy Ants
Photo courtesy of Scott Nolen, Truly
Nolen of America, Inc.

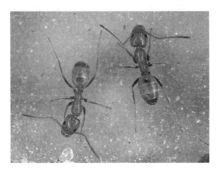

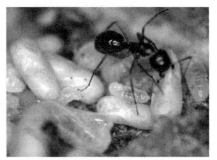

FIGURE 13.9   Odorless House Ant
Photo courtesy of Scott Nolen, Truly
Nolen of America, Inc.

FIGURE 13.10   Carpenter Ant
Photo courtesy of Scott Nolen, Truly
Nolen of America, Inc.

Biology

Ants can be distinguished from other insects by the narrow pedicel
or hump just past the thorax and by their elbowed antenna. Ants
undergo a complete metamorphosis: egg, larvae, pupa, and adult.
They have three distinct castes: workers, queens, and males. Workers perform the duties of constructing the nest and foraging for
food, while the queens and males produce offspring. The head of an
ant can vary greatly in size and shape, with the mandibles or teeth
being very important body characteristics. Ants use their mandibles
to cut, gnaw, carry, and build. However, ants don't eat with their
mandibles. Instead, workers regurgitate food in tiny liquid drops
and feed it to fellow workers. For general identification purposes,
ant body coloration ranges from black to brown to yellow and red.

Control Strategies

The procedure used to control ants includes a five-step process:

1. Identify the ant.
2. Locate the nest(s) by following the workers.
3. Direct the treatment at the place they live, whether by baiting,
   liquid applications, or use of a nonresidual insecticide aerosol
   for cracks and crevices.
4. Control conditions contributing to the infestation (sanitation,
   harborage removal, exclusion, etc.).
5. Follow-up to evaluate the treatment.

Cockroaches

Cockroaches are probably the most prevalent pests found in food-service facilities nationwide. They are not only a nuisance; they are also known to carry disease pathogens with the potential to cause allergic reactions in people. These common disease pathogens include: Salmonella (food poisoning), Bacillus, Clostridium, Coliform, Streptococcus, and Staphylococcus. Plus, cockroaches can carry the bacteria Escherichia coli, which causes diarrhea, and Shigella dysenteriae which causes dysentery. There are over 7,000 species of cockroaches worldwide, with about 70 species found in the United States. The most common include: the American, Brown banded, German, and Oriental. Each species has its unique habits and preferences for food and shelter. The locations the cockroaches inhabit help with proper identification. For example, the American roach (*Periplaneta americana*) is found primarily in sewers and comes into a dwelling through the drains. However, it cannot reproduce inside a dwelling and, therefore, you most likely see only adults and no immatures.

Biology

Cockroaches reproduce by simple metamorphosis from egg, to nymph, to adult. Immature nymphs are smaller versions of the reproductive adult. Because they are gregarious, they are usually located in groups with nymphs and adults occupying the same location. They are generally nocturnal in their foraging habits. Occasionally, they are seen in the daylight if all of the harborages are filled and they are forced to move into alternative hiding places. Females produce egg capsules, or **oothecae,** that contain eggs arranged in two parallel rows that each contain up to 60 eggs. The egg capsule is either carried around until just before the nymphs hatch or is cemented to a surface (generally near a food source). Depending on the temperature and humidity, developmental time can be as little as 2 months or as long as several years, depending on the species. In a controlled environment, such as a foodservice facility, cockroaches can become established in a very few months.

Control Strategies

It is always assumed that a cockroach problem will develop at some point in time in a foodservice facility. Therefore, a good plan is essential. The procedure used to control cockroaches includes a six-step process:

1. Prevention—inspect all incoming food items for egg capsules and live cockroaches inside/outside the facility.
2. Good sanitation focused on harborages, food, and water.
3. Inspection of the facility using valuable tools like flushing agents and monitoring traps.
4. Control conditions contributing to the infestation (sanitation, harborage removal, exclusion, etc.).
5. Baiting with a gel bait or use of a nonresidual insecticide aerosol for cracks and crevices.
6. Follow-up to evaluate the treatment.

Flies (Non-Biting)

Non-biting flies are a worldwide problem not only because they are a nuisance but because they harbor diseases that impact humans. For example the house fly, *Musca domestica*, has been reported to carry over 100 different pathogenic organisms both within the body and externally. Flies prefer food sources with high moisture, such as fermenting and decaying organic matter, for egg laying and habitat location. Control is difficult because of this pest's ability to fly significant distances from its original source. Of over 18,000 fly species, about 200 are associated with human environments within which selective and specific breeding and harborage are required.

Biology

Flies undergo four different changes in their life stages— egg, larvae (maggots), pupa, and adult. Adults are generally good fliers but not always, and the female can lay upwards of 1,000 eggs in her lifetime. Eggs are laid near or on the food source. White, legless maggots emerge in days, depending on temperature and humidity, and undergo three to four instars

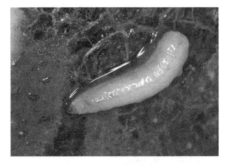

FIGURE 13.11 Maggot
Photo courtesy of Scott Nolen, Truly Nolen of America, Inc.

before pupating. Upon emerging, the adults feed on a sugar source such as nectar, then mate, and the cycle begins again, in many cases all within a confined space such as a food facility or warehouse.

Control Strategies

The most fundamental and critical factor in a successful fly control program is sanitation. All fly species need moisture and a food source. Identifying and controlling the environment through good sanitary practices will significantly lower fly populations. The proper identification of the type of fly will help suggest locations in need of special attention. Drain flies, also known as moth flies, are usually a problem in drains, grease traps, and general sewage lines. Use of the new bio-enzymes in the drainage system can help alleviate a drain fly problem.

Phorid flies can be found almost anywhere. However, remember that they need moisture and decaying organic matter. Inspect accordingly and remove potential sources of these conditions conducive to phorid flies. House flies usually originate on the outside and enter a building through open doors, poorly screened windows, etc. A good outdoor program to control flies would include moving trash receptacles or dumpsters from 50 to 75 feet away from all building entrances. The introduction of light traps, which utilize an ultraviolet light (UV) source, will also help to control house flies indoors.

The use of insecticides represents the least desirable and least effective control method for flies. Further, food handling establishments must follow strict regulatory requirements due to the potential for contaminating food products with insecticide residual.

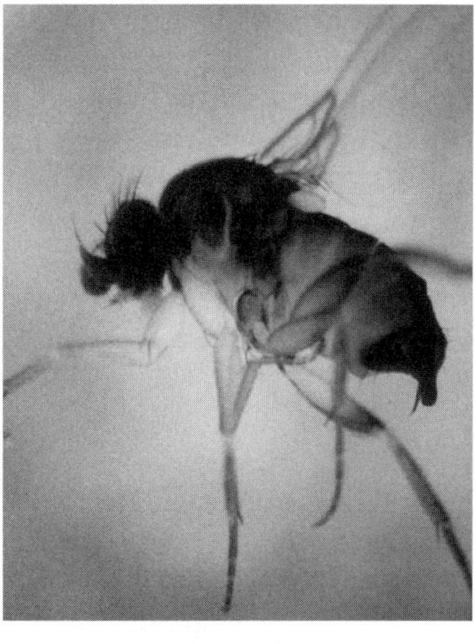

FIGURE 13.12 Phorid Fly
Photo courtesy of Scott Nolen, Truly Nolen of America, Inc.

Stored Product Pests

Stored product pests or pantry pests on a worldwide basis account for nearly 35% of all losses to food and food products once the food has been harvested. These pests are comprised of a large group of beetles, moths and mites, some of which are not only difficult to see but to identify. They vary in size from $\frac{1}{16}$ to $\frac{3}{4}$ of an inch. They walk, hitchhike, or fly into a warehouse, restaurant, or food facility. What makes them difficult to control is that they have the capacity to produce thousands of offspring in confined spaces, even under control environments, particularly if areas are not inspected frequently enough. The end result is the loss of all kinds of food commodities.

Biology

The two primary pests are beetles and moths, both of which have complete metamorphosis consisting of egg, larvae, pupa, and adult. Depending on the species of beetle, they can feed on dry dog food, dried fruits and vegetables, whole grains, and spices, producing anywhere from one to six generations a year. Because many of these beetles are extremely small, usually $\frac{1}{16}$ of an inch, they can be difficult to find and identify. In addition, some of these beetle adults, such as the red flour beetle, are good fliers and can spread an infestation in a relatively short time. Adult moths, on the other hand, are usually a little larger at $\frac{1}{2}$ inch or so, light brown to gray in color, and are generally attracted to lights. The adults do not cause damage but are the mode of distribution within the facility. The larvae are usually off-white in color with a distinct head capsule. Depending on temperature and relative humidity, they can produce 3 to 12 generations per year.

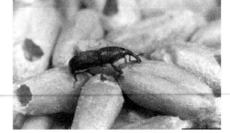

FIGURE 13.13 Granary Weevil
Photo courtesy of Scott Nolen, Truly
Nolen of America, Inc.

Control Strategies

The keys to minimizing stored product pests are: prevention/monitoring; sanitation; proper storage; stock rotation and ventilation; and control options. A good preventive program includes keeping the pest out by caulking and reducing their potential entry points. Good sanitation is of primary importance. Without it, insecticide control options are extremely difficult. All products should be properly stored, inspected, and rotated out of the system as soon as the product is purchased. A good ventilation system will keep the airflow moving and the temperatures within good operating range. Correct pest identification is critical to any insecticide application. Therefore, all control strategies should be focused around the biology of the pest. If an insecticide is necessary, it must be labeled for the targeted pest and treatment location. It should also be selected for minimum toxicity. The treatment program should be re-evaluated on a regular basis.

Rodents

Rodents are among some of the most notorious mammals on earth because they are so prolific and adapt well to almost any environment. They have the ability to feed on a wide range of food, can survive under difficult conditions, and use sophisticated behavior patterns that enable them to avoid danger from predators, specifically people. The family **Muridae**, to which the commensal rats and

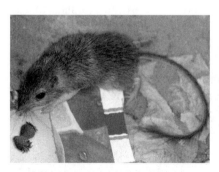

FIGURE 13.14 Field Mouse
Photo courtesy of Scott Nolen, Truly Nolen of America, Inc.

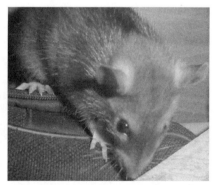

FIGURE 13.15 Norway Rat
Photo courtesy of Scott Nolen, Truly Nolen of America, Inc.

FIGURE 13.16   Roof Rat
Photo courtesy of Scott Nolen, Truly
Nolen of America, Inc.

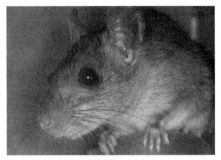

mice belong, has approximately
500 species and, in most cases,
can be found worldwide. The
problems with rodents are well-
documented, from having an affinity for gnawing on electrical
wires with disastrous results, to contamination of food, to the spread
of disease (Bubonic plague and Hantavirus). In addition, if the
rodents and humans are in close confines, rodent attacks are not
uncommon, with potentialy serious effects, particularly if the victims are babies or the elderly.

Biology

The type of rodent most likely to be encountered in a foodservice
facility is commensal rodents. These consist of the Norway rat, black
roof rat, and the house mouse. In general, the Norway and black
roof rats have litters almost monthly with up to 6 to 12 young per
litter. Depending on food, shelter, and the environment, a female rat
in the wild usually lives less than 1 year but can have upward of
five litters during this lifetime. Their diurnal activity at dawn and
dusk can be modified by human activity, competition, and the availability of food. Rodent harborages consist of a network of burrows
and runs that connect primary and secondary food sources in which
they are opportunistic omnivores. Their home range consists of the
area which the rodent covers in its day-to-day travels for food,
mating, and caring for its young. Research has demonstrated that
the home range of rats is about 100 feet, whereas a mouse has a
home range of about 20 feet. When food and shelter are abundant,
it is not unusual for different rodent species to coexist in the same
area or building, utilizing the same food resource.

Control Strategies

The integration of all the key aspects of rodent control is critical in
maintaining a rodent-free environment. The five key elements to a
rodent IPM control strategy include:

1. Inspection and monitoring
2. Exclusion
3. Sanitation
4. Nonchemical controls
5. Rodenticides

The most successful rodent control plans begin with a thorough inspection of the facility. The inspector is looking for runways, burrows, tracks, urine stains, feces (droppings), gnawing damage, grease marks, and visual signs.

The most common indications of a rodent problem are fecal droppings and visual sign of nesting materials. A good detection device is a UV light under which urine stains glow blue based on the intensity and frequency of runway use.

A monitoring program should follow that will enable the professional to identify the rodent. Once identified, a plan can be established to include an exclusion program with a major emphasise on sanitation. Nonchemical controls consist of physical trappings. If that has limited success, then a rodenticide application may be appropriate. The primary chemical control is the use of anticoagulant baits; the rodent feeds on the bait and dies from internal bleeding. These rodenticides are strategically positioned around the facility in secured, tamper-resistant bait boxes that are checked frequently depending on the level of infestation. These baits are slow to act.

Summary

Management in the foodservice industry is a dynamic process by which owners and operators are constantly evaluating and re-evaluating the way they do business. Pest control in the food industry is just one aspect that needs constant attention. Therefore, pest control strategies within a food handling establishment are primarily

> **Learning Point:** Keys to a sound IPM Plan are to have a working knowledge of the pests one is likely to encounter and to know what actions are appropriate to reduce and eliminate those pests.

focused on maintaining low levels of pests with limited use of pesticides to ensure a low-risk chemical environment. Maintaining pests at low levels takes a plan and requires a commitment by the management.

Following the guidelines in this chapter, a manager within the food handling establishment should now be able to recognize when a pest problem exists and be aware of some of the control options that are available. He should also have a working knowledge of the IPM principles that are critical in any control strategy. The objective of the control strategy is to minimize pesticide exposure by employing IPM principles that include physical, mechanical, cultural, biological, and educational tactics to maintain pest numbers at extremely low levels. By maintaining pests at low numbers, the need for chemical controls is minimized. However if a pest is present in sufficient numbers to warrant action, the least toxic chemical controls are used as a last resort. An understanding of pest biology enables a manager to make an informed decision as to whether to attempt pest control himself or to have a professional perform the service.

The case studies give the manager not only an opportunity to see the various situations he might encounter at a food establishment but what solutions were available and how successful they were in controlling the pest problems. While an individual involved in the foodservice industry will very likely encounter pest problems, the key to a successful resolution of these problems is to recognize the problems early and have a plan to minimize the impact to business.

CASE STUDY #1: CHAIN RESTAURANT

The owner of five fast food chains in Tucson, Arizona, didn't want the expense of regular, professional pest control services and opted to have only occasional special services performed. These services were erratically scheduled, and no pest control maintenance efforts were made between special services. A German cockroach problem in all five restaurants eventually became so severe that roaches had collected in the ceiling and were visible to customers during daylight.

Evaluation

Due to concerns by the food manager, another pest control service company was engaged to evaluate the situation and recommend the best course of action. A commercial pest control technician inspected all locations and interviewed restaurant personnel including managers, cooks, and counter staff. He learned that previous companies had sprayed but had not employed the most up-to-date roach baiting techniques. He determined that the primary pest problem was German cockroaches and that there was also a minor infestation of American roaches adjacent to the hot water heater.

He detailed a number of sanitary issues that needed to be corrected including the collection of grease, a roach food source, under most fixed fryers. Further, some structural items needed to be addressed in several of the restaurants such as broken tiles which can act as harborages (hiding places) for pests. He also evaluated each location in terms of the most likely cockroach pathways and harborages throughout the facility. This is important because cockroaches tend to develop habitual patterns of activity. If pest materials are applied outside of the range of customary cockroach pathways, they cannot be effective.

Treatment

Once a thorough inspection and evaluation of each restaurant had been completed, the pest control commercial technician met with the manager

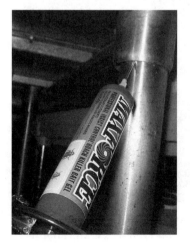

FIGURE 13.17 Baiting a Plumbing Joint
Photo courtesy of Scott Nolen, Truly Nolen of America, Inc.

continues

of each restaurant and discussed the corrective sanitary and structural repair measures that needed to be taken before the initial intensive service could be performed. Then, the initial service involved the inside application of a roach bait product containing a non-repellent; that is, its chemical makeup attracts the roaches to the bait rather than repelling them. This bait was applied selectively in areas that had previously been identified as the most likely cockroach harborages and pathways.

The initial service also involved an outside perimeter spray of a product containing the **pyrethroid cyfluthrin.** This material has a residual effect that acts as a barrier to many types of pests and discourages them from entering the premises.

The initial service was followed by routine monthly services, scheduled outside of restaurant operating hours, and callback services as needed. During each service visit, the commercial pest control technician communicated with restaurant personnel concerning their observations of pest activity.

The selective baiting procedure worked well, and the cockroach population was reduced significantly over a period of about 6 months.

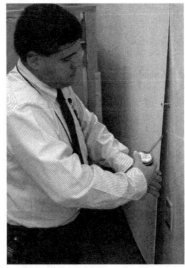

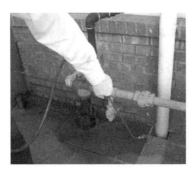

FIGURE 13.18 Exterior Treatment
Photo courtesy of Scott Nolen, Truly Nolen of America, Inc.

FIGURE 13.19 Dusting Behind Kitchen Wall Panel
Photo courtesy of Scott Nolen, Truly Nolen of America, Inc.

Eventually, the efficacy of the baiting reached a plateau. Then, baiting was augmented by the application of a borate-based dust in voids and other possible harborage areas. This dust acts as a desiccant (it dehydrates an insect by abrading the waxy exoskeleton), and it is also a stomach poison. Monitoring stations were used to track cockroach activity and identify additional pathways. These stations are made of heavyweight paper formed into a pyramid shape, open on both ends. A roach sees them as a harborage, enters the station, and is trapped by a sticky substance on the floor of the station. These stations not only help identify areas of activity but also identify which direction the roach was coming from, pointing out additional possible harborages.

Outcome

After 1 year of regular service, each of the restaurants was clear of cockroach infestation. Essential to this successful outcome were the willingness of restaurant management to comply with sanitary recommendations and the requested structural repairs as well as good ongoing communication between the commercial pest control technician and restaurant personnel.

Questions for discussion:

1. Was the treatment appropriate for the result?
2. Should the manager go on a scheduled monitoring program?
3. What were some of keys to the success of the program?

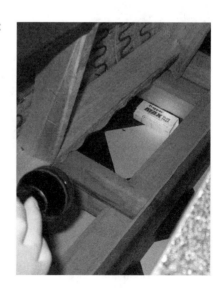

FIGURE 13.20 Insect Under Booth Seat
Photo courtesy of Scott Nolen, Truly Nolen of America, Inc.

CASE STUDY #2: LARGE FOODSERVICE FACILITY

The new owners of a large restaurant establishment in the Southwest were alarmed by what seemed to be a significant infestation of cockroaches as well as mice. They called in a pest control company to evaluate the problem.

Evaluation

A pest control sales inspector performed a thorough inspection of the premises and identified a large German cockroach infestation. The building was old and, over time, had been expanded by a number of additions and building add-ons. Some of these had developed cracks where they adjoined the original structure. There were exterior holes in the structure. In some instances, interior upgrades had been installed over old materials, new carpeting had been installed over old, chipped tiles, etc. There were numerous nooks and crannies within the structure, all pest havens. The inspector suspected that this structure had long been a pest control service problem, but the new owners did not know the service history.

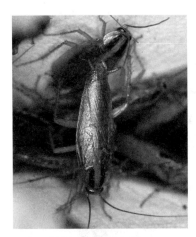

FIGURE 13.21   Significant Pest Pressure
Photo courtesy of Scott Nolen, Truly Nolen of America, Inc.

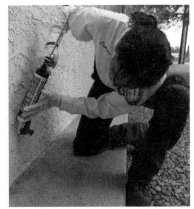

FIGURE 13.22   Caulking Around the Spigot
Photo courtesy of Scott Nolen, Truly Nolen of America, Inc.

Treatment

Because of the abundant pest harborages in this building as well as the many structural impediments to good access to pest hiding places, the pest control company decided that the best tactic was a heavy application of synthetic pyrethroid aerosol spray. A team of pest control technicians went in after normal business hours to perform this initial service. The effect of pyrethroid is to drive pests out of their harborage areas. They can then be eliminated out in the open.

However, as the commercial pest control technician assigned to the monthly service of this establishment discovered, this initial treatment strategy was a mistake. Pyrethroids are a repellent—they drive pests away. For many months after the initial service, roach baits were not effective because they were tainted by the pyrethroid residue, and the roaches were repelled from the bait rather than wanting to take it. The commercial pest control technician shifted his focus to the use of a spray material containing cyfluthrin, which is both a barrier treatment and a contact kill material. He also advised management on the many mechanical alterations to the structure that would help decrease the cockroach infestation. These included repairing the holes in the exterior walls, caulking cracks and crevices throughout, fixing broken tiles, caulking a back splash in the kitchen that had separated from the wall, etc.

To address the problem with mice, the technician placed tamper-resistant bait

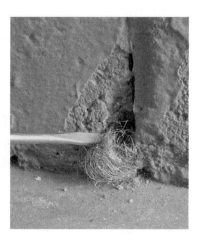

FIGURE 13.23 Stainless Steel Wool Exclusion
Photo courtesy of Scott Nolen, Truly Nolen of America, Inc.

continues

boxes with an anticoagulant bait in strategic locations around the restaurant. These bait boxes were checked on each service visit and moved if there was no activity. He also placed glue boards in some areas to monitor mouse activity.

Outcome

There has been a significant reduction in cockroach infestation, despite the error of overusing synthetic pyrethroids initially. However, given the structural anomalies, the facility will likely never have more than 70% effective control for German roaches. The mice problem has abated. The commercial pest control technician continues to communicate closely with facility management on further mechanical alterations that might help. The technician also continues to attempt the use of nonrepellent baits, anticipating that the pyrethroid residual effect will eventually dissipate.

Questions for discussion:

1. Was the control management appropriate for what was achieved?
2. What was learned from the application of the pyrethroid?
3. As a manager of a foodservice facility, is 70% acceptable for control?

CASE STUDY # 3: COMMERCIAL FOOD STORAGE WAREHOUSE

A 100,000-square-foot food storage warehouse in Salt Lake City, Utah acted as the centralized food product distribution center for a supermarket chain operating in a tri-state area. Warehouse management became concerned with increasing mice and stored product pests. Indian meal moths and flour beetles had infested a broad range of stored products including dog foods, bulk grains, and flour. Upper management could not tolerate a situation that could lead to the shipment of products contaminated by these pests and/or mice urine and feces. A team of pest control professionals, including their company's national technical director, came in to evaluate the situation.

Evaluation

The obvious difficulty for the pest control professionals was how best to address a pest problem on such a large scale given the size of the facility, the levels of stored product, (pallets were stacked five stories high by computerized lifts), and the broad range of products affected. Aiding in the analysis was the fact that the stored products were very well-organized due to a computer tracking system that could identify when items had been placed in the warehouse, where items were located in the warehouse, etc.

The pest professionals consulted with warehouse management and the department heads in various sections of the warehouse. The plan that emerged from these conversations was to grid the warehouse, breaking down the immense area into smaller, easily identifiable sections. A log sheet was developed and posted in each section upon which employees were instructed to describe signs of the various infestations, logging approximate location within the section, and the time and date of the observation. Each section was then evaluated as a separate entity to determine the specific pests within that section and devise the most effective initial service plan. After initial service, the plan was to treat, evaluate, and re-inspect as necessary within these grids on a predetermined, organized schedule.

To prevent infestation of new product coming into the warehouse, warehouse management proactively elected to hold each pallet of incoming product outside the warehouse until it could be inspected for pest infestation and, if none was found, the pallet was shrink-wrapped before storing in the warehouse so that the product was protected from the ongoing infestation.

continues

FIGURE 13.24   Pheromone
Trap
Photo courtesy of Scott Nolen,
Truly Nolen of America, Inc.

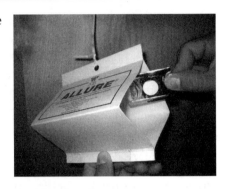

Treatment

Treatment methods varied depending on what was being stored in a particular section and what kind of pest problem was present. The approach in each section was to introduce mechanical alterations that would help reduce the possibility of infestation, such as making sure stock was rotated and keeping the product on the pallets as opposed to on floor. Where stored product pest problems were encountered, pheromone traps were used to identify and gauge the intensity of infestation. Then the infested product was removed for disposal. Before any new product could be stored in that area, the section was cleaned, vacuumed, and a crack and crevice treatment, a pyrethroid-based product called cyfluthrin, was rendered. This treatment killed any remaining pest larval activity in the cracks and crevices.

For the mice infestation, glue boards were placed and UV techniques employed to help define patterns of mouse activity. While running along their "trails" or runways, mice frequently urinate. A UV light, commonly known as a "black light," will cause the urine to fluoresce, thereby identifying the

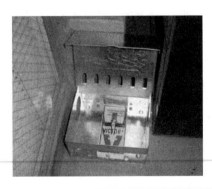

FIGURE 13.25   Mechanical
Mouse Trap in Station
Photo courtesy of Scott Nolen,
Truly Nolen of America, Inc.

mouse runways. When mice runways were found, they were baited with an anticoagulant approved for use in these locations and contained in tamperproof bait stations. Due to regulatory constraints concerning the use of pesticides in other areas of food storage, mechanical trapping was used instead of the anticoagulant; the types of traps used were snap traps repeating mouse traps capable of catching multiple mice. Because of the variety of infestations, detailed inspection and treatment records were essential. Teams of pest technicians were on-site multiple times a week on a prescheduled basis to treat, review incident logs, and re-inspect previously treated areas for evidence of any continuing infestation.

Outcome

It took the better part of a year to restore the warehouse to effective control and then maintain a low level of infestation within acceptable guidelines. In this type of environment, a 100% sterile situation is impossible. Some eggs will still hatch, there will be the occasional stray mouse, etc. A good realistic outcome in this situation is effective control, which was achieved in this case.

This positive outcome was due to a high level of cooperation and communication between the warehouse management, several hundred warehouse employees, and the teams of on-site pest professionals. Another key to success was breaking the warehouse down into unique, identifiable sections of manageable size through the grid process and then bringing effective control to each section in a manner appropriate to the type of products stored in that section and its particular array of pest problems.

Questions for discussion:

1. Was the control plan appropriate for what was achieved?
2. What is the value of log sheets?
3. Discuss the role of communication in the pest control plan.

CASE STUDY #4: ELEMENTARY SCHOOL CAFETERIA

A 250,000-square-foot elementary school in Brevard County, Florida, consisting of eight concrete block buildings connected by overhead walkways, had a significant German cockroach, American cockroach, and Pharaoh ant infestation throughout the facility. Rooms were constructed on true floating slabs with dropped, acoustical tile ceilings throughout. Each classroom had a kitchenette that included a sink, a small refrigerator, and a microwave. Each classroom also had two bathrooms and a supply storage area. In addition to the mini-food facilities in each classroom, the school had a main cafeteria with food preparation and serving areas. The auditorium building had a huge storage area under the wooden stage.

Evaluation

After a thorough inspection of the entire property, and conversations with faculty, administrative staff, and maintenance staff, the pest management company found that the entire school had signs and many sightings of all three pests.

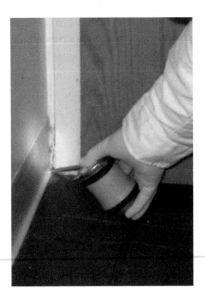

The primary difficulties in treating this facility were the time frame (service had to be rendered when children were not present), the many harborage areas (many cracks and crevices, some of which were not visible due to cabinets being directly on top of them), the numerous storage areas jammed with paper products, and pest food sources

FIGURE 13.26 Dusting Cove Base
Photo courtesy of Scott Nolen, Truly Nolen of America, Inc.

that were readily available all over the school (students who brought lunches and snacks, the kitchenette areas in each classroom, the main cafeteria, and the accidental spills and dropping of food by young children). Also, the pest professionals were limited by law as to what type and class of chemical material they could use to treat pests in a school environment.

Treatment

In close coordination with school officials, a treatment plan was developed to commence at the end of the school year. A key component of the plan was the removal of all stored paper products from classrooms, under the auditorium stage, and in the cafeteria. These items were removed and loaded into a tractor trailer unit stationed on the school's parking lot. The stored items were then treated with a total release pyrethrin aerosol which constituted a virtual fumigation, using pyrethrin in lieu of a **fumigant**.

Crews of pest technicians then implemented the treatment plan for the facility itself. A boric-acid based dust was placed in all accessible cracks and crevices throughout the facility, including the cafeteria. The school maintenance staff worked alongside the technicians, caulking cracks and crevices to seal in the dust. Baits of two types were used to control the German roach problems, an avermectin-based product in powder form and a gel bait containing hydramethylnon. Boric acid granular bait was used under the auditorium stage

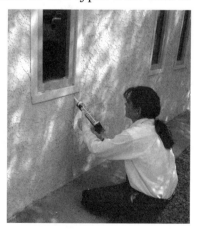

FIGURE 13.27 Caulking Below Window
Photo courtesy of Scott Nolen, Truly Nolen of America, Inc.

continues

to address the American roach problem. Boric-acid based ant syrup and a hydramethylnon-based bait were also used to control the Pharaoh ants.

Cracks and crevices on the exterior of the facility were treated with a boric-acid based dust and then caulked to seal in the material. A band of bifenthrin was sprayed to a height of 2 feet and to a distance of 10 feet out from each exterior wall.

Insect monitoring stations were placed throughout the facility and five stations were placed in each classroom: one in each of two classroom bathrooms, two in each kitchenette, and one in each classroom storage unit. Using these monitoring stations to guide further applications, follow-up services were rendered until the school was back in session. Additional treatments were rendered as needed.

Outcome

The facility was brought under effective control due to the ability to establish control while the school was not in session, children were not constantly bringing in new food sources, the fastidious treatment of pest harborages (applying dust in cracks and crevices which were then sealed), and the application of the appropriate baits. Throughout, close communication between the pest control professionals and school personnel helped ensure a successful outcome. Further, the school personnel were advised to keep all food products in containers—whether in the classrooms or cafeteria area—so these items would not act as an attractant to pests or be exposed to pests.

Questions for discussion:

1. Why would classrooms have pest problems?
2. Is a crack and crevice treatment appropriate?

CASE STUDY #5: RESTAURANT IN A MINI-MALL

The new owner of an Italian restaurant in a mini-mall in Broward County, Florida, requested the services of a pest professional due to a large population of German cockroaches. The previous owner had made little effort to control the pest problems. Some of the previous owner's equipment was left on the site for use in the new restaurant, and much of it was infested with roaches as well. The new owner expressed his willingness to cooperate in any way possible, which is always an important part of any pest control program.

Evaluation

After arriving for the first inspection of this facility, the pest control inspector noted that the roach infestation was primarily emanating from a wall shared by the Italian restaurant and another food-handling establishment next door. After asking for permission and then performing a brief inspection of the other facility, the inspector determined that this facility also had serious pest problems. In addition to pest problems, this restaurant had numerous sanitation issues that needed to be corrected. The inspector offered the services of his company to this establishment as well because it would be an ideal way to insure effective pest control for both restaurants. However, the other owner refused pest control assistance. In the Italian restaurant, more pockets of roach populations were found inside several of the pieces of equipment which were used by the previous owner. There were additional problem areas identified around the dish washing area.

After the inspection, a sanitation report was provided to the owner of the Italian restaurant to alert him to certain deficiencies which were contributing to the pest problems. These deficiencies included a large amount of moisture accumulating around the entire dish washing areas due to several leaks that needed to be fixed. Also, several base-

continues

Commercial Sanitation Report
Commercial Pest Management Program

Inspector: D. Perkins	Branch: 210	Date: 6/7/06

Account Name: Ma's Diner	
Address: 333 3rd Street	City/St/Zip: Anywhere, AZ 85000
Contact: Joan Smith	Phone: 555-5555
Type of Account: PC	Service Freq: monthly

Full inspection done? ☑ Yes ☐ No

✓	Service for-	Location of Infestation / Notes
	Rats	In food prep area. Mouse droppings from food prep cabinets must be removed.
✓	Mice	
	Ants	
✓	Cockroaches	
✓	Silverfish	
	Pigeons	
	Scorpions	

Sanitation Report

Yellow Zone
Windows/Ext. Doors — Y N
Insect/rodent harborages in walls? ☑
Pipe/conduit entries sealed? ☑
Doors rodent-proof? ☑
Doors kept closed? ☑
Windows screened & tight? ☑

Red Zone
Food Preparation — Y N
Equipment clean? ☑
Floors clean? ☑
Deli area clean? ☑
Bakery clean? ☑
Meat prep area clean? ☑

Red Zone
Public & Employee Areas — Y N
Restrooms clean? ☑
Locker rooms clean? ☑
Employee lounge clean? ☑

Red Zone
Storage Areas — Y N
Floors clean? ☑
Floor drains screened? ☑
All areas accessible? ☑
Wall space accessible? ☑
Food stored in sealed containers? ☑

Red Zone
Display Areas — Y N
Gondolas clean?
Produce area clean?
Spillage in candy/nut area?
Pet food spillage?
Spillage in flour/cereal area?

Green Zone
Exterior — Y N
Dumpster/compactor area clean? ☑
Lot free of rodent harborages? ☑
Loading dock clean? ☑
Wall space accessible? ☑
Lot free of trash/weeds? ☑

Other: Recommend sealing rodent access points + removing clutter behind equipment to reduce harborages.

Special Notes

Needed special materials to service account: N
Account has special policies/requirements related to service: N

Time needed to service: 40 mins	Additional time needed for special requirements: N

Additional details regarding account's general condition:

Customer's signature: J. Smith	Date: 6/7/06

FIGURE 13.28   Commercial Sanitation Report
Photo courtesy of Scott Nolen, Truly Nolen of America, Inc.

boards and metal coverings were in disrepair and needed to be replaced. Other baseboards were detached from the wall, creating harborage areas for insects. Several areas had numerous cracks and crevices that needed to be caulked. The owner was very receptive to these recommendations and agreed to take corrective measures immediately.

Treatment Plan

The primary goal of the initial pest control service was to treat the wall shared by the Italian restaurant and the restaurant next door to prevent roaches from accumulating in the wall. The technician drilled several areas of the wall and placed a fine film of a boric-acid dust product inside to prevent the migration of roaches from one restaurant to the other.

Then, control efforts were transferred to all of the equipment in the restaurant. Every piece of equipment was inspected and baited, using cockroach gel bait (containing hydramethylnon and fipronil) that would control the existing population. Particular attention was paid to the casters on each piece of equipment. Then, other areas were also treated with a gel bait product where permissible, and the areas which were likely to get hot when in use, such as equipment motors, were treated with dry bait (containing the active ingredient avermectin) that would not run when heated.

After the initial treatment, the pest control technician scheduled a follow-up visit with the owner of the facility in 2 weeks. On the second visit, all areas were inspected again and a reduction of about 85% of the roach population was noted. More bait application was performed, and additional insect monitoring stations were installed to assist in evaluating the effectiveness of the control efforts.

continues

Outcome

The location was visited in about a month, and no new roach activity was found. The owner of the restaurant was very pleased with the results and expressed his gratitude to the technician. The pest control company also expressed their appreciation to the owner for his willingness to cooperate and implement all of their recommendations to help make effective control achievable.

Questions for discussion:

1. Can control be achieved despite having common walls?
2. Was the role of baiting adequate?

Student Activity

1. Have students make an informal field trip to a few local restaurants, particularly ones identified in the newspaper as not quite meeting the required standards for sanitation. The students should look for pests or potential places pests can harbor and make a plan of action to resolve the problem.

Web Sites

EPA USA
http://www.epa.gov/pesticides/

USDA
http://www.csrees.usda.gov/ProgView.cfm?prnum=5257

Florida: http://edis.ifas.ufl.edu/IG095

California: http://www.co.el-dorado.ca.us/emd/envhealth/guide_food.html

North Carolina: http://ipm.ncsu.edu/getsubs2.cfm?TopicID=8

Indiana (Purdue): http://news.uns.purdue.edu/UNS/html4ever/
010910.B.Pest.Center.html

Nebraska: http://entomology.unl.edu/courses/ent407.html

References

1. Photos courtesy of Scott Nolen, Truly Nolen of America, Inc.
2. Mallis, Arnold. *Handbook of pest control* (9th ed.). (2005). Richfield, OH: Pest Control Technology (PCT).
3. Smith, E. & Whitman, R. (1992). NPCA field guide to structural pests. Dunn Loring, VA: National Pest Control Association.
4. Ebeling, Walter. Urban entomology. http://www.entomology.ucr.edu/ebeling/index.html.
5. Baur, F. (Ed.) (1984). *Insect management for food storage and processing.* St. Paul, MN: American Association of Cereal Chemists.
6. Hedges, S.A. & Moreland, D. (1995). *PCT field guide for the management of structure infesting flies.* Richfield, OH: G.I.E., Inc.
7. Hedges, S.A. & Moreland, D. (1994). *PCT field guide for management of structure infesting ants.* Richfield, OH: G.I.E., Inc.

PART IV

LONG-TERM PLANNING

## CHAPTER 14

MANAGING QUALITY IN FOOD AND NUTRITION SERVICES

Cheryl Koch, MS, RD, LD, FADA, CNSD and Carmen Roberts, MS, RD, CDE

Reader Objectives

After reading the objectives and reflecting on them, the student will be able to:

1. Identify key drivers behind health care and medicine today.
2. List key concepts of quality management.
3. Define benchmarking and how it can be applied to health care organizations.
4. Name important elements of regulatory compliance.
5. List major regulatory agencies that have an impact on nutritional care.
6. Identify main components of performance improvement and the steps involved in implementation.

Key Terms

Benchmarking: methodologies of quality and process improvement.

Joint Commission on Accreditation of Healthcare Organizations (JCAHO): a voluntary accreditation body that measures quality for healthcare companies.

Performance improvement: specializing in process, control, machinery, metering, automation, and energy solutions.

Quality management: a method for ensuring that all the activities necessary to design, develop, and implement a product or service are effective and efficient with respect to the system and its performance.

Health Care in the Twenty-First Century

The face of health care is changing. In contrast to a system that has historically structured itself to meet the needs of providers, payers, and insurers, health care now has the patient's needs and interests as its focus. In 1996, the Institute of Medicine (IOM) initiated a quality initiative focused on assessing and improving the nation's quality of care. In addition, the IOM issued a definition of quality that has become the foundation for much of the quality work that exists in health care today: "The degree to which health services for individuals and populations increase the likelihood of desired health outcomes and are consistent with current professional knowledge." Since this time, the IOM has focused on implementing its vision and completing a literature review in an effort to document the current challenges to providing quality health care today. By 2001, the IOM had issued two landmark reports: *To Err is Human: Building a Safer Health System* and *Crossing the Quality Chasm: A New Health System for the 21st Century*. The latter report defined six aims for improving health care quality by improving safety, effectiveness, timeliness, efficiency, and equity and by implementing patient-centered care. The IOM identified these changes in quality as being critical to improving health care. Ten years since the onset of the IOM's initiative, we have seen progress toward meeting these goals and a trend toward basing payment decisions on quality care and medical evidence. Payers are aligning reimbursement with outcomes and creating payment systems that recognize the cost of care when the care is provided using accepted standards of practice. One example is the change in nutrition reimbursement for diabetes management. Most payers will fully reimburse nutritional professionals for providing diabetes self-management training when specific guidelines are followed and standardized care is based on outcomes evidence. These trends are increasingly important as nutrition plays a role in programs such as the Hospital-Consumer Assessment of Health Plans Survey initiative, the Health and Human Services Medicare Quality Initiative, and the Hospital Compare Web site.

What Is Quality Management?

Quality management is the process of ensuring that all necessary activities are in place to design, develop, implement, and evaluate products and services. The quality management process is one of ongoing evaluation and constant readiness that is being driven by the new millennium's educated and demanding consumer.

All businesses and organizations are renewing their focus on *the customer*. Without the customer, organizations cannot sustain themselves and remain financially viable. Therefore, the focus of running a successful business, department, or facility should be to meet both the perceived needs of the customer and customer satisfaction. The quality and effectiveness of services provided to customers must be systematically evaluated and revised to produce the best overall outcome and to remain competitive within the marketplace.

Focus on Customer-Centered Care

Since the 1990s, health care has seen the evolution of customer-centered care, forcing providers and regulators to adapt to an environment of continual quality improvement and readiness. As health care providers view problems from the patient's point of view, they become more effective at recognizing and solving problems, allowing them to provide safe, quality care in an even more cost-effective manner. As nutrition professionals, it is essential to become actively engaged in this healthcare quality management effort.

Quality measurements are changing, as is the approach to **benchmarking** quality in health care. In 1987, the US Congress first developed a quality award named after Malcolm Baldrige who served as the Secretary of Commerce from 1981 until his death in 1987. The award is a tribute to his long term contributions toward improvement in the efficiency and effectiveness of government. This is a highly coveted award traditionally presented to business and educational organizations. Until recently, it had not been awarded to healthcare organizations; however, by 2004 there were four hospitals that had been recognized by this award. Healthcare facilities that have sought this

> **Learning Point:** Healthcare providers should view problems from the patient's point of view and become more effective at recognizing and solving problems, allowing them to provide safe, quality care in an even more cost-effective manner.

honor have taken the time to ask the questions: "What is important to our business, how do we address these needs, and what results are we achieving?" This reflects the desire of healthcare organizations to be recognized for excellence.

Measurement of Quality

In food and nutrition management, services and products are continuously evaluated in an effort to improve customer satisfaction and clinical outcomes. Examples include patient satisfaction with meals served, patient comprehension of nutrition education by a dietitian, and a variety of foods served in a clinical or retail food service environment. Outcome measurements can be used to improve the quality of delivered services in an institution. Examples of quality improvement initiatives include reducing patient wait time, management of inventory supply, promptness of tray delivery, and effectiveness of dietitian education.

Performance Improvement: Why Is it Important?

In the environment of health care today, it is essential for all managers to ensure that quality services and products are provided to all customers to remain competitive within the marketplace. Performance improvement, the process by which a problem is identified, analyzed, and resolved, can be used to track and evaluate processes and outcomes within a healthcare organization. Examples of performance improvement topics include *customer satisfaction, financial gains and losses, clinical outcomes, efficiency,* and *employee productivity.* Ideally, performance improvement initiatives are executed by a team within an organization that can identify a problem and work toward its solution to achieve an optimal outcome. The performance improvement team is often comprised of employees and managers who are closely tied to the initiative identified and will have the greatest impact on the desired outcome. Healthcare organizations are often required by regulatory agencies to develop, execute, and report results on performance improvement initiatives in an effort to continually improve clinical and process outcomes.

Why Implement a Performance Improvement Initiative?

There are many reasons to initiate the performance improvement process. Initiatives can be aimed at improving customer satisfaction, achieving improved clinical outcomes or public health objectives, or providing a quality product or service. Performance improvement projects are often customer- or client-driven in response to an identified problem or opportunity for improvement. Once a goal is achieved, the performance improvement process is used to continuously improve a process or to maintain a level of quality. The process can be motivating and rewarding to both managers and employees because the focus is outcome-oriented and positive results can be achieved. It enables staff to collaborate within their department and with other healthcare professionals. The process allows employees to become involved in identifying and working toward a solution in which they have a vested interest. The process can be beneficial for both the organization and employees alike.

The Performance Improvement Process

The performance improvement process is ongoing in that once a problem is identified and a solution is implemented, the process to maintain the desired outcome is monitored and evaluated on a continual basis to ensure that the level of quality is maintained. The analysis is customer-focused; it identifies a process and examines the key players who will have an impact on it. The process must include the ability to benchmark data in an effort to make improvements and repeat it if necessary.

There are multiple models for the quality improvement process that organizations can adopt to guide them through each step of implementation. All include the steps of *planning and organization, data collection and analysis, development and execution of a resolution,* and *ongoing evaluation* to ensure that the resolution is effective.

> **Learning Point:** Initiatives should be aimed at improving customer satisfaction, achieving improved clinical outcomes or public health objectives, or providing a quality product or service.

Many decisions need to be made before the project is implemented. Who will initiate the process improvement? How, where, and when will it be piloted? What data will be collected to measure the effect of the process improvement, who will collect it, and for how long? In identifying a quality improvement initiative, selection of the problem identified or a process to improve upon is the first step in implementation. The following steps should be identified in the initial stages of the process.

Team Involvement

It is essential to identify all stakeholders involved in the process. For example, if a food service manager wants to improve the efficiency of tray delivery in a hospital, he would not only want to involve the food service staff in problem resolution but also include nursing staff and facility personnel in the project because it may also impact their job flows and routines.

Identifying the Problem and Process

In order to have a better understanding of how a process works, the performance improvement team will map out the current process to more effectively examine the problem identified. There are multiple tools that are used to measure and monitor performance improvement. The team may use a flow chart (Figure 14.1) or a workflow diagram to map out the current process. The team may then use brainstorming or utilize a cause and effect diagram (Figure 14.2) or a fishbone diagram (Figure 14.3) to generate ideas about how to tackle the problem identified.

Once a problem is identified, the team will decide on a process or portion of the process to improve. The team will decide where, when, and how the data will be collected and measured. This is the active phase of the project and could vary from days to even months or years to complete, depending on the scope of the initiative. If the scale of the project is very large, the team may choose to pilot it on a smaller area, such as one medical unit or department, or on a smaller population for ease of implementation. Once the project is complete, the team may choose to roll out the improvement initiative to other areas in future phases.

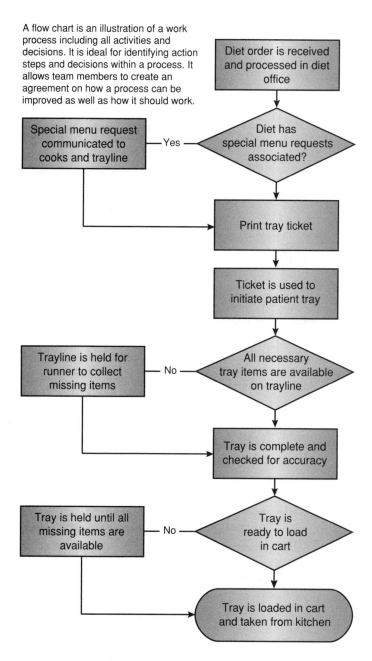

A flow chart is an illustration of a work process including all activities and decisions. It is ideal for identifying action steps and decisions within a process. It allows team members to create an agreement on how a process can be improved as well as how it should work.

Diet order is received and processed in diet office

Special menu request communicated to cooks and trayline — Yes — Diet has special menu requests associated?

Print tray ticket

Ticket is used to initiate patient tray

Trayline is held for runner to collect missing items — No — All necessary tray items are available on trayline

Tray is complete and checked for accuracy

Tray is held until all missing items are available — No — Tray is ready to load in cart

Tray is loaded in cart and taken from kitchen

FIGURE 14.1 Risk Assessment Matrix Combining Likelihood of Hazard Occurrence with Severity of Consequences of Hazard Occurring

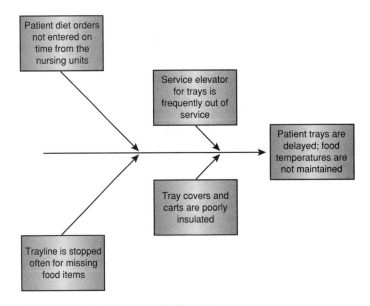

FIGURE 14.2   Cause and Effect Diagram

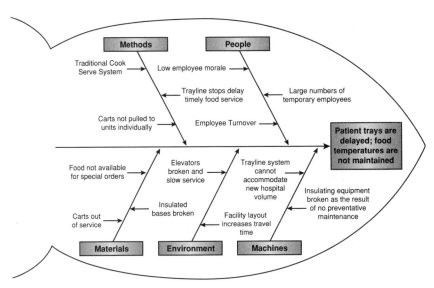

A fishbone diagram is essentially a pictorial display of a list. Each diagram has a large arrow identifying a problem. Lines off the large arrow represent main categories of potential causes or solutions for the problem. The most typical categories used for this diagram are equipment, people, machines, environment, and materials. You can create the categories that work best for the problem you are working through.

FIGURE 14.3   Fishbone Diagram

Measurement and Data Collection

After the team has decided on a performance improvement initiative, the data collection and analysis process begins. The team will make decisions about the factors that will be measured, what standards will be set, how the process will be carried out, and how the process will be reported in an effort to impact future decision making. It is important to remember that while benchmark or survey data may have assisted in identifying the need for a performance improvement process, additional data may need to be collected to supplement or provide additional information. Types and sources of data that may be collected in a healthcare environment include retrospective chart reviews, patient surveys, and open medical record reviews.

Multiple tools can be used in the data collection process, depending on the type of data collected. A simple checklist or questionnaire can be used for data gathering; in some cases, a more complex spreadsheet may be used to gather data for multiple variables. Data are then analyzed to make conclusions about the identified problem. Analysis tools include a workflow diagram, Pareto analysis, scattergram, histogram, and a control or run chart. This enables everyone involved to visualize the results and make conclusions about problem or process resolution.

Putting a Plan into Action

Once data are summarized and results are analyzed, the team proposes a solution to the problem identified based on the outcome of the data. If a solution is unclear at this time, the team may need to go back to the brainstorming and data collection phases of this process to drill down to find other causes and potential solutions to the problem identified.

Analysis and Ongoing Evaluation

The pilot should be evaluated for success utilizing data collection and analysis. Did the process improve as expected, and did data support the improvement? Often the performance improvement initiative may uncover additional project ideas and surprising results, which is why the process is ongoing. The team should evaluate the success of the pilot, and at that time evaluate whether or not the proposed change will be adopted by the organization, modified to better meet the needs of the project, or rejected in an effort to discover a new proposal for improving the process. Discussion among all stakeholders in the performance improvement initiative with regard to the program's successes and opportunities for improvement is a critical part of the process and a key step in starting the process improvement cycle again. Unlike older models for quality assurance, which focused on a problem and a threshold that must be met to resolve the problem, the model for performance improvement emphasizes raising the bar above problem resolution to ongoing and continued quality services. The performance improvement process is essential for all management staff to adopt to remain competitive for services in today's healthcare environment.

What Is Benchmarking?

Quality in health care is about achieving and maintaining excellence. The way both health care providers and patients view quality has changed significantly. It is part of our professional performance obligation, and our patients are demanding it. As one considers the **quality management** process, one of the most important tools that can be employed is benchmarking. Most simply put, benchmarking is the process of comparing the performance of one organization against others providing the same service or product. Benchmarking compares like products or services and is effective only if measurement is consistent and complete. Benchmarking is one of the most effective ways to understand performance, identify best practices, and assist in resource allocation to keep up with a constantly changing healthcare environment. Benchmarking allows an organization to identify top performers and to review practices or processes that can be adapted to meet specific organizational goals.

Benchmarking can occur as part of an internal departmental or institutional process or as part of an external data collection and analysis process. In many instances there are outside companies that are contracted to provide benchmark data for individual processes. Examples of internal data collection include collection of data by a department that is submitted to the hospital's quality management team who will then trend data between departments and services. External benchmarking for nutrition services may be done by a contract management company who is benchmarking between accounts and regions of the country, or by an association such as the Health Care Foodservice Management association which has a benchmarking service for its members. Tables 14.1 and 14.2 illustrate benchmarking monitors in foodservice and clinical nutrition.

Table 14.1 Example of Foodservice Benchmarking Monitors

Employee Sanitation and Safety	Benchmark	Outcome	Action
1. Change into a clean uniform or overgarment before service	100%	90%	Not met: It is mandatory that every employee has a clean uniform or cover while working. This quarter, the department was short of clean uniforms and will order more from the cleaners. This monitor will be followed up and ongoing.
2. Completed training in food service & customer care	80%	50%	Not met: Due to employee turnover and when training classes were offered, new employees were not able to meet this benchmark. Classes will be offered more often to accommodate the turnover. This monitor will be followed up and ongoing.
3. Completed food hygiene training	80%	70%	Not met: Due to employee turnover and when training classes were offered, new employees were not able to meet this benchmark. Classes will be offered more often to accommodate the turnover. This monitor will be followed up and ongoing.
4. Completed nutritional awareness training	50%	60%	Met: As a result of meeting this benchmark, the benchmark will be raised to 60% in ongoing monitors.

Table 14.2 Example of Clinical Nutrition Outpatient Clinic Benchmarking Monitors

	Benchmark	Outcome	Action
I. Criteria: Diabetes Medical Nutrition Therapy			
Indicator 1: Patients with Gestational diabetes who receive diet counseling will improve their blood glucose values and not require insulin.	90%	100%	Met: Continue diet counseling for referred patients. Recommend increased use of diet counseling. This monitor will be followed up and ongoing.
Indicator 2: Nutrition counseling for patients who are overweight will result in weight loss.	80%	67%	Not met: Continue diet counseling for referred patients. Ask patients to request follow-up counseling. This monitor will be followed up and ongoing.
Indicator 3: Nutrition counseling will improve blood glucose level.	80%	55%	Not met: Continue diet counseling that promotes glucose control. Overweight patients should continue weight loss. This monitor will be followed up and ongoing.
Indicator 4: As a result of diabetes counseling, patients will get an annual eye exam.	75%	50%	Not met: Continue to encourage eye exams, even if no symptoms are present for baseline data. This monitor will be followed up and ongoing.

Indicator 5: As a result of diabetes counseling, patients will get an annual foot exam.	75%	25%	Not met: Newly dx'd pts may not require a foot exam while under 40 years of age unless symptomatic. This monitor will be followed up and ongoing.
II. Criteria: Diabetes Complications Data Indicator 1: Patients who receive diabetes counseling will have a low incidence of ER/hospital visits or admissions.	75%	94%	Met: Continue diabetes education to promote self care and early signs that indicate medical care that can be managed as a non-emergency. Benchmark will be increased to 85%. This monitor will be followed up and ongoing.
Indicator 2: Patients who receive diabetes counseling will have a low incidence of foot infection.	80%	97%	Met: Continue diabetes education to promote self care and early signs that indicate medical care that can be managed as a non-emergency. Benchmark will be increased to 90%. This monitor will be followed up and ongoing.

Organizational Benchmarking

When starting the benchmarking process, it is important to consider data that can be provided by industries outside of your own. While benchmarking within your own industry is beneficial, it may not be desirable to limit benchmarking only to your competitors. If your competitor is unable to provide relevant data, it would not be valuable to include that company in the process. Take time to consider all providers of the service, especially those who serve as a model for quality service. For example, if you are converting to a room service delivery model, there may be some benefits in benchmarking yourself against hotel room service operations. While it is true that hotels do not deal with the same complexities in preparing a meal as a healthcare operation (therapeutic/modified diets and modified textures), wouldn't it be a great marketing tool to say that you can deliver meals to patient rooms in the same time frame as a five-star hotel's room service department?

One specific example of benchmarking that is utilized by all hospitals that are accredited by the **Joint Commission on Accreditation of Healthcare Organizations (JCAHO)** is the ORYX® initiative. This initiative integrates outcomes and other performance measurement data assisting organizations with their quality improvement efforts and assisting JCAHO with the accreditation process. While this initiative began in the late 1990s, the benchmarking initiative has evolved into collaboration between JCAHO and the Centers for Medicare and Medicaid Services, where common measures referred to as "hospital quality measures" were developed. These measures are important in assisting in alignment of quality care and in enabling comparisons with other healthcare facilities, resulting in national benchmarks.

Finally, managers of nutritional processes need to be careful not to fall into the trap of collecting data that either do not provide them with the information they need or that are not fully utilized. Data collection is time-consuming and often challenging. Benchmarking is beneficial only if the data analysis is completed and **performance improvement** planning and implementation take place. As we see health care continuing to strive for improved patient, employee, and physician satisfaction, we observe an increasing amount of cross-industry benchmarking and adaptation of tools. Hospitals are now employing companies like Ritz Carlton and

> **Learning Point:** The performance improvement process must include the ability to benchmark data in an effort to make improvements and repeat if necessary. The performance improvement process includes the steps of planning and organization, data collection and analysis, development and execution of a resolution, and ongoing evaluation to ensure that the resolution is effective.

Disney to provide training and service analysis to assist them in meeting their goals.

Regulatory Compliance

The health care arena is regulated by multiple agencies that have an increasing interest in provision of nutritional care, both clinically and operationally. As a result, agencies that previously have not paid close attention to the provision of patients' nutritional care are now incorporating new standards targeted specifically at nutrition services in healthcare facilities.

As this trend has evolved, regulatory guidelines with regard to nutrition have become more specific and outcome-focused. One example of this shift is the 1998 directive from President Clinton to improve care in nursing homes, called the Health Care Financing Administration (HCFA). This initiative resulted in an unprecedented effort to improve the nutritional status of nursing home residents, attaching financial penalties to those who failed to comply.

Similarly, JCAHO has integrated stronger nutritional standards into its survey process. Since compliance with JCAHO standards is linked directly to reimbursement of Medicare and Medicaid, healthcare facilities have tremendous incentive to comply. While these standards are less prescriptive and are more open to interpretation than the standards outlined by HCFA, they provide guidelines for nutrition education, clinical care, and safe storage and provision of food and nutritional products.

Regulatory Review

Regulatory review is important to ensure that excellent patient care is being provided and that the organization is committed to optimal outcomes. In the past, regulatory agencies have focused on compliance with policy and interpretation of standards; however. the process of ensuring compliance is changing. Current agency reviews attempt to validate institutional measures and performance improvement methods in order to improve patient safety and health, care quality. For example, JCAHO no longer wants to look at the organization's final survey score (did the facility pass the "test" by having all the right policies in place). Instead it has a focus toward achieving and maintaining excellence in health care as it evaluates the facility's commitment to improving patient outcomes.

JCAHO's shift toward excellence and continual readiness was most noticeable in 2004 when it implemented a tracer methodology to assist in reviewing organizations. This methodology requires surveyors to identify 10 to12 patients within the primary clinical service's groups, review the patients' medical records, and validate the care the patients received. Throughout this process, surveyors evaluate flow of information from one area to the other, identify system disconnects, and assess relationships between disciplines involved in the patient care process. JCAHO's findings will now result in a pass/fail recommendation with "requirements for improvement," which are items for which the organization must submit an action plan to correct.

While many regulatory reviews are mandatory, healthcare facilities and programs may select to be reviewed for a variety of reasons including peer recognition, financial implications, and to assist in identifying opportunities for change and improvement.

Regulatory review can be prestigious for a facility, providing high visibility and assisting in marketing the facility or service that is being reviewed or accredited. This type of review is typically optional and may only affect a specific service or area of the hospital. One example would be designation as a disease specific "center of excellence." Achieving this designation may not affect reimbursement but can ultimately affect the bottom line by attracting additional patients for services provided.

Regulatory review can also lead to financial gain, and many facilities or programs undergo regulatory review to assist in securing managed care contracts or to receive federal or state funding. In some instances a third party reviewer may substitute surveys for Medicare and Medicaid for federal certification. More commonly these reviews are mandatory; opting out may result in lack of funding or diminished resources. The HCFA example cited previously is a prime example of this type of review.

Finally, a facility may select to undergo a review process to facilitate change. The review process can assist an organization in supporting and enhancing programs and implementing strategic initiatives. For example, many healthcare organizations participate in quality patient surveys that will allow them to benchmark performance with indicators such as safety or patient satisfaction. The data from this benchmarking process are frequently used to assist with development of performance improvement initiatives.

Another way to facilitate change is through an internal review by either a facility or department. Internal reviews may utilize regulatory standards as part of their effort, or internal reviews may focus more on facility specific indicators or opportunities for improvement.

Regulatory Agencies

The following quality-related organizations may have some impact on nutritional standards and reviews that are completed in the healthcare environment. They should all be considered resources for nutrition professionals. Regulatory agencies and standards will vary by institution, patient population, geography, and level of accreditation.

Agency for Healthcare Research and Quality (AHRQ)

The AHRQ, which is governed by the Department of Health and Human Services, is an agency that supports research design that will ultimately improve health care quality, reduce costs, improve patient safety, decrease medical errors, and improve access to healthcare services. The goal of the AHRQ is to provide healthcare professionals, leaders, and policy makers with the outcomes research and information that are essential to providing informed decisions regarding healthcare quality.

The American Health Quality Association (AHQA)

The AHQA represents quality improvement organizations and professionals who are working collaboratively to improve healthcare quality in the United States. Through identifying opportunities for improvement and interpretation of data, the AHQA is able to provide assistance to health providers, hospitals, and nursing homes as they strive for quality improvement.

The National Association for Healthcare Quality (NAHQ)

The NAHQ is an organization of healthcare quality professionals that is focused on improving the quality of health care in all healthcare settings.

The National Guideline Clearinghouse™ (NGC)

The NGC is an initiative of the AHRQ in partnership with the American Medical Association and American Association of Health Plans. The NGC is a public resource for evidence-based clinical practice guidelines and other related materials produced by the AHRQ.

The Institute for Healthcare Improvement (IHI)

The IHI is a resource for healthcare organizations that assists them in making lasting quality improvements that result in enhanced clinical outcomes and cost-effective care.

The Institute of Medicine (IOM)

The IOM works to disseminate knowledge with the goal of improving the health of the nation. The institute has a body of publications that is evidence-based and provides health and science information and advice to policy makers within the government, corporate sector, and the public.

The Joint Commission on Accreditation of Healthcare Organizations (JCAHO)

JCAHO maintains standards that focus on improvement of quality and safety within healthcare organizations. The JCAHO evaluates over 15,000 healthcare organizations through an extensive on-site triennial survey, which is performed by a team of JCAHO healthcare professionals.

National Committee for Quality Assurance (NCQA)

The NCQA assesses and reports on the quality of the nation's managed care plans. The council provides an accreditation process that includes a survey conducted by teams of physicians and other healthcare experts to examine specific quality standards.

Summary

As the healthcare environment continues to become more focused on quality patient-centered care, nutrition professionals must meet the market demands to provide high-quality nutritional care in a cost-effective manner. Through quality management, an emphasis on continued performance improvement, and benchmarking against other organizations within a competitive marketplace, high-quality nutritional care can be successfully achieved.

Student Activities

1. Locate the Web site for the JCAHO's ORYX® initiative and describe it more fully.
2. Call a local hospital's foodservice department and discuss meeting a JCAHO regulation. What is the regulation and how is it monitored and documented?
3. Call a local health maintenance organization and discuss meeting a JCAHO regulation. What is the regulation and how is it monitored and documented?
4. Call a local hospital's clinical nutrition department and discuss meeting a JCAHO regulation. What is the regulation and how is it monitored and documented?
5. Locate several other regulatory agencies mentioned in this chapter and give specifics on their regulations.

Resources

American Dietetic Association. ADA quality management page. Retrieved July 17, 2006, from http://www.eatright.org/cps/rde/xchg/ada/hs.xsl/advocacy_354_ENU_HTML.htm.

Berwick, DM. (2004). *Escape the fire: Designs for the future of health care.* San Francisco, CA: Jossey-Bass.

Institute of Medicine Committee on Assuring the Health of the Public in the 21st Century, Board on Health Promotion and Disease Prevention. (2003). *The future of the public's health into the 21st century.* Washington, DC: National Academics Press.

Institute of Medicine. *IOM health care & quality page.* Retrieved July 17, 2006, from http://www.iom.edu/CMS/3718.aspx.

Joint Commission on Accreditation of Healthcare Organizations. JCAHO ORYX for hospitals page. Retrieved July 17, 2006, from http://www.joint commission.org.

Kovner, A.R. & Neuhauser, D. (Eds.). (2004). *Health services management: Readings, cases, and commentary.* (8th ed.). Chicago, IL: Health Administration Press.

Press, I. (2006). *Patient satisfaction: Understanding and managing the experience of care.* (2nd ed.). Chicago, IL: Health Administration Press.

Roizen, M.F. & Oz, M.C. (2006). *You, the smart patient: An insider's handbook for getting the best treatment.* New York, NY: Free Press.

Studer, Q. (2003). *Hardwiring excellence: Purpose, worthwhile work, & making a difference.* Gulf Breeze, FL: Fire Starter Publishing.

## CHAPTER 15

DISASTER PLANNING FOR FOODSERVICE OPERATIONS

Candace A Stewart, MS, RD, LD/N

Reader Objectives

After studying this chapter and reflecting on the contents, the student should be able to:

1. Understand the key steps in the development of an effective disaster plan (research, hazard analysis, policy and procedure development, task identification, writing of the disaster plan, and drill/critique/revision).
2. Understand that, through the development of a facility-specific disaster plan and implementation, successful outcomes in disaster management can be achieved.
3. Support the role of the food and nutrition services manager as a catalyst to champion the development of an effective disaster plan in his or her work environment.

Key Terms

Enteral feeding: a method to feed, in which a tube is placed through the body wall into the intestine, and a nutritious liquid is forced through the tube into the intestine.

FEMA (Federal Emergency Management Agency): an agency of the federal government having responsibilities in hazard mitigation.

Hazard analysis: identification, studies, and monitoring of any hazard to determine its potential, origin, characteristics, and behavior.

Nonperishable food: food that will not decay rapidly if left unrefrigerated.

Perishable food: food that will decay rapidly if not refrigerated.
Policy and procedure development: a guiding principle designed to influence decisions; a particular course of action intended to achieve a result.

Introduction

There is no question that events in recent history have intensified the focus on disaster or emergency preparation and response. Food and water are primary needs in the event of a disaster. But, what is the status of disaster planning in foodservice management today? How good are foodservice disaster plans when disasters really happen?

For the purposes of this chapter, "disaster" will be defined as any event that produces a serious interruption of electricity, gas, water supply, or labor that interferes with the preparation and distribution of food and water.

Guidelines and Regulations Regarding Disaster Plans and Resources

In many practice areas and geographical areas of the country, multiple government and regulatory organizations have established criteria regarding the requirements for disaster plans.[1-2] An institution frequently is obligated to comply with federal, state, and county requirements as well as private regulatory criteria. These various regulations and guidelines are extremely helpful in defining disaster plan practices. Additionally, the institution may have corporate guidelines and requirements.[6,7] Very typically, multichain institutions create generic policies that are intended to be individualized to each facility's specific needs. Each individual facility is responsible for crafting a plan specific to the environmental risks and the individual facility characteristics as well as adaptation for local applicable regulations.

Designated emergency feeding centers may additionally be guided by requirements from the Federal Emergency Management Agency (FEMA).[2] FEMA is a comprehensive source of information applicable to all practice environments.

Although many guidelines do exist to facilitate the development of a facility-specific disaster plan, too often little time is dedicated to crafting a facility-specific plan that will actually be useful in the event of a disaster. The development of disaster plans often becomes mere paper compliance, resulting in a disaster plan that is only an afterthought when the disaster actually strikes. As a manager in food and nutrition services, you may be the catalyst to ensure this process happens in your facility, with the potential for profound impact in the event of a disaster.

Developing a Life-Saving Disaster Plan

Where to Start?

An important concept in disaster management is that all areas of the facility must function as a team. A disaster plan for food and nutrition services in the absence of a facilitywide disaster plan is pointless. The process begins with the designation of a facility disaster committee. An effective disaster committee needs management support and time to complete a thorough examination of the disaster risk their facility and community may face, as well as the best approaches to address a disaster in the event that it becomes reality. The following are the necessary steps in developing a life saving disaster plan:

1. *Step One: Search for previous facility disaster plans and current regulatory and company requirements.*

   The prior experiences of the facility are extremely important in the evaluation of future risks. A facility disaster plan best functions when it is an accumulation of previous plans, review of experiences, and subsequent revisions. As previously mentioned, various levels of requirements exist regarding disaster plans, and the requirements frequently change. Ensure that you have the most current version of any requirements.

2. *Step Two: Hazard Analysis*

   This process begins with a disaster committee meeting, including representatives of all departments. Committee members begin by brainstorming the likely scenarios their facility may experience (see Table 15.1). Sample questions to ask include:

Table 15.1   Sample Hazard Analysis

The potential hazards that Smith's Nursing Center is vulnerable to are:

- Hurricanes
- Tornadoes
- Thunderstorms and lightning
- Power outages during severe hot or cold
- Hazardous materials incident from Crystal River Nuclear Power Plant
- Bomb threat
- Explosions from gas tank or propane tank storage companies
- Chemical spills
- Fire

- What are the potential hazards that this facility is vulnerable to experience?
- What disaster situations has the facility experienced in the past?
- Is this a facility that would likely be called upon to evacuate in the event of a weather event or would this facility be more likely to be receiving evacuees from elsewhere? Are both of these scenarios plausible?
- What disasters unrelated to weather are a potential?
- Does the facility have a generator?
- What risks does the facility face related to geographical location?
- Are there environmental factors that impose a potential risk?

3. *Step Three: Key Disaster Policy and Procedure Development*

Gather existing policy and procedures regarding attendance and role delineation in a disaster setting. The committee again brainstorms on application and identifies the need for a new policy (see Table 15.2).

Sample questions to ask here are:
- What is the chain of command in the absence of the administrator, etc?
- What will the expectations be regarding attendance?
- Are attendance practices different for staff not responsible for direct care?

Table 15.2   Policy and Procedures—Disaster Preparedness

It is the policy of Smith's Nursing Center that all department managers are required to report to duty in the event of a hurricane or any other type of a disaster situation. All managers are expected to remain throughout the duration unless the administrator determines otherwise. Positions that are considered department heads are Administrator, Director of Nursing, Maintenance Director, Medical Records Director, Therapy Director, MDS Coordinator, Food and Nutrition Services Manager, Housekeeping Director, Activities Director, and Social Services Director.

It is the policy of Smith's Nursing Center that staff may bring family members to the facility if needed. The therapy department will be set up to accommodate family. All family members must bring their needed personal items, clothing, bottled water, and medications.

It is the policy of Smith's Nursing Center that the administrator's office will be designated as the News Center. The News Center will be equipped with radio and backup supplies in the event of a power outage. In the event of a disaster, department heads will be updated hourly and will communicate updates to staff.

The news room will additionally be equipped with a cell phone for emergency use only.

- When will lockdown situations exist?
- Can staff bring family or pets to the facility?
- How are staff compensated for disaster hours?

4. *Step Four: Task Identification*

   Next, committee members are assigned to develop a list of tasks needed to prepare for an impending disaster–tasks to be completed during an active disaster and tasks to be completed during recovery (see Table 15.3).

   Sample questions to ask here include:
   - What types of supplies and services may be needed in each plausible situation?
   - Who will be responsible for purchasing and storing supplies?
   - Who will be responsible for maintaining an active phone list?

Table 15.3   Task Identification—Hurricane Preparedness

Eight hours before anticipated landfall:

Dietary

1. Relocate emergency supplies to accessible area within the facility.
2. Review the emergency menus and prepare to implement.
3. Ensure that a printed copy of all resident diets and allergy is available.
4. Print a 3-day supply of tray and nourishment tickets.
4. Direct staff to begin filling collapsible containers with water.
5. Begin limiting unnecessary water usage.
6. Adjust staff arrival times to avoid travel during the storm.
7. Notify all dietary staff of attendance expectations during the storm and confirm contact numbers.

- What are the primary roles of each department head and staff?
- Who will maintain news contact and inform staff of status?
- Who will coordinate relief efforts for staff?

5. *Step Five: Disaster Plan Is Written for Each Likely Event*

   The information developed from the previous steps is written in simple, specific terms for each potential disaster event (see Table 15.4). The comprehensive plan is developed, and copies of the plan are positioned in highly visible areas of all departments.

6. *Step Six: Staff Training*

   A sometimes forgotten essential element of the process is staff training. Very often disaster policies and procedures are briefly reviewed at the time of hire. Frequently, updates to the disaster plan are not reviewed with staff. Subsequently, years later when the disaster plan is activated, the staff are unprepared to take on their roles and responsibilities. Policies and procedures, unique to a disaster event, should be reviewed in detail followed by a test to ensure comprehension and frequent repetition.

7. *Step Seven: Disaster Drill, Critique, and Revision of Disaster Plan*

   A drill is conducted by notifying staff of the disaster plan policy. Staff are advised that a specific disaster drill is being conducted

Table 15.4   Hurricane Plan (Introduction)

Purpose: To provide an effective plan for the Smith's Nursing Center to be used in time of emergency to prevent, minimize, and to the extent possible overcome the effect of emergency circumstance and/or natural disasters.

Situation: Smith's Nursing Center is located in Hudson, Florida, in Pasco County. Based on historical data, the occurrence of a hurricane is likely. This center is located 19.75 feet above sea level, with risk for flooding from coastal water surges.

Scope: This plan is designed to be used to prevent loss of life from the hazard discussed above. The size and severity of the hurricane will dictate the preparation and response that must be coordinated with this effort. This hurricane plan will address expectations of the facility and staff for their own well-being and possibly for evacuees who will be brought into the facility. This plan is organized to correspond to a sequence of probable events that would normally take place as a hurricane approaches, when it reaches the facility, and the aftermath of recovery after the storm has passed.

and they are to report to work and perform their tasks as directed by the disaster plan. Staff are expected to perform as if the conditions were real. Following the conclusion of the drill, observations and comments are recorded and utilized to drive indicated revisions in the plan.

Learning Point: In many disaster settings, electrical outages, gas outages, water outages, sewer line backups, and equipment failure are immediate consequences with direct impact on the Food and Nutrition Services Department. As a manager in Food and Nutrition Services, a significant role you will play will be to promote a controlled, organized approach to feeding your population. Your composure will impact your staff significantly. Prepare yourself for this role through detailed review of your department's roles in the event of a disaster. Consistently and fairly implement the disaster policies and procedures regarding staff tasks and attendance. Model the team approach through your support of other departments during this crisis.

Disaster Policies and Procedures for Food and Nutrition Services

Food and Nutrition Services disaster policies and procedures should address the various circumstances that may present to your department. For example, a policy and procedure should address if the facility has a functioning generator and designate key outlets in the food and nutrition services department that should be connected to the generator. This may be the only change necessary when the facility is under generator power, and no other changes in procedures may be necessary. However, if your facility does not have a generator, or your department is not included on the facility's main emergency generator, or the generator fails, many subsequent procedures should follow.

Key procedures should also center on refrigeration, storage, and use of **perishable** items. Refrigerated and previously frozen items that have been maintained in the appropriate temperature range are utilized before utilizing the **nonperishable** menu items. Policies and procedures should be written simply with an indication of when they are put in place. Reference to these procedures will prevent the unnecessary discarding of safely served food items.

Additional information included in the department's emergency food and nutrition services manual should include current contact numbers for all staff and vendors.

Many managers also prepare a disaster food order in coordination with their food vendor and include this as a component of their disaster plan. This order includes additional snack food items, nonperishable items, and paper supplies to be ordered in addition to their existing disaster supply stock. Should a pending disaster occur during the absence of the manager, the order may be submitted by anyone available in the facility.

Emergency Food and Water Supply

In the absence of other regulatory requirements, MyPyramid may be utilized to determine quantities of foods needed to feed your population for a specific time frame. Basic water needs are often planned to provide a minimum of 1 gallon of water per resident per day for drinking purposes only.[3] Significantly more water will be required

> **Learning Point:** Unfortunately, vendor contracts are of limited benefit because they frequently are unable to be honored in the event of an actual emergency due to available supply and delivery issues. It would be wise to contact smaller, local vendors that have supplies on hand for emergencies. Do not rely on one vendor for an emergency.

for bathing and other care issues. Storage of sufficient water to supply the recommended volume is challenging for many facilities. Plastic collapsible containers can be obtained from most foodservice suppliers. These containers are stored flat and are available to be filled with water when a disaster warning is issued. Most facilities enter into contractual agreements with vendors to supply water in the event of an emergency.

In most areas of practice, regulatory guidelines mandate the food supply that must be maintained by the facility.[1] Typical minimum requirements are 3 days of nonperishable food items, but in some cases, the requirements are for a 7-day supply.

Disaster or emergency menus should be written simply and be easy to follow (see Table 15.5). The disaster menu determines the food items and amounts necessary to ensure adequacy of non-perishable food items. From the menu, disaster food needs can be estimated and procured (see Table 15.6). In the event of a disaster, policies allow for residents to be placed on the least restrictive therapeutic diet possible; consistency restrictions remain for safety.

Frequently disaster plans fail to anticipate needs for feeding and hydrating staff and sometimes families and even pets during a disaster. Independent of the regulatory requirements for food and water supplies for your population, additional food and water supplies must be available for staff. If the facility allows for family or pets to be brought into the facility, supplies must also be available to accommodate both family and pets.

Also frequently forgotten are replacements for nutritional supplements. A sufficient supply of canned supplements not requiring refrigeration or dry milk products to prepare an alternate supplement must be included in the emergency supply stock.

Table 15.5   Sample Menu: Non-Perishable Food Items

Regular Diet	Mechanical Soft Diet	Pureed Diet
Breakfast		
6 ounce Orange Juice	same	same
¾ cup Cold Cereal	same	¾ cup Cream of Wheat
2 ounce Canned Ham	2 ounce ground ham	2 ounce pureed ham
2 pkg Saltines	2 pkg moistened crackers	2 pkg moistened crackers
8 ounce Reconstituted Dry Milk	same	same
8 ounce Beverage	same	same
Sugar, salt, pepper	same	same
Lunch		
½ cup Tuna Salad	same	½ cup pureed tuna salad
1 sl Bread	same	1 slice pureed bread
or 2 pkg crackers	same	or crackers
½ cup Carrot salad	same	½ cup purred carrots
½ cup Pears	same	½ cup pureed pears
8 ounce Reconstituted Dry Milk	same	same
8 ounce Beverage	same	same
Sugar, Salt, Pepper	same	same
Dinner		
1 cup Ravioli	same	1 cup pureed ravioli
½ cup Green Beans	same	½ cup pureed green beans
1sl Bread	2 pkg moistened crackers	2 pkg moistened crackers
or 2 pkg crackers		
5 Vanilla Wafers	same	5 pureed vanilla wafers

8 ounce Reconstituted Dry Milk	same	same	
8 ounce Beverage	same	same	
Sugar, Salt, Pepper			
HS Snack			
3 Graham Crackers	same	3 pureed Graham Crackers	
6 ounce Juice	same	same	

Table 15.6 Guidelines for Calculating Servings Per Can Size

Size of Can	Net Weight	Serving Size		
		Number of 4 ounce (½ cup) servings	Number of 6 ounce (¾ cup) servings	Number of 8 ounce (1 cup) servings
#10	105 ounces	26	17	13
#5	46 ounces	11	7	5.75
#303	16 ounces	4	2.6	2
#300	14 ounces	3.5	2	1.7

Volunteers and Their Role in Food and Nutrition Services

The use of volunteers or family in food and nutrition services should be encouraged. Policies should allow for cross training of other department staff and/or family members to complete simple food preparation or cleaning tasks. Participation of volunteers will both spare fatigued dietary staff of these tasks and allow volunteers to feel a part of the facility's efforts to feed residents and staff.

Disaster Paper and Chemical Supplies

An often underestimated need in the Food and Nutrition Services Department is the need for paper products and chemicals. Assuming no ability to utilize a dish machine, paper products will be required to replace all plates, dishes, cups, feeding utensils, and trays. Additional paper products will also be necessary for patient hydration passes, snacks, and medication administration. Clarification as to which department purchases and stores what for these shared tasks is essential in the disaster planning process.

An additional basic item often overlooked is the need for trash bags. Because garbage disposals are nonfunctioning and trash pick-up services are disrupted during disaster conditions for lengthy periods of time, trash accumulation is excessive and the use of trash bags skyrockets.

Trayline pans, bowls, utensils, and scoops will require sanitizing by chemical solution. The need for chemical sanitizer is often underestimated, especially in facilities that typically sanitize via a high temperature dish machine not requiring chemical sanitizers.

The need for hand sanitizers is also essential because hand washing sinks may be unavailable. Lastly, the need for batteries, flashlights, and radios is often forgotten in the dietary supply inventory; these essential items are invaluable.[5,8]

Food and Nutrition Services Resident or Patient Information

The ability to access resident or patient information regarding dietary orders and allergies is often challenging during a disaster. Frequently, computerized tray ticket systems are unavailable. A policy and procedure designed to ensure that a current paper listing of all diet orders and allergies is available at all times is an essential component of a food and nutrition services disaster plan. Blank tray tickets must be included in the disaster supply to allow for the provision of handwritten tray tickets.

Clinical Issues in Disaster Planning in Foodservice Management

Many clinical nutrition issues are impacted in the event of a disaster. As the focus switches to surviving the present moment, very often the interruption of the usual daily routine results in a decline in interest in consuming foods and beverages. Especially in the case of the elderly, guarded hydration and nutritional status may already exist and may become quickly exasperated even after only a few days of minimal intake of food and fluids. The unavailability of air conditioning or heat can rapidly impact hydration status. The profusely sweating or shivering frail elderly in a disaster environment is a clinical challenge for everyone. As the Food and Nutrition Services Manager, another important aspect of your role will be to refocus staff on the priority of feeding and hydrating your population, as well as themselves.

At particular risk are the special needs population residents, such as dialysis dependent residents, tube fed residents, and dependent diners. Comprehensive disaster plans should include a component to ensure dialysis residents are dialyzed when possible and that, if appropriate, more stringent fluid and diet restrictions are put in place. For residents receiving tube feedings, a sufficient supply of enteral products, as well as delivery systems and water for flushes, must be included in the emergency supply.[11] As previously noted, a comparable replacement for nutritional supplements that require refrigeration is frequently forgotten in the facility's disaster food supply inventory. Dependent diners require lengthy assistance to consume meals. Facility staff may be undermanned and exhausted. Policies and procedures to utilize families and volunteers to assist with dependent diners are essential in a complete disaster plan.

A factor, also not often anticipated, is the potentially poor acceptance of room temperature food items served per the disaster menu. Chili at room temperature may meet the infection control guidelines and nutritional analysis, but will anyone actually consume it? Alternate food items such as peanut butter crackers or cheese crackers may be of less value from a nutritional standpoint; however, they will result in more value to the resident because they will be consumed. The availability of snack foods and beverages may greatly enhance the intake of your population.[8,10]

Recovery Post Disaster

Often, very little emphasis is placed on recovery. However, as a manager you may find that a return to usual practices and systems is more difficult than anticipated. In this phase, your department may have full use of electricity, water, and other supplies, but your employees are still operating at a reduced capacity. The impact of the realization that perhaps their home has been destroyed or their spouse's income is lost may contribute to significant stress, resulting in changes in behavior and performance of your staff. Human Resources can assist you in providing staff with information regarding resources, such as FEMA, the Red Cross, or other relief efforts. As a manager, your *positive approach* to recovery and compassion will further build staff's support of your leadership. The American Dietetic Association has fostered the involvement of nutrition professionals in relief efforts through active Web site postings (www.eatright.org) during the relief efforts and has established a fund for members most in need.[9]

Barriers in the Development of Successful Disaster Plans

Managers may suffer from complacency, assuming, for example, that they are immune to disasters or that they will be taken care of by their generator. During recent weather disasters, generators were unable to continue to function after days and weeks of use. A second fallacy is the belief that a disaster can't happen at your facility because you are a large hospital with very ill patients; you believe your facility is a priority and that you'll have power restored very quickly in the event of a disaster. Again, history has shown us that in a large disaster there are simply too many critical areas to be prioritized and serviced promptly.

Disaster plans require effort and foresight. Often in today's work environment of cost controls and labor management, many facilities just don't take the time to work out the process of emergency

> **Learning Point:** As a Food and Nutrition Services Manager, your responsibility is to ensure that policies and procedures are in place to nourish and hydrate your population in any anticipated situation. To accomplish this in the event of a disaster requires a management team committed to the goal. You are in a position to advocate for your population on an issue crucial to their care. Assume the role of catalyst in your work environment and spearhead the move to develop a disaster plan that will make a crucial difference in your facility!

planning. The current status of disaster plans and disaster preparedness in many facilities is of serious concern.

Summary

Events in recent history have focused attention on disaster preparations and response. The delivery of food and water is a primary need in the event of a disaster. Multiple layers of government authorities, voluntary certifications, and corporate policies direct the requirements for disaster plans in healthcare facilities. Each facility is responsible for developing and implementing a plan that meets the established criteria. Due to time constraints and complacency, disaster plans are often seen as mere paper compliance. Developing an effective disaster plan requires:

1. Research regarding the regulations specific to the institution
2. **Hazard** analysis
3. **Policy and procedure development**
4. Task identification
5. Writing of the disaster plan in simple terms
6. Staff training
7. Drill, critique, and revision

Disaster policies and procedures for Food and Nutrition Services should address the specific circumstances that may happen in the facility, for example, what employees should do if there is no power and no generator. Standard guidelines and practices regarding food safety must be practiced at all times.

Emergency food and water supply requirements vary in practice, setting, and geographic area. Storing adequate water is difficult; collapsible containers are frequently utilized to conserve storage space. Emergency or disaster food supply corresponds to the written menu and is replaced at frequent intervals to prevent spoilage.

Food and Nutrition Services disaster policy and procedures frequently do not account for the food and fluid needs of staff, families, and possibly pets in addition to residents or patients. Failure to account for these needs can result in significant inadequacies of supplies. Disaster supplies of paper products and chemicals are another area typically underestimated.

A key component of the Food and Nutrition Disaster Plan is a provision to ensure that a record of all resident diets and allergies is available. Special needs residents, such as those requiring dialysis, **enteral feedings**, or assistance with feeding, are at high risk of nutrition and hydration-related complications and need special planning.

Post disaster recovery is rarely a component of disaster plans. A positive approach and compassion toward staff will further build staff's support of your leadership.

Student Activities

1. Telephone a healthcare work environment and inquire of staff if a written disaster plan exists for the facility and where it would be located. If staff are unable to answer this question, ask the manager. How many people did you have to ask before you located the plan?
   a. Once you have located the disaster plan, evaluate the plan based upon what you have learned in this chapter.
   b. Is the plan current? What date was it last revised?
   c. What are the regulatory guidelines applicable to the facility?
   d. Is the plan specific to the facility or is it a generic plan?
   e. Does it appear that the facility followed the seven steps outlined in the chapter to develop the plan?
   f. How useful do you feel this plan would be if a disaster were to occur at this facility today?

    g. Are the policies and procedures easily understood?

    h. Is the disaster menu practical?

    i. What would you do differently?

2. Select a healthcare environment and investigate the regulatory guidelines regarding this type of facility. Apply the seven steps outlined in the chapter and develop a sample disaster plan applicable to the facility for one specific scenario. Develop a policy and procedure specific to disaster menus for the facility.

References

1. American Health Care Association. (1999). *The long term care survey: Regulations, forms, procedures, interpretive guidelines.* Washington, DC.
2. Federal Emergency Management Agency. (2001). State and local guide 101: Guide for all-hazard emergency operations planning. Retrieved October 1, 2005, from http://www.fema.gov/pdf/rrr/allhzpln.pdf.
3. Florida Health Care Association. (2005). *FHCA disaster preparedness guide.* Tallahassee.
4. Joint Commission on Accreditation of Healthcare Organizations. (2005). Standing together: An emergency planning guide for America's communities. Retrieved January 15, 2006, from http: www.jcaho.org.
5. U.S. Food and Drug Administration. (2005). FDA offers valuable food safety information for hurricane aftermath. Retrieved October 1, 2005, from http://www.cfsan.fda.gov.
6. Diversicare Management Services. (2005). *Foodservice policy and procedure manual.* Brentwood, TN.
7. HCR-Manor Care. (2006). *Dietary procedures manual: Foodservice guidelines.* Toledo, OH.
8. Centers for Disease Control. (2006). Hurricane recovery: Keeping food and water safe. Retrieved October 1, 2005, from http: bt.cdc.gov.gov.disasters.
9. Molt, M. (2005). *Food for fifty* (12th ed.). Saddle River, NJ: Prentice Hall.
10. Stein, K. (2006). Will you be ready to help when disaster hits? *Journal of the American Dietetic Association, 106*(2), 190–194.
11. Sysco Foodservices. (2002). *Disaster plan.* Palmetto, FL.
12. U.S. Department of Health and Human Services. (2005). *2005 Food Code.* College Park: Public Health Service, Food and Drug Administration, Center for Food Safety and Applied Nutrition.

CHAPTER 16

FOOD SAFETY AND BIOTERRORISM

Sam Beattie, PhD, and Beverly McCabe-Sellers, PhD, RD

Reader Objectives

After studying this chapter and reflecting on the contents, the student should be able to:

1. Describe the scope of the bioterrorist threat to the food supply.
2. Identify organisms that may be disseminated by ingestion.
3. Describe the foods most at risk of intentional contamination.
4. Compare and contrast the challenges in distinguishing an intentional food contamination from an unintentional food contamination.
5. Recommend actions foodservice managers may take to promote preparedness.

Key Terms

Bioterrorism agents/diseases:
Category A
- Can be easily disseminated or transmitted from person to person;
- Result in high mortality rates and have the potential for major public health impact;
- Might cause public panic and social disruption; and
- Require special action for public health preparedness.

Category B
- Are moderately easy to disseminate;
- Result in moderate morbidity rates and low mortality rates; and
- Require specific enhancements of the Centers for Disease

Control and Prevention's (CDC's) diagnostic capacity and enhanced disease surveillance.

Category C: emerging pathogens that could be engineered for mass dissemination in the future because of availability, ease of production, and dissemination; potential for high morbidity and mortality rates and major health impact.

Terrorism: includes the unlawful use of force or violence against persons or property to intimidate or coerce a government, the civilian population, or any segment thereof, in furtherance of political or social objectives.

Introduction

Historically, the concept of food security has been in the context of an adequate, nutritious, and acceptable food supply for individuals and families. Recent events have given the phrase food security new meaning: food defense. Food defense means protection of food from *intentional adulteration* by aggressors who are intent on harming a population of people either physically, psychologically, or economically. This concept is different than food safety, which involves the natural or unintentional contamination of foods by physical, chemical, or biological hazards. Food **terrorism** then is the intentional adulteration of food to affect a political, economic, social, or other type of change.

Foodservice establishments, whether they are for-profit or nonprofit, serve an incredible number of meals each day and have a tremendous economic impact in the United States. The United States Department of Agriculture (USDA) Economic Research Service and National Restaurant Association estimate that approximately 500 billion dollars were spent on food consumed away from home in 2005 with nearly half of all food dollars (over a trillion dollars) going to purchasing food that is eaten away from home.[1] This involved over 70 billion experiences outside of the home.[2] The commercial foodservice industry employs over 12 million people, making it the largest private employer sector in the United States.[2] These statistics show the sheer size of the foodservice industry and how difficult it may be to ensure food defense within such a large and diverse sector.

The recognition that food could be used as a threat preceded the events of September 11, 2001. There have been several incidents of tampering with food with the intent to cause illness or economic disruption throughout history. Several of these are outlined in Table 16.1. Prior to 2001, assessment of the security of the food supply had been addressed by several think tank research groups, including the Rand Corporation. The incident on September 11, 2001, caused the U.S. government to assess the national security and look for vulnerabilities existing in the country. In response to this, the U.S. Congress passed and the president signed the Public Health Security and Bioterrorism Preparedness and Response Act of 2002 (The Bioterrorism Act). This act mandated that regulatory agencies such as the Food and Drug Administration (FDA) and the Food Safety and Inspection Service of the USDA implement specific provisions regarding the food supply. These provisions were directed at all aspects of the food supply chain and started with the registration of all food processing facilities, feed mills, and distributors of foods. The four provisions and their implementation dates are:

- Registration of Food Facilities (December 12, 2003) requires that all *domestic and foreign facilities that manufacture/ process, pack, or hold food for human or animal consumption in the United States register with the FDA.* This excludes restaurants, farm stands, retail grocers and establishments, and nonprofit food establishments as well as those food processors exclusively regulated by the USDA (mainly poultry and meat processing). The rationale of registering a food facility is that rapid notice could be given if a food processing sector is identified as a target for terrorist groups.
- Prior Notice of Imported Food Shipments (December 12, 2003) requires that all shipments of food to the United States from other countries be registered with the FDA *before* the food arrives in the United States. Historically, importers were required to report to the Bureau of Customs and Borders Protection only after the food arrived. The new requirement allows for increased inspection prior to a food arriving in the United States.
- Administrative Detention of Foods (published June 4, 2004 but took effect in 2002) gives new power to the FDA to detain foods that are suspect and of possible health concern for humans or animals. Effectively, if the FDA has credible evidence that a food was adulterated to make it a health

hazard for humans or animals, that food could be impounded for up to 30 days while an investigation goes forward to determine its safety.

- Establishment and Maintenance of Records (December 9, 2005 and other dates depending upon size of facility) requires that all companies involved in the food chain maintain records on manufacture, transportation, and distribution of their foods. Specifically, any manufacturer or processor, transporter, packager, distributor, and importer must be able to track who was the immediate previous supplier or transporter and who is the very next recipient of the food. An example of this would be a grocery store that receives food from distributor XYZ, and the food is shipped by trucking company ABC. The grocer would be required to track that the food was shipped by XYZ by means of ABC. However, the grocery would not be required to document what consumer received the food. This record-keeping requirement is commonly maintained by many companies. The new rule requires that all who process, handle, or transport food maintain these records for a minimum of 2 years. The rationale for this rule is to allow rapid and complete traceability and recall of a suspect adulterated food.

Table 16.1 Specific Examples of Food Tampering in the US and World

1978 Militant Middle Eastern group claimed injection of mercury into Israeli oranges imported into Europe

1984 Salmonella in salad bars. Oregon1989 Claim that Chilean grapes were contaminated with cyanide resulted in loss of millions of dollars to the Chile produce industry – claims were never substantiated.

1993-4 Intentional use of banned pesticide on millions of bushels of oats destined for breakfast cereal. Loss to cereal company $167 million.

1994 Intentional Shigella contamination of pastries by unhappy employee – 12 made ill.

2003 Intentional contamination of hamburger with a nicotine-based pesticide. 92 ill customers.

These new laws help expand the ability of the FDA to recall and detain a suspect adulterated food. The USDA implemented similar rules specific to the meat and poultry processing sector.

In addition to the Bioterrorism Act of 2002, the President of the United States has issued Homeland Security Directives in the intervening years. Directive Nine (2003) specifically addressed food and agriculture sectors and mandated several action steps:

- Identify and prioritize sector-critical infrastructure and key resources to establish protection requirements.
- Develop awareness and early warning capabilities to recognize vulnerabilities.
- Mitigate vulnerabilities at critical production and processing nodes.
- Enhance screening procedures for domestic and imported products.
- Enhance response and recovery procedures.

Through cooperative efforts involving the local, state, and federal agencies, the defense of the food supply has changed over the past several years. However, as this chapter will demonstrate there are key defense measures that a foodservice operator can utilize to ensure the food that they produce is safe.

Threats to Our Food Supply

History has shown that there are several types of hazards that can be introduced to foods. However, for an adulterant to be effective several criteria must be met. Importantly, the adulterant or threat of adulterant does not necessarily have to cause mass illness but may cause economic or psychological damage to the population. Important factors to consider when identifying whether an agent can be used as a food adulterant are 1) dissemination either from person to person or through food; 2) the number of casualties it produces; 3) the impact on public psyche and economies; 4) requires an investment in health care, social services, food defense, and other types of planning. The CDC has placed specific agents in categories (A is the highest; then B and C) based upon the matching of these criteria (Table 16.2). In all cases, preventing these agents from entering the food supply is the most effective way to protect health.[3]

Table 16.2   Categorization of Bioterrorism Weapons for Use in
                 Foods or Water

Category A Diseases/Agents

The U.S. public health system and primary healthcare providers must be
prepared to address various biological agents, including pathogens that are
rarely seen in the United States. High-priority agents include organisms that
pose a risk to national security because they can be easily disseminated or
transmitted from person to person; result in high mortality rates and have
the potential for major public health impact; might cause public panic and
social disruption; and require special action for public health
preparedness.

Specific Agents that could be disseminated in foods:

Anthrax (Bacillus anthracis)

Botulism (Clostridium botulinum toxin)

Plague (Yersinia pestis)

Smallpox (variola major)

Tularemia (Francisella tularensis)

Category B Diseases/Agents

Second highest priority agents include those that are moderately easy to
disseminate; result in moderate morbidity rates and low mortality rates; and
require specific enhancements of the CDC's diagnostic capacity and
enhanced disease surveillance.

Specific Agents that could be disseminated in foods:

Brucellosis (Brucella species)

Epsilon toxin of Clostridium perfringens

Food safety threats (e.g., Salmonella species, Escherichia coli O157:H7,
Shigella)

Q fever (Coxiella burnetii)

Ricin toxin from Ricinus communis (castor beans)

Staphylococcal enterotoxin B

Water safety threats (e.g., Vibrio cholerae, Cryptosporidium parvum)

Category C Diseases/Agents

Third highest priority agents include emerging pathogens that could be
engineered for mass dissemination in the future because of availability;
ease of production and dissemination; and potential for high morbidity and
mortality rates and major health impact.

Specific agents that might be used in the food supply by aggressors include:

- Biological
- Chemical
- Physical
- Radiological

The least likely of these agents to be found in foods are radiological or radioactive compounds. These are difficult to obtain, produce, and handle, which makes them unlikely to be used in an intentional contamination of large quantities of foods. Either chemical or radiological agents would have an immediate effect on the targeted population. On the other hand, biological agents disseminated in foods would take potentially days before the targeted population felt an effect.[4] This makes the biological agents a particular concern. These agents are categorized into specific priority levels A, B, C and are defined in Table 16.2. Highest priority agents—**Category** A—are identified as causing high mortality if used on the population. Category A agents include the toxin produced by *Clostridium botulinum* and several bacteria that could be spread through food. Foodborne pathogens such as *Salmonella*, *E. coli* O157:H7, and *Vibrio cholerae* and chemical toxins from castor bean (ricin) and *Staphylococcal enterotoxin* are considered moderate to high risk. These would cause considerable illness but limited numbers of deaths. It should be noted that **Category B** agents are relatively easy to obtain or isolate, which gives them a higher probability of being used but with less mortality than Category A agents. **Category C** is reserved for emerging pathogens, viruses, and potentially genetically engineered microorganisms.

The Aggressors: Requirements and Motivation

The mere threat of an intentional adulteration of food may be sufficient to cause widespread concern and economic loss. In order for an aggressor to successfully complete an actual attack, several conditions must be met. By understanding these conditions, it is much easier to institute controls that will help prevent the occurrence of an attack.

In order to successfully tamper with a food product, an aggressor must:

- Have access to the food for a sufficient amount of time.
- Obtain or produce a contaminant.
- Introduce a sufficient quantity of the agent into the food.
- Commit the crime without discovery.

The ability of an aggressor to commit an act of food adulteration requires that the aggressor have access to the targeted food. This is as simple as access to an unmonitored salad bar that would impact relatively few individuals. Access to a large amount of food as in a storage tanker or silo would be more difficult but is not inconceivable. In fact, one of the largest intentional adulterations of food was by a pest control operator who had permission to fumigate tens of thousands of pounds of oats stored in a grain elevator. He used a fumigant pesticide that was not approved for use on oats but saved him money.

In order for an attack to be successful, sufficient quantities of the agent must be produced and placed into the food. These are the most difficult aspects of food bioterrorism. New regulations are in place to restrict the availability of purified cultures of foodborne pathogens. A skilled microbiologist or chemist might be able to isolate the agent from raw materials. Growing or obtaining enough raw material to contaminant a large amount of food may be difficult. In the case of toxins from *Clostridium botulinum*, it is difficult to grow the anaerobic organism and to produce toxin. Once produced, the toxin must be isolated from the growth medium and concentrated—both procedures are extremely hazardous and difficult. Ricin, a deadly toxin, can be isolated relatively easily from the castor bean and concentrated. In the United States, it is a felony to isolate ricin.

If an aggressor were able to adulterate a volume of food, the toxin or organism must go undetected for sufficient time to get the food into the population. If a compound or bio-agent is detected immediately or during processing, then the scale of the attack may be reduced because of limited distribution of the impacted food. Simulations show that an intentional adulteration of a food product manufactured in the Midwest would reach the coastal areas of the United States in less than 3 days, with illness occurring in 4 to 5 days post-manufacture.

Motivation for an attack may be derived from several sources with the end goals varying in severity from mild disruption of business to causing mass casualties. The general goals of most aggressors may include:

- Cause economic disruption or devastation
- Increase cost of security
- Cause death
- Loss of productivity
- Loss of confidence
- Loss of trade and commerce

There are four general types of actors that could be considered aggressors in the sense of intentionally adulterating the food supply. Each of these types of aggressors would have a specific reason for causing illness or disruption of the food supply:

1. Disgruntled employees
2. Criminal actors
3. Extremists/terrorists

Disgruntled employees are those who feel that they have reason to be upset with their employer or some aspect of their work. It is possible that the individual had been laid-off or fired. These actors are most difficult to stop because they may have ready access to the food and be able to introduce a significant amount of agent into the food. The employee may be able to escape detection. An example of an actual attack by a disgruntled employee occurred in 2003. A grocery store employee who had disagreements with other meat department employees added a nicotine-based pesticide to around 200 lbs. of hamburger. Approximately 100 people were made ill by nicotine poisoning within 2 hours of consuming the meat. The reason that the employee gave for contaminating the meat was that he hoped the other meat department employees would get into trouble for the adulteration.

Criminal actors are those who benefit either emotionally or monetarily from the intentional adulteration or disruption of the food supply. This would include actors who falsely claim that the food supply will be or is contaminated in an attempt to extort money from the company. An example of this type of activity was demonstrated by a pest control operator responsible for fumigating large grain elevators containing oats. The operator used a pesticide that was not approved for use on oats and was less expensive. The end result was a massive recall of an oat-containing breakfast cereal, which in the end cost the food processing company $167 million dollars. The pest control operator saved around $80,000 but was sentenced to jail for his precipitating the fraud. Another example of intentional adulteration of food for criminal intent occurred in China in 2002. The criminal actor in this case used the rat poison tetramine to contaminate water and flour of a competing pastry shop. Forty-two deaths occurred and over 300 people were hospitalized in this criminal action. The criminal was executed. Several other incidents using tetramine have occurred in China.[5]

Extremists and *terrorists* are those who have a political, social, religious, or other type of cause. Terrorists are often loose networks of individuals working in independent cells that may plan and con-

---

The First Documented Food Bioterrorism Act in the United States.

In the first documented food bioterrorism act in the United States, members of a cult experimented with using *Salmonella typhimurium* to cause illness in a community. In the early 1980s, followers of a religious guru established a large commune in a sparsely populated county. The cult members were successful in dominating the local township elections, and they changed the name of the town. As they grew in numbers and power, there was an effort to change county zoning laws to allow the commune to expand. In order to achieve this goal, it was proposed that members of the cult would run for county commission seats. However, non-cult voters would have outnumbered the cult members, so a plot was developed to cause a mass outbreak of illness in the county seat. The commune was successful in obtaining cultures of pathogenic bacteria such as *Salmonella typhimurium, Francisella tularemia,* and others that could be used to contaminate the water supply of the county seat. Select individuals of the commune proceeded to cultivate *S. typhimurium* and developed an easily distributed bio-weapon. This weapon was tested in 11 restaurants in the county seat. Within 1 week, medical facilities were overwhelmed by the ill. Fortunately, no one died in the incident although over 700 people were made ill. Importantly, it took a cult insider to alert the authorities to the fact that the cult was responsible for the illnesses; otherwise the true cause of the outbreak would have gone undetected.[5,6]

duct an action. It should be noted that in most cases, terrorists work without official approval from any government. Support is, therefore, from third-party sources rather than directly from any government. Generally, a government-sanctioned terrorist activity would be considered an act of war by the affected country. Extremists may be very sophisticated in their ability to produce and disseminate a biological or chemical weapon. An example of this is the outbreak of *Salmonella* in Oregon caused by a religious group (*see the side bar*).

An example of terrorists threatening to cause economic loss occurred in 1989. Grapes were used as the food and cyanide as the chemical contaminant. A group or individual sensitive to issues occurring in the Middle East and angry with United States and Japan contacted the media with the claim that Chilean grapes had been injected with cyanide. There were no deaths, illnesses, or evidence that this was true; however, Japan, the United States, Canada, and several other countries placed an immediate embargo on Chilean fruit. The economic loss caused by the Chilean grape threat was estimated to be in the hundreds of millions of dollars with dozens of growers going out of business.

Tactics of Aggressors and Methods to Protect Food

Aggressors need to have access to the food for a successful attack to occur. The methods used to achieve access are varied and can be controlled by the foodservice; however, it is difficult to recognize employees who may have the desire to cause harm to either the company or the population. The four methods most likely used to attempt an act of terrorism are insider compromise, covert entry, exterior attack, and forced entry.

Insider compromise involves an employee or someone who has legitimate reasons to be in the food facility. Insiders include truck or delivery drivers, sanitation crew, production workers, vendors, regulatory personnel, contractors, and service employees. Thus, a control for insider compromise is to compartmentalize the foodservice as much as possible. For example, delivery drivers do not need to be in production areas but rather they should be segregated to the receiving areas. Access to areas where food is stored should be controlled and limited to only production personnel who require access and the occasional cleaning crew. In schools, teachers and students should be restricted from entering the foodservice and food storage areas without supervision. If the school foodservice is used after serving hours, foods should be secured and unavailable for adulteration.

In multipurpose facilities such as schools, many different people may have access to the foodservice. These employees and visitors may also have access to chemical supply rooms such as pesticides or herbicides, science laboratory chemicals, and janitorial cleaning compounds. In situations such as this, both the access to the chemicals and access to the foodservice must be restricted. Employees should be instructed to report unauthorized personnel in production areas.

Disgruntled employees are a significant potential threat to foodservice operations. This type of aggressor has demonstrated the means and the wherewithal to create an attack. If given the time and the opportunity, an unhappy or vengeful employee could easily contaminate foods with a variety of chemical, biological, and physical hazards.

Controls for insider attack include doing background checks on potential employees with consideration of their basic constitutional rights. It is U.S. law that all potential employees be verified for eligibility to work in the United States. An additional background criminal check may be desired if allowed by local law. For current employees, management must be diligent in keeping staff in the area to which they are assigned. Any employee who is asking sensitive questions about the food flow or how it is received or distributed should be considered a potential threat. Employee attendance should be monitored closely with respect to early or late arrivals. Access to sensitive documents must be restricted to personnel who need to see these. These documents may include such materials as delivery/shipping schedules, employee contact information, formulas or recipes, and other information. Finally and possibly most importantly, personnel issues must be addressed to ensure that an employee does not become disgruntled or unhappy to the level of aggression.

Covert entry is the use of forged or falsified credentials to gain access or entry into a facility. Aggressors could pose as regulatory personnel or vendors to gain access to the facility. Regulatory personnel carry identification papers and are usually known to the foodservice employees. Vendors may not carry that level of identification; they may be kept from the production areas by meeting in the dining area or offices.

Prevention of covert entry involves being able to either keep the actor away from food or rapidly identify the actor once in the production facility or near foods. Staff identification in the form of uniforms or nametags can assist in detection of unauthorized individuals. Verification of visitors' identity and logging in visitors is an important prevention step as is restricting entrance to production and warehouse areas. When visitors do have to be in the production areas, briefcases, backpacks, and other items should be restricted to nonproduction areas. In all cases, visitors must be accompanied in the facility at all times—this includes regulatory personnel. Once again employee diligence in reporting unknown or unauthorized individuals is an important control.

Vehicle access and parking in nonpublic areas should also be controlled. Loading docks are potential entry points for aggressors. In public areas, visitors lurking near salad bars or self-service areas should be reported or challenged. These areas should be under constant watch because they are easy targets for potential threats.

Exterior attack occurs when a contaminated food enters the facility rather than being produced in the foodservice facility. Thus, the aggressor has adulterated the food prior to receipt by the foodservice employees. The food may be contaminated during transportation or during manufacture at the supplier.

The controls to prevent an exterior attack include purchasing food from reputable vendors and legitimate businesses. There is the potential for receiving counterfeit or mislabeled product from either criminal actors or terrorists. A "good deal" in a reduced price product could become a significant problem if the product is counterfeit, contaminated, or mislabeled. A reputable supplier will have a food defense plan in place at its operation and can guarantee the product is safe. Products from reputable vendors should be delivered in clean trucks by drivers who have proper identification and correct bills of lading for goods being delivered. A delivery schedule should be arranged with the vendor. Deviations in delivery time could indicate time and opportunity for a tampering incident. Delivery should be observed by an employee, and inspection of the delivered products must occur before the driver leaves.

Once the product reaches the foodservice area, packaging must not be damaged or appear to have been tampered with in any way. Package integrity must be determined by receiving personnel and standards for unacceptable damage established. Receiving and production personnel should be made aware of product quality and sensory characteristics. An odd aroma or appearance in a food could suggest tampering. Canned goods should be inspected for label integrity. Labels are glued onto the can rather than loosely wrapped around the can. Tamper evident seals on salad dressings and other products must be intact. Properly trained receiving employees are the first barrier to prevention of exterior attack.

Forced entry involves gaining access to a food facility by forcibly breaking doors, windows, roofs, or ventilation systems. This could occur in the production area, seating area (salt shakers have been contaminated with rat poison), and warehouses. Breaking and entering a food facility can be prevented by installation of locks, alarms, video surveillance, and by hiring guards. While any one of these actions may not prevent access, when used together they are more effective.

In addition to the production area, utilities such as gas, electricity, water, and airflow systems must be secure. Loss of food caused by a temporary power outage will have an economic impact upon the viability of the foodservice industry. Access to the water supply could allow an aggressor an opportunity to add a biological or chemical agent.

Schools should be aware of foodservice areas that have dual purposes such as activities in the dining area that would provide access to the production areas. Surveillance or other security measures to prevent tampering with food and equipment is necessary in these situations.

Developing Food Defense Plans

A systematic review of all phases of the foodservice operation must be undertaken to determine the vulnerability of the facility to the activities of an aggressor. A self-assessment should be done with action plans developed to correct identified weaknesses. Self-assessments must cover all aspects of the operation that are listed in Table 16.3.

Table 16.3   Food Defense Measures That Should Be Considered in Foodservice Assessment Checklists

Management
  Develops food defense plan or designates team to do so
  Develops specific protocols in case of aggressor attack (when and who to call, recall, how to handle suspicious materials, etc.)
  Ensures team is trained in provisions of the food defense plan
  Conducts inspections associated with food defense
  Develops emergency contact list of first responders and posts where employees can have access
  Delivers food defense training to employees
  Verifies that suppliers are legitimate and conscious of food defense
  Verifies and validates food defense plan

Personnel
  Application procedure includes background check and verification of right to work
  References are validated
  Trained in food defense upon hiring
  Trained to recognize and report any suspicious activity or food
  Control of personal items in production area
  Protocol developed on sick leave and requirement to inform management of illness
  Terminated employees relieved of all access means to facility (keys, electronic access, etc.)
  Must have means of employee identification (name tags or uniforms)
  Employee schedule must be followed
  Only authorized personnel in production areas
  Positive identification required for all visitors, regulatory, and other personnel

Property and Storage
  Physical security includes working locks on all access points (doors, windows, etc.)
  Loading dock is secured
  Food storage areas have limited access during production day

continues

Table 16.3 (continued)

Food storage areas are locked when facility is closed

Chemical storage areas always locked with restricted access

Avoid propped open doors or windows

Maintain inventory control looking for unexplained additions

Food and Production Areas

Only approved, validated vendors may supply food, chemicals and other supplies

Food is code dated by vendor and upon arrival at facility

Unloading of received materials is supervised

Bill of lading must match invoice, which must match purchase order

All incoming supplies must be inspected and verified against invoice

Access to production areas is limited to authorized workers only

Personal items are not authorized in production area

Shipping or catering vehicles secured and locked

Public areas

Self-service areas such as salad bars must be monitored

Prevent access to production, warehouse, and chemical storage areas

Sealed or tamper evident condiment displays

Staff understand requirement to report people lurking around foods

Hazard Analysis and Critical Control Point (HACCP) methods are used to determine where potential inadvertent or known food-related hazards may be controlled in the flow of food through a processing or foodservice operation. HACCP is a systematic approach to ensure food safety. Operational Risk Management (ORM) is a similar approach for food defense except, instead of a natural or inadvertent food adulteration, ORM looks for the places where an intentional adulteration could take place and then institutes specific controls for that vulnerability. As a risk assessment tool, ORM is integrated into all decisions made by management. Risk is defined then as a hazard for which the likelihood of occurrence and severity of damage has been determined. ORM is a modification of military operational procedures for determining and addressing the risk associated with field operations during times of war and for reducing the losses associated with potential failures.

The concept of ORM is predicated upon four key rules.

1. Accept no unnecessary risk. This indicates that risks are a way of life; however, critically assessing what risks are and prioritizing risks will ensure that those most likely to occur receive the most planning and action. Unnecessary risk comes about when a hazard is either overlooked or underestimated in the level of severity and probability of occurrence. Adequate risk assessment is therefore critical to ORM.
2. Make the risk decision at the appropriate level of management. Decision making is one of the most important aspects of management. Translating the decision into action may involve several layers of employees with appropriate accountability for actions.
3. Accept risk when benefits outweigh the cost. A decision must be done on a risk benefit analysis. The classic example is a lock rather than a 24-hour guard. The guard will provide more security than the lock but will be prohibitively expensive.
4. Integrate ORM planning into all levels of operations. This is critical because all potential vulnerabilities must be explored throughout planning processes. For example, the type of door lock or window placement should be considered when developing plans for new establishments. Another example is the screening of potential vendors to ensure that they are aware of food defense requirements.

These four rules are designed to assist in mitigating the risks associated with identified hazards. As in HACCP, ORM is a systematic way to look at the entire operation including the management, people, equipment, and facilities' design and layout. The causes of failure are most likely that a hazard was not identified; therefore, management and employees could not control the steps to prevent a hazard or risk. An example of this would be a management decision to not track lot numbers of food used in production. In the event of a recall, there would be no way to know which foods are contaminated by a specific hazard. The probability of a recall occurring is relatively high. Therefore the risk of this hazard being passed on to consumers is relatively high. This risk could be mitigated by requiring that a lot tracking system be in place when receiving and producing foods within a facility.

The basic steps to ORM are:

1. Identify the hazards that exist in the facility and food flow. The entire operational theatre must be evaluated, including facilities, management, employees, and food flow. As in HACCP, a flow diagram of the process of food procurement and production should be made. At each point in the flow, a systematic "what if" scenario might be played to highlight vulnerabilities in the specific step. These vulnerabilities are the hazards that could occur in the step. Examples of this process are:

   Receiving
   What if the drivers are unmonitored during delivery?
   Hazard is that driver could contaminate foods.
   What if the truck has been left unattended without being locked?
   Hazard is that aggressors could enter the unlocked truck and contaminate the food.
   What if no lot tracking is available for received foods?
   Hazard is that an intentionally contaminated ingredient could not be tracked in produced foods.

   Food Production
   What if access to production areas is not controlled?
   Hazard is that an aggressor could contaminate food.
   What if employees are allowed to bring personal items into production areas?
   Hazard is that an employee could carry a contaminant to foods.

2. Assess the risk of each hazard. A hazard becomes identified as a risk when the severity and probability of the hazard have been determined. Each hazard that is identified will have a probability of occurrence and, if it does happen, a level of severity to the operation and customers. A matrix of severity and probability is shown in Figure 16.1. In the risk assessment, both probability and severity must be taken into account. A hazard that has been identified as having a severe consequence and is frequently present must be considered a serious risk to the operation. An example of a hazard that falls into the high category of the risk assessment matrix would be the lack of a lot tracking system. The inability to adequately recall or stop production because of an intentionally adulterated ingredient could result in large numbers of people becoming ill and/or

dying and cause significant economic loss in the amount of food that would have to be destroyed. For this hazard the severity is Category I (catastrophic) or Category II (critical), and the probability is Category B (high) or C (recalls are not infrequent), which results in a risk level of extremely high to high.

Being able to evaluate hazards and assign a specific risk level is critical to having an accurate ORM program. Just as in HACCP, severity and probability of occurrence of a hazard are

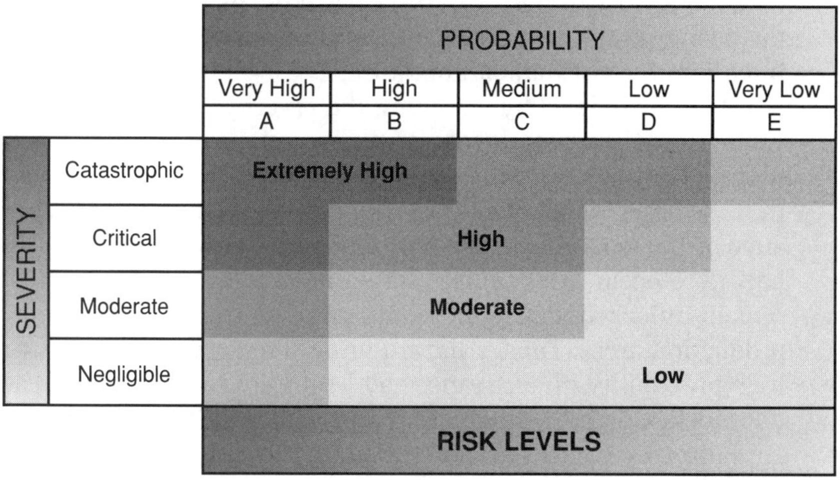

		PROBABILITY			
		Very High	High	Medium	Low	Very Low
		A	B	C	D	E
SEVERITY	Catastrophic	**Extremely High**				
	Critical			**High**		
	Moderate			**Moderate**		
	Negligible				**Low**	
		RISK LEVELS				

Probability definitions

Very high — hazard is continually present in the population and occurs often to individuals

High — hazard is present in the population with individual occurrences

Medium — hazard occurs sporadically but may occur in individuals

Low — hazard is rarely present but may occur in individuals

Very low — hazard occurs extremely rarely in either population or individuals

Severity definitions

Catastrophic — deaths occur with business failure

Critical — severe illnesses with business decline

Moderate — mild illnesses with minor business interruption

Negligible — very mild or no illnesses with no business interruption

FIGURE 16.1   Risk Assessment Matrix Combining Likelihood of Hazard Occurrence with Severity of Consequences of Hazard Occurring

fundamentally important to establishing control points and corrective actions. Once the risks have been categorized, they must be prioritized as to the immediacy of action to establish the control measures. For example, a high-risk level hazard would be evaluated and controlled before a medium- or low-risk level hazard.

3. Establish control measures for each identified risk. In HACCP, critical control points are defined as measures that control the identified hazard. In ORM, the same concept applies in that control measures for the identified risk must reduce or eliminate the identified risk. Specific steps must be taken to protect the business and the customer from the consequences of an intentional act of food adulteration. These steps effectively reduce the risk level by changing the severity or probability categories. There may be cases when a risk has been defined as highly likely to occur and will be catastrophic if it does occur. In these cases, it may be necessary to completely reject acceptance of the risk and establish procedures that will not allow the hazard to occur. An example would be to allow the facility to remain unlocked during off-hours or allow free access to food production areas. Thus, a hazard (unfettered access) that has a high probability of occurring may be mitigated by installing a door lock, which then reduces the probability of an intruder.

For many of the risks identified in a foodservice establishment, control may be exerted at the planning stage for construction or renovation of the facility. Planning in food defense is much more economical than retrofitting the facility. The security of salad bars and other self-service areas can be significantly enhanced (with the concomitant reduction of risk) by placing these areas where they can be constantly monitored. Doors and windows can be placed to minimize intruder entrance to processing and storage areas. In renovations, application of security devices such as video cameras, door locks, alarms, and window locks decreases the risk of attack. Finally, in existing facilities, development of new procedures and adequate training of staff in these food defense procedures will help with control of identified risks.

For the "what if" scenario of no lot tracking, the hazard has been identified with the risk level placed at a minimum of high. The control measure for this risk then becomes establishment of a lot recording method that includes the vendor, transporter, usage level, and products made from the ingredient. This then allows for trace back of a recalled ingredient with forward trace capabilities to end users.

An important consideration in establishing control measures is the risk to benefit analysis. If a specific hazard has a control that will be expensive to institute, then the management must consider this and possibly look for alternatives or other modifications to mitigate the expense. However, the resultant safety is difficult to quantify in real costs, but failure to ensure safety can result in catastrophic losses.

4. Make risk control decisions. Each of the controls that were identified in the risk assessment should be evaluated for feasibility, cost, and likelihood of successful implementation. Each of these aspects requires that all levels of management and staff are engaged because they will be involved in the day-to-day aspects of the controls. While most of the risk associated with a hazard may be reduced, this residual risk should be considered and deemed acceptable. Successful control measures must have the acceptance and understanding of all staff who are involved in the implementation. The cost analysis of a control measure becomes primarily a management decision while feasibility relies upon the input of staff who must implement the control.

5. Implementation of control measures. Once determined to be feasible without unacceptable expense, then implementation should be undertaken. In some cases, this will be immediate while other measures may take a period of time before implementation is complete. An example would be the immediate installation of door locks to secure storage areas, while changing vendor delivery patterns may take a period of time.

Critical to implementation of control measures is the concept of accountability for the control. Understanding "who" is to be responsible for ensuring that the control is in place and being monitored is part of the accountability for the control. A useful tool is the development of standard operating procedures that outline the policy and who is responsible for carrying out the measure. These written documents can form the basis for a training program in food defense and the controls that the establishment is using to ensure safety. Training allows for refinement of the control and assists with employee understanding of the measure. Failure in control measures is most likely to come from personnel.

6. Supervise and review. HACCP requires verification of monitoring and validation that the monitoring is effective. These are the same requirements as for ORM. Once in place, the control measures for a risk must be validated that they are working as they should. Monitoring verification is difficult when dealing with how employees might handle an intruder, observation of wrongdoing, or other employee-specific control measures. Through testing and questioning, the understanding that a staff member has for the control measure might be ascertained. For other, less subjective control measures, checklists can be used to verify that doors are locked, access is restricted, chemicals are secured, etc.

In the event that a verification check of a control measure shows persistent deficiencies, the control measure must be evaluated and the root cause of the failure determined. Should this be the only known control measure for an identified risk, then it is crucial that management identify the mechanism to correct the control measure so that it is effective. Communication with the staff responsible for the measure may help identify why there are problems with the control measure. Continual assessment of control measures in light of changing world and local events should also be done. As new threats are identified, federal and state officials will contact the pertinent industries as to their vulnerabilities. New threats may result in significant changes to the ORM program of a food establishment.

Attendant Programs

In addition to the four key rules and the six steps just listed, ORM requires a set of prerequisite checklists to ensure proper functioning. These steps are outlined in Table 16.3 and help set a framework for the rest of the ORM program. Daily, weekly, and annual checklists of food defense measures could be developed from these lists of important considerations in securing a facility.

Summary

An intentional act of food tampering could be devastating for both customers and the foodservice involved. The general thought is that an intentional large-scale adulteration of food is likely to occur. When this adulteration might happen is not known, but if it does happen there are specific measures that must be taken once the act is discovered by either regulatory authorities, health professionals, or the company involved. Crisis communication guidelines are designed to ensure rapid and accurate reporting of the action and the steps that are being taken to mitigate the amount of illness associated with the agent. It should be noted that in certain cases the facility may be closed and all foods destroyed, surfaces decontaminated, and employees monitored closely for health reasons.

The general steps that must be taken in the event that a company recognizes an intentional act of aggression are:

1. Have one or two designated persons who are trained in crisis communication handle all regulatory, media, and consumer requirements. A team approach should be taken to the crisis, but these one or two are the communicators.
2. Communicate the problem to regulatory and law authorities. Normally first responders include fire and law enforcement; public health may be called in as needed. The Federal Bureau of Investigation is responsible for domestic terrorism enforcement.
3. Cordon off the facility and point of attack must be cordoned off with evidence preserved to the best of abilities.
4. Be aware that law enforcement agencies will be looking for witnesses to the crime. It is imperative that the foodservice employees identify potential witnesses in either employees or customers.
5. Work with public health authorities to identify the consumers who may have been contaminated or may have consumed the contaminated foods.
6. Work with public health authorities to decontaminate the facility and any areas that were contaminated in the attack.
7. Upon approval of authorities, reopen the establishment for business.

These steps begin the process of solving the crime and protecting consumers from further exposure to the contaminants. Specific measures may be required to prevent the future occurrence of the incident. These corrective actions should be documented and clearly communicated to regulatory and law enforcement agencies. The actions taken and the lessons learned will add to a base of knowledge that will help prevent future attacks.

Issues for Class Discussion

1. How well prepared are foodservice departments to provide food to individuals in the event of an intentional attack on the food supply? In the event of an attack that compromises access to food? In the event of a quarantine?
2. What research is necessary to identify a foodservice department's capacity to use food on hand in the event of food shortages?
3. What priority should food security be in the foodservice department's preparedness efforts?
4. What level of investment is appropriate for security of the food supply, and who should provide the funding in foodservice facilities?
5. Are foodservice managers involved in preparedness activities? What role should foodservice managers assume for risk assessment, surveillance, planning, response, and recovery in the event of an attack?

References

1. Economic Research Service, United States Department of Agriculture. Food away from home: Total expenditures. Retrieved November 15, 2006, from http://www.ers.usda.gov/Briefing/CPIFoodAndExpenditures/Data/table3.htm.
2. National Restaurant Association. (2006). 2006 restaurant industry fact sheet. Chicago, IL: National Restaurant Association.
3. Centers for Disease Control and Prevention. Retrieved October 10, 2006, from http://www.bt.cdc.gov/agent/agentlist-category.asp.
4. Shea, D.A. & Grottron, F. (2004). Small-scale terrorist attacks using chemical and biological agents: An assessment framework and preliminary comparisons. CRS report for Congress. Washington, DC: Library of Congress.

5. Croddy, E. (2004). Rat poison and food security in the People's Republic of China: Focus on tetramethylene disulfotetramine (tetramine). *Archives of Toxicology, 78,*1-6.
6. Torok, T., Tauxe, R.V., Wise, R.P., Livengood, J.R., Sokolow, R., Mauvais, S., Birkness, K.A., Skeels, M.R., Horan, J.M. & Foster, L.R. (1997). A large community outbreak of salmonella caused by intentional contamination of restaurant salad bars. *Journal of the American Medical Association* 278, 389–395.

## CHAPTER 17

ENTREPRENEURSHIP: WRITING A BUSINESS PLAN FOR ESTABLISHING YOUR OWN RESTAURANT OR PRIVATE PRACTICE AND REIMBURSEMENT FOR REGISTERED DIETITIAN SERVICES

Bradley Beran, MBA, PhD, Michelle Easterly, BS, MS, and Mary Angela Miller, MS, RD, LD, FADA,

Reader Objectives

After studying this chapter and reflecting on the contents, the student should be able to:

1. Understand and identify the components of a business plan.
2. Find research and information references in developing a business plan.
3. Provide a basic self-analysis to employees to see if they have the personal characteristics to operate their own business.
4. Understand basic forms of small business ownership.
5. Identify and find the rules, codes, and other regulatory requirements to small business operations.
6. Understand the importance of accurate financial planning, assessments, and statements.
7. Identify how a registered dietitian (RD) can get reimbursed for medical nutrition therapy counseling.

Key Terms

Business plan: a summary of how a business owner, manager, or entrepreneur intends to organize an entrepreneurial endeavor and implement the necessary and sufficient activities in order for the venture to succeed.

Dietetic Practice Group (DPG): a group of dietetic professionals whose goal is to support and expand a network of dietetics professionals and share information and experiences on nutritional management.

Entrepreneur: a person who undertakes and operates a new enterprise or venture and assumes some accountability for the inherent risks.

Franchise: an authorization to sell a company's goods or services in a particular place.

Income statement: a financial statement that contains a summary of a business's financial operations for a specific period of time. It shows the net profit or loss for the period by stating the company's revenues and expenses.

LLC (Limited Liability Company): a legal form of business offering limited liability to its owners. In that respect, it is similar to a corporation and is often a more flexible form of ownership, especially suitable for smaller companies with a limited number of owners.

Market niche: a specialized portion of a market.

Partnership: a type of business entity in which partners share with each other the profits or losses of the business undertaking in which they have all invested.

Payor: the legal term for a person, institution, or government who is required to make a payment on an income stream, such as a promissory note.

Sole proprietorship: a business that legally has no separate existence from its owner.

Introduction

Writing a **business plan** is the culmination of an intense and thorough analysis of a concept or idea. The plan represents the level and depth of an **entrepreneur**'s knowledge and understanding of a proposed endeavor. In this chapter, the authors will present and discuss entrepreneurship and the business plan from a three-point approach. First, the chapter will discuss what running your own business is like, such as the commitment, the dedication, and the demeanor (does the entrepreneur have what it takes to run his or her own business?). Second, the chapter will discuss the business plan itself, which includes preplanning

> **Learning Point:** Writing a business plan is the culmination of an intense and thorough analysis of a concept or idea.

information, what the plan contains, what an entrepreneur should know, how to assemble the plan, and how to present the plan. Third, the authors interviewed several business owners, restaurateurs, and nutritionists in private practice. Their views, opinions, and advice will be presented. This chapter is not an all-inclusive "how to" on writing a business plan but rather provides an overview, insights, and resources to continue research into developing a business plan.

Owning a Small Business—Do You Have What It Takes?

Owning a restaurant or consulting business can be very rewarding. It is also a considerable amount of work requiring time, dedication, perseverance, good planning and organization skills, an understanding of costing, pricing and financials, physical and mental stamina, and much more.[1]

The restaurant industry in the United States is enormous and reached over $511 billion in sales in 2006.[2] Yet, with all this revenue, the average restaurant will net less than 5% of this total, which is split among the nation's 925,000 restaurants.[2] Additionally, a small business typically does not make any profit for just over the first 3 years. This leaves little room for error. An entrepreneur must be a highly motivated self-starter possessing a wide array of talents, knowledge, and technical skills. *Often, if the entrepreneur doesn't do it, it doesn't get done, and seldom are there available finances to hire someone else to do it.*

> **Learning Point:** A critical self-evaluation is an important step in confirming that you have the characteristics and drive to be an entrepreneur.

The dedication required to start and run a business is extraordinary. Before beginning, the prospective entrepreneur should ask, "Why do I want to start my own business?" Many people believe that starting their own business frees them from the Monday through Friday, 9-to-5 daily routine and increases their independence and flexibility. In most cases, restaurateurs starting a new business work 12- to 16-hour days, 6 to 7 days per week, just getting the business started.[1] Once the business gets going, the time commitment doesn't decline much, if at all. Your business is your life. Like a child, it requires constant attention, care, and nurturing to succeed. This is especially true for practitioners in private practice; if they are not working, they are not making money. Make sure to ask these additional questions when thinking about starting your own private practice:

1. Do you mind working alone or are you willing to work alone?
2. Do you have the knowledge or skills to work independently? Or do you need some professional support?
3. Do you have the skills to manage the stress supervision of owning a private practice?
4. Do you have the understanding of the people and the community in which you would operate a private practice?[1]

Starting and running a business are not for everyone. The authors recommend visiting the U.S. Small Business Administration (SBA) Web site and reviewing the article "Do You Have What It Takes?"[1]

If the entrepreneur has the dedication, drive, and ambition to start a restaurant or consulting practice, it will be necessary to review and evaluate skills, abilities, and experience. Fairly and accurately assess your strengths and weaknesses. This will determine where additional expertise is needed to fill shortcomings.[3] No one can do everything well all by himself or herself. An honest assessment is as critical as procuring the necessary expertise to support weak areas. A business' support network should have a team of experts that includes a banker, an accountant, insurance professional, and a lawyer.[4] These experts will have the knowledge to efficiently assist with business organization and planning, finance and banking, and protecting the business.

Where to Start—Initial Planning

When considering opening a restaurant or private practice, a few general questions need to be answered, especially with regard to the total market, **market niche,** competition, and finances. Who is the market and what are its demographics? A single market is often too large to be considered as a potential group of customers.[1] Begin by break-

> **Learning Point:** Sound initial planning will help identify your niche and determine an underserved customer demand area.

ing down a market into manageable segments, and analyze a potential segment, gleaning relevant demographic data that can support a proposed business. This will help determine if the business can be supported by the chosen market niche, determine what check averages could be supported, further define the client or customer base, and help assess what services may be required or desired. Depending on the type of restaurant or private practice, different income levels, professions, ethnic backgrounds, commute times, and job locations will all influence how a niche is filled. Consider this simple general information analysis: In 2005, an estimated 28 meals per person were consumed in a vehicle (up from 21 in 2002), and in 2002, $910 per person was spent on meals away from home.[2] With takeout and delivery accounting for about 58% of this, that segment took in about $528 per person. This is a growing market. Detracting from that growth is the current price of fuel at about $3 per gallon in April 2007. The increase in energy costs reduces the amount of discretionary income available for dining out, takeout, and delivery meals. How could this affect the business, and can the business take advantage of this situation?

Trends in nutrition or health usually dictate the market niche for practitioners in private practice. Consider these trends in health: In 2005, the new Food Guide Pyramid was unveiled as an interactive Web site that personalizes nutrition plans. As stated on the Web site (www.mypyramid.gov), "One size does not fit all," and the MyPyramid plan chooses foods and amounts that are right for each individual. Additionally, it puts a particular emphasis on physical activity, one factor that the Food Guide Pyramid had not even mentioned in the past. Personalized nutrition with the combination of physical activity is here to stay. *Trends need*

> **Learning Point:** Staying on top of trends and market conditions will keep your business current, relevant, and interesting to your clients.

to be incorporated into a private practice. These trends without a doubt will be in the media, and potential clients will see and hear them. It is the nutritionist's responsibility to know them, understand them, and be able to explain them to the client.[5]

What niche will I fill? This is a refinement of a market analysis. As a restaurant, what type of food will be served, what meal periods will be covered, how many days per week will the business be open, what hours of operation, is takeout available, is delivery available, will home replacement meals be offered, and many more general questions about the operation need to be asked and answered. If consulting in private practice, define the scope and level of services that will be offered, and use this to develop a vision and philosophy statement to guide the practice. When looking at filling a niche, it is important to identify an unfilled or underfilled need or demand in the marketplace. With many more two-income families, time to cook meals at home is decreasing, and the market for home replacement meals is increasing. Takeout and delivery accounted for 58% of the total restaurant revenues in 2001, and this figure continues to grow.[2]

With the nutrition crisis and obesity epidemic on the rise among children, Diabetes mellitus type 2 is becoming more prevalent and a common problem associated with children. One out of three children born in 2000 in the United States will become diabetic. The odds are nearly 50% higher for African- or Latin-American children. By knowing the community and clientele, it is easier to find and define a niche and fill it.[6]

Who is the competition? This will help identify an underserved or overserved niche and identify who is filling that niche. By assessing the competition, points of difference can be planned for to set one business apart from another. When assessing the competition, determine if they are busy, possibly too busy, demonstrating excess demand for the supply? What are the customers saying, both good and bad? This information can help define a niche with points of difference that may include, for example, menu items and styles, service differences, more convenient locations, curbside delivery/takeout, Internet ordering, and others.

How will I fund the business? Regardless of an entrepreneur's personal characteristics, ideas, marketing, niche, and competitive advantage, if the funding to start and operate the business is not in place or available, a restaurant, consulting practice, or other business will not get off the ground. There are several funding and investment sources available, but nearly all will require a payback, often with interest or dividends. While grants are available, there are very few, and they are difficult to obtain.[1] Credit cards are often a poor choice due to their high interest rates. The SBA, banks, and similar traditional sources of funds do not like to make loans for restaurants due to their failure rate. This leaves personal savings, friends, relatives, venture capitalists, and few others. With a sufficient amount of personal or private funding, the SBA and other institutions will make loans. The amount depends on several factors that vary by area and many other factors too numerous and variable to mention here. How much money is needed to open and operate? Generally, a business should have enough money to open and operate for at least 6 months.[3]

> **Learning Point:** Accurate and complete financial information is critical to planning a successful endeavor.

For private practice, funding is less critical in the beginning mostly because there are fewer and less costly capital outlays and capital investments than a restaurant would have. Even though the start-up expenses are not as steep, it is pertinent to fully understand the complexity of the financial situation for starting your own private practice. This includes fundamental knowledge on revenue sources, payers, and reimbursement guidelines.

Payers are insurance companies, third-party administrators, self-funded employers, managed care organizations, or federal health benefit programs (Medicare/Medicaid) that reimburse claims. **Payor** coverage requirements can be so confusing, complicated, and change so frequently that it often deters RDs from even reaping the benefits of coverage. Some choose to forgo payor coverage or insurance coverage altogether. These dietitians require their clients to pay fees and costs out-of-pocket.[7,8] If choosing to get payor coverage, a complete understanding of coverage guidelines is imperative. This includes understanding Medicare Medical Nutrition Therapy (MNT) and Diabetes Self-Management Training benefits, how to become a provider, benefit coverage and reimbursement guidelines, and patient eligibility. Additionally, keep up to date with all frequent changes, and be able to translate confusing payment requirements into clear, simple language. Following those guidelines should maximize reimbursements from payers.

Assembling the Information

As mentioned in the beginning of this chapter, writing a business plan is the conclusion to all of the necessary *research, planning, analysis,* and *concept development.* There are no short-cuts, but there are alternatives, each with different costs and constraints. In restaurant planning, once a niche has been identified, how the restaurant will fill that niche can be approached in a few different ways. A restaurant could be a stand-alone property, part of a strip mall, an enclosed mall location, part of or housed within another business (a coffee and pastry shop inside a bookstore or a café inside a department store), or other form. Also, the restaurant could be an independent, a **franchise**, a new start-up, or the purchase of an existing business.

> **Learning Point:** How you form your business will have major implications on liabilities, taxes, control, and organization.

When planning a private practice, once the vision/mission/philosophy has been developed and the scope of services has been defined, the business plan can proceed in many ways as well. A stand-alone practice can be in a private house (if zoning allows), in a storefront, as a part of another medical practice (nutrition counseling as part of family practice), or a shared space with another practitioner (share an office with a physical therapist or personal trainer), as examples.

Basic Forms of Ownership

Ownership of the business is another consideration. The three most common choices are **sole proprietorship, partnership,** and **Limited Liability Company (LLC).** Sometimes restaurants will form as S Corporations or Corporations. Those definitions will not be listed here because 70% of all U.S. eating and drinking establishments are small businesses with 20 or fewer employees.[9] Private practices also typically have few employees and are commonly set up as LLCs where recognized. Table 17.1 lists the major business ownership types.

Table 17.1 Major Business Ownership Types

Sole Proprietorship—A sole proprietor is simply a person who is engaged in business as an individual. Sometimes the individual uses his own name in the name of the business, e.g., "Jones Auto Repair." However, in many cases, the sole proprietor will want to use an "assumed name" such as "Brandon Auto Repair."

While doing business as a sole proprietor may seem fairly simple, there is one very serious adverse consequence, especially if the business involves products, which could cause harm or injury to other persons. As a sole proprietor, you are personally liable for any and all debts and liabilities of the business. Whether a claim is made against your business by a customer, an employee, a competitor, or a trade creditor, you will be personally "on the hook" for any such claim. As a result, all of your personal assets, home, motor vehicles, savings accounts, jewelry, household goods, etc. will be subject to the claims of all such creditors. While certain jointly owned property (e.g. a residence) of a husband and wife may be exempt from liability to the creditors of only one of the spouses, even these joint assets may be jeopardized if both the husband and wife are involved in the operation of the business. Obviously, these are risks that many persons engaged in business would like to avoid.[10]

Partnership—A partnership occurs when two or more persons combine to operate a business. Normally, the allocation of profits and losses, management and operation of the partnership is set forth in a written "partnership agreement" that is signed by all of the partners. Also, the partners of a partnership do have some very limited protection from the claims of creditors [for example] under the Mississippi Partnership Act. Under the applicable law, a creditor must first seek recovery against the assets of the partnership before seeking recovery against the personal assets of the individual partners. Nonetheless, it is clear that the personal assets of the partners are ultimately exposed to the claims of partnership creditors.

Unlike the corporation, the earnings of the partnership are not exposed to "dual taxation." Under the Internal Revenue Code, all of the earnings of the partnership are allocated and taxed directly to the individual partners. This is one of the principal reasons why many individuals choose to operate in the partnership form, rather than as a corporation.[10]

continues

Table 17.1 (continued)

Limited Liability Company (LLC)—The Limited Liability Company or "LLC" is a relatively new form of doing business, which is now recognized in most states. The LLC has grown in popularity because it combines the best features of a corporation and a partnership. Like a corporation, the owners (called "members") of the LLC are not personally responsible for the debts of the LLC. Like a partnership, there is no dual taxation, and the earnings of the business are taxed directly to the members. The LLC is also preferable in many ways to the "S corporation," which also avoids personal liability and dual taxation. The LLC is not subject to most of the limitations, which are imposed on S corporations by applicable law. For example, while an S corporation is not allowed to have more than one type or class of stock ownership and is not allowed to have more than 75 shareholders, the LLC is not subject to such limitations. Overall, the LLC simply allows more flexibility in the structure, operation, and management of the business than does the S corporation.[10] The primary advantage of LLCs is the limitation of personal liability in the event of a business failure or liability claim. Personal assets of the owners are not available to the creditors. A second advantage afforded by LLCs is that income is taxed at personal income tax rates. Corporations also provide protection of personal assets; however, a corporation is an entity unto itself. This means that the income from a corporation is taxed twice, once as the income of the corporation, and a second time as income to the shareholder who receives a dividend from the corporation.

Note: All persons interested in establishing their own business should consult an appropriate professional.

Know the Rules of Operating Restaurants and Consulting Practices

All businesses operate under various rules. Zoning defines where businesses of various types may operate. In some areas, consulting practices can be run out of a home in a residential area. This is seldom the case for a caterer. Restaurants must also comply with fire codes, health codes, building codes, and possibly special permits, zoning changes, labor laws, employment laws, and more. Some-

Learning Point: Without knowing all of the rules that affect a business, the operation could run illegally and possibly be closed down or exposed to fines and liabilities without the entrepreneur knowing the problem. Ignorance of the law is no excuse.

times variances (nonpermanent changes) to zoning are given to businesses that want to open in areas not zoned for that particular use. This often involves public hearings and other approvals and can be very time-consuming and frustrating. Be prepared for many meetings, questions, and challenges to your plan. Building codes set the requirements for parking, ingress and egress, rest rooms, construction and renovation requirements, and more. Compliance issues with the Americans with Disabilities Act, the Civil Rights Act, and others could occur. It cannot be stressed enough: Learn all of the rules that regulate how you operate.

Operations Planning

If a restaurant operation is the focus of the business plan, everything revolves around the menu. While location is important, for many quality operations, customers will also seek out the restaurant. The menu and supporting recipes are the control point of operations. They determine equipment needs and options, purchasing specifications, level of labor skills and training, production style, and more. Without a menu, none of the equipment and labor needs can be defined.

Once a menu is set, several questions in support of the menu need to be answered. If the menu is based on scratch preparation, extensive use of convenience items, or something in between, what skill levels do you need in your employees; how many employees do you need, and where will you get them? Also, is the food necessary to support the menu available, within target cost parameters, and on a consistent basis? This follows with what equipment is required to support the menu. If specialized equipment is required, can it have multiple uses or support many items? Equipment loads must be sufficient to meet expected demand. Energy efficiency and availability along with equipment types need to be determined. For example, heat-generating equipment selections include natural gas, steam, electric, and induction generation. to name four. Each has different efficiencies, purchase costs, ventilation requirements, and operation costs. Kitchen space must be adequately balanced with the dining room so that the kitchen is not too small to be efficient, nor too large to take away from dining room seats that could bring in revenue. The discussion so far has not included tables, chairs, lighting, textiles, colors, flatware, glassware, and other items. *All of these decisions are made in the context of market niche and demographic decisions made early in the project.*

After all of the operations decisions have been made, it is necessary to put the support network into place. What is needed for training, payroll, benefits, business filings, taxes, and more? Who does the purchasing, checks in the food, pays the bills, and does the advertising? These are only a few of the many details to be planned.

Planning for Unplanned Expenses

Many Web sites, texts, and other resources fail to consider nonprimary business expenses. Community groups, youth groups, the chamber of commerce, and a host of others often ask new and existing businesses for donations, gift certificates, membership fees, dues, and other items. Seldom are expenses like these even thought of when planning a business. Entrepreneurs often are so focused on planning an operation that external, noncritical influences are overlooked. A business in a community must also operate as a good and supporting citizen of the community. As mentioned previously, this could include joining and participating in the chamber of commerce, local, state, and national organizations like the National Restaurant Association, the American Culinary Federation, or the state and local chapters of these organizations, to name a few.

As a practitioner in private practice, it is even more important to operate as a good supporting citizen in the community. Networking is essential to get the business name out in the community. Joining the American Dietetic Association (ADA), the largest organization of food and nutrition professionals, would be an automatic step.[7,8] Additionally, joining a division of the ADA called **Dietetic Practice Groups (DPGs)** is the next reasonable step to take. These are professional interest groups. DPGs stay consistent with the views, missions, philosophy, and position of the national organization or the ADA.

Nutrition Entrepreneurs is a DPG of the ADA.[11] According to its Web site, the main objective of this practice group is to assist members to achieve their professional and financial potential by providing the tools to build and maintain a successful nutrition-related business. The DPG members consist of chief executive officers (CEOs), business owners, consultants, speakers, writers, chefs, educators, spokespersons, and more. These members are typically RDs or dietetic technicians who may:

- Provide professional nutrition consultations in private practice.
- Write books, newsletters, or magazine articles.
- Implement nutrition programs for employee wellness programs.
- Design nutrition software or nutrition education tools.[10]

Volunteering at local organizations that associate within your discipline or speaking at support groups are additional ways to make a name for the business and get referrals.

A small "rainy day fund" for other unexpected expenses should be planned for and maintained. A business cannot be so cash strapped that an equipment failure, like a cooler breakdown, creates excessive hardship. Another positive aspect of having a contingency fund is the opportunity to take advantage of occasional deals that come along. It affords a business the flexibility to buy when it wants to, to take advantage of market conditions, sales, etc. You will not be at the mercy of "I need it now" pricing and delivery.

Assembling the Numbers

Many hopeful entrepreneurs like to start with cost and finances or look at them early in the planning process. Usually, entrepreneurs who work with numbers first have in mind a budget or amount they can afford and try to make the business fit the budget. The problem with this approach is that often critical components are overlooked, cut, or ignored with the idea that "we can get that later," leaving the business to struggle without all of the resources needed to be successful. The finances should be done last after all other planning has

> **Learning Point:** Collecting and evaluating the financials is the last step, not the first, in completing a business plan.

been done; the numbers should be extracted and assembled from all of the individual components. If all is done completely and accurately, a good picture of how much money is necessary to start the business on a good resource foundation is developed. *The numbers should present a good financial picture of the proposed business and, at a minimum, should include a pro forma* income statement *for at least 3 years, pro forma cash flow statement, pro forma balance sheets, a break-even analysis, and all appropriate sub-schedules including expected capital expenditures, food costs, labor analysis, and operating expenses.*[12]

Writing the Plan—Assume Nothing

A formal business plan is a document that details many points about a business. It also tells the reader, who may be a venture capitalist, banking institution, SBA, or another unfamiliar with the details of a particular enterprise, how well the entrepreneur has thought out his or her business and how deep an understanding he or she has.

The business plan should be an honest and fair representation of what is really expected if the business plan is implemented. It is not a document that is created in order to receive funding. Funding should be the result of a well thought-out, rea-

> **Learning Point:** The business plan should be an honest and fair representation of what is really expected if the business plan is implemented.

sonable plan. The topics presented earlier are only the beginning of many details and concerns that need to be planned. These details force the entrepreneur to develop a clear understanding of many pieces of the business and present his or her level of understanding and accuracy to potential financial backers. On questioning, an applicant should never have to reply to a question with "I don't know. I never thought of that." A potential investor should not be able to ask an applicant/expert a relevant question about something they never thought about. Table 17.2 lists all of the essential parts of a business plan.

Table 17.2 Essential Components of a Business Plan

ELEMENTS OF A BUSINESS PLAN
1. **Cover sheet**
2. **Statement of purpose**
3. **Table of contents**
  I. **The Business**
     A. Description of business
     B. Marketing
     C. Competition
     D. Operating procedures
     E. Personnel
     F. Business insurance

  II. **Financial Data**
     A. Loan applications
     B. Capital equipment and supply list
     C. Balance sheet
     D. Breakeven analysis
     E. Pro-forma income projections (profit & loss statements)
        Three-year summary
        Detail by month, first year
        Detail by quarters, second and third years
        Assumptions upon which projections were based
     F. Pro-forma cash flow

  III. **Supporting Documents**
  Tax returns of principals for last three years personal financial statement
        (all banks have these forms)
  For franchised businesses, a copy of franchise contract and all
        supporting documents provided by the franchisor
  Copy of proposed lease or purchase agreement for building space
  Copy of licenses and other legal documents
  Copy of resumes of all principals
  Copies of letters of intent from suppliers, etc.

Startup Basics. Retrieved April 12, 2006, http://www.sba.gov

Really Knowing Your Business—The Details

An entrepreneur, when reviewing a restaurant's business plans, should be able to answer at least the following:

1. What five menu items have the highest margin?
2. What five menu items have the lowest margin?
3. What is the most expensive item on the menu? The least expensive?
4. Approximately how many guests, based on average check, are needed to break even every day/week/month/quarter/year?
5. At your maximum capacity, how many employees need to be working?
6. What is the minimum number of employees you can operate with if the day is slow?
7. What is the value of the inventory on average and how often do you expect to turn your inventory?
8. What is the monthly fixed cost of operation?
9. What is the expected prime cost, food cost, labor cost?
10. What credit cards will be accepted and what are their fees?

While these may seem like obvious questions, they represent the level of detail and understanding that the applicant really has to have of a prospective business. *When consulting, reviewing business plans.* When working with restaurateurs, it is always surprising how many of them have such a lack of knowledge regarding the basics of their product, menu, cost, profitability, and volume.

For nutritional professionals in private practice, knowing your business is your business. The nutritionist is the nutrition expert and needs to know your nutrition science and metabolism, understand current trends in nutrition, keep up on current research, and be able to interpret and relay this information to the client in a way that he or she will be able to understand complex terms and concepts. Often the information that clients obtain from the media is generalized summaries from

> **Learning Point:** A complete and detailed understanding of a business's operation at detailed levels is important in understanding the level of complexity and detail necessary to successfully run that business.

larger research studies and misinterpreted or misapplied by the clients. The RD must understand the conceptions or misconceptions presented by the media and be able to relay correct scientific information the client will understand and be able to put to practical use.

Advice from the Professionals

Getting into business is one thing; staying in business is quite another. The restaurant business has a high failure rate, with most failures attributed to poor planning.[1] Several professionals were interviewed—restaurateurs and private practice nutritionists—for their tips, thoughts, ideas, and recommendations. Their answers have tremendous consistency even though their styles and types of operations vary greatly.

The Restaurateurs

Several restaurateurs were interviewed with the understanding that they and their businesses would remain anonymous. With this assurance, the owner/operators agreed to give details about their restaurants that would not be available if they were identified. The restaurateurs are a broad group of operators, one starting his 36th year in the same restaurant and the rest with 10 to 20 years of experience. All have planned, opened, and operated successful restaurants.

The group of restaurateurs identified several areas as critical, with all being equally important. Each said a failure in one area could doom the business. The primary areas each restaurateur identified were:

- Know your costs, menu, and clientele to contain and minimize costs.
- Take advantage of opportunities and enhance revenues.
- Employ quality and trustworthy employees.
- Do whatever it takes to meet customer requests.
- Create an attitude and aura of customer service and satisfaction.

It should be noted that none of the restaurateurs talked specifically about a business plan but rather the operations that provide or result from the information that drives the business plan. All of the discussions focus on operations and planning with the goals of providing consistency, satisfied customers, a strong revenue stream, and a positive bottom line for the present and future.

Know your costs, menu, and clientele to contain and minimize costs.

The restaurateurs grouped these three areas together, considering them to be intertwined and inseparable. The general consensus was that each area supports the other and meets customer demands while remaining profitable. Knowing your clientele, their likes, dislikes, styles, spending patterns, and the like is the basis for providing a menu of items that meet their needs at their price points. By maintaining price points and the associated costs to provide a positive gross profit, the restaurant remains profitable, provides jobs and incomes for its employees, contributes to the community, provides a service for the customers, and remains a viable business. Also, it guides the chefs and managers in making menu and purchasing decisions. One said, "There is no such thing as a good buy on something I can't sell. If it sits in the cooler or storeroom because my customers don't like it and won't buy it, it's money I've thrown away that could have been used to generate sales." All restaurateurs indicated that knowing cost limits is critical. A comfortable contribution margin must be maintained in order to pay the bills and provide profit to the restaurant. Purchasing products to run as specials or new menu items may continue to create customer interest and reduce menu boredom, but it can't come at a cost that requires a selling price above or below the clientele's expectations.

Another restaurateur pointed out that he purchased an item at a good price, created a special out of it, and "priced it at the lower end of the menu scale" to move the items quickly and get a good return. The item didn't sell. Upon analysis, he said that the problem was the item was too cheap and perceived by the clientele to be an inferior product. He modified the recipe, created a new item, raised the price, and sold out in 4 days. "Knowing what your customer will pay and what they expect to pay is important in pricing. We have menu items that return very good margins that we could reduce the price on. But if we did, the customers wouldn't buy them; they would be too cheap."

Take advantage of opportunities, and enhance revenues.

Several of the restaurateurs indicated good opportunities are few and far between. All said a good opportunity was more than a good price. A good opportunity had to meet operational goals and needs, which was the problem. Many products are on sale, many advertising opportunities exist, there are good deals on equipment, uniforms, and the like, but few actually fit a restaurant's parameters. One restaurateur summed it up this way, "There is no such thing as a good buy on something you can't use or don't need."

Many indicated this was one of the most creative ways to improve the restaurant's bottom line; keep customers and employees from becoming bored with the same static menu and day-to-day operations. One operator has changed and adapted his restaurant in his three plus decades of owning his restaurant. "When we started out, we were a steak house. We have also gone though several phases, a full menu, Italian focused, seafood focused, and now we're back to primarily a steak house again, all adapting to trends, customers, and the economy, to keep the restaurant going." He also has seen a shift in the type of business, indicating that when the restaurant first started it was common to turn 600 to 800 covers on a Saturday and again on a Sunday. Now, special functions are 75% of the business. This includes banquets and catering (weddings, office parties, and receptions), Sunday brunch, and a seafood buffet 2 nights per week. Buffets were seldom done when the restaurant opened, and they rarely did any type of catering or banquets. Now, the restaurateur indicated that without adapting and becoming primarily a banquet and catering restaurant, he probably wouldn't be in business.

Another restaurateur indicated that his predecessor was a good example of how to go out of business. This operator purchased his restaurant out of bankruptcy court at substantially less than what the previous owner had accumulated in debts. He explained that the last owner had a great idea but no planning. "If he saw it and needed it, he bought it. He basically overextended and couldn't generate enough income to pay his bills. A good plan would have told him, based on the size of the property and the expected business, he couldn't get enough sales, even at maximum capacity, to pay the debt load." Knowing what you can afford, and sticking to it, will help you stay focused on what's immediately important and what can be put off for a while until the cash reserves are better.

Employ quality and trustworthy employees.

All restaurateurs agreed that an operation is only as good as its employees. This goes far beyond the servers and chefs and includes human resources, office and support staff, and everyone else. Several operators said by having quality, trustworthy employees freed up time from direct day-to-day oversight to allow for planning and managing operations, giving them the opportunity to "look down the road," rather than get too tied up and distracted in things that should be "automatic." While all restaurateurs expressed similar thoughts, one said it best.

> Instead of wondering if the salt and pepper shakers are filled, if there is enough ketchup, and tracking down the backup case of coffee, my employees and I have an honest and trustful relationship. They know what needs to be done and proactively do it without me having to constantly check up on them. We create an environment where they have responsibilities and the authority to make decisions, and I support them. Finding my staff was not easy, but it was well worth the effort. We reviewed over 500 applications, interviewed over 200, hired 150, and ended up with 45 very good team members. We are all a team and work together. They don't work for me; they work with me.

This level of trust is not easily attainable or maintainable. Another restaurateur indicated that she strived for the team effort and was generally successful, but also indicated that regardless of how good your employees are, you still need to watch them and check on what's going on. Keep the controls in place and monitor. She cited an example where an executive chef continued to take on more responsibility for ordering, billing and receipts, scheduling, and so on. After 5 years of increasing business, the restaurant was still barely running at break-even. Several other employees complained to the restaurateur about the executive chef's actions and activities, and it was discovered the chef was embezzling from the business. A final audit showed a minimum loss of nearly a quarter of a million dollars. The restaurateur said she let her guard down and was really taken. Here was a good person with good abilities whom she trusted. She indicated that the chef offered to take on an additional responsibility here and another there and slowly made her job easier by taking on these duties. She said that if the chef had offered to take on all of the responsibilities at one time she would have been suspicious, but over the course of 3 years she thought nothing of it.

Do whatever it takes to meet customer requests.

The restaurateurs indicated that meeting customer requests is important for a few reasons. First, they want to let the customers know that they will work with them to create a special product or event designed specifically for them. Second, the opportunity to increase revenues for the restaurant and incomes for the employees should not be passed over if the request is possible. Third, it's free market research. If customer tastes are changing, special requests and things that are outside of the restaurant's normal items could indicate a change in client tastes and a shift in consumer demand. Fourth, successful events, especially ones done to meet customer requests, are venues to the best form of advertising—word of mouth. One restaurateur said that he would consider just about anything but would only accept when he felt he could do the job well. While word of mouth is the best advertising if you do a good job, it's also the worst for your operation if you do a poor job. Fifth, doing new and different things changes the routine for the staff. Something new alleviates boredom and creates interest and excitement for the staff.

Create an attitude and aura of customer service and satisfaction.

This is the "feel" of an operation. Many variables go into this ideal, including staff, communications, décor, atmosphere, cleanliness, orderliness, presentation, and product quality. It's all of the details that come together to create the effect of the operation. Do customers feel comfortable and welcome when they arrive? Is this supported by their treatment? Ultimately, do the customers perceive a good value for what they spend? While this sounds simple, it is difficult to teach, train, and maintain.

The Private Practitioners

Recognize your needs and lifestyle, and be honest with yourself.

Before starting a private practice, you need to be honest with yourself. What are your needs? What are your financial responsibilities? Are you independently responsible for retirement and other benefits? How are you going to financially support yourself? For instance, if the money does not flow in right away, are you prepared to handle that?

Make yourself available.

Not only do you have to make yourself available to your clients, but you also need to make yourself available to your community. Many people get the wrong idea when you start your own private practice. That is true; however, it's not as luxurious as you may think at first. You are at the mercy of your clients. You may have clients intermittently throughout the day; you may have a 12-hour day one day and a 2-hour day the next. There is never a regimented schedule to follow or set hours. Make yourself available to your clients with the time that you spend with them. Make yourself available by listening to your clients, understanding their needs, and then knowing how to properly direct them to be able to achieve the results they want. If by chance what they need is beyond your scope of practice, then refer them to someone who can help.

Know medical nutrition therapy and its practical application to food.

It is your obligation as a private practice dietitian to know appropriate MNT and be able to direct a client to foods that are available in the community. For example, if you are consulting with a patient who has celiac disease, you should know the appropriate food to recommend, where it is available to them, and how it tastes.

If you tell your client to increase his or her fruit and vegetable intake, recommend fruit that he or she will be able to find in the community. If you tell a client to eliminate some fat from his or her diet, be able to explain different cooking methods that will cut out the fat. It's important to be able to relate to clients on their own terms, so they understand more clearly.

SPECIAL SECTION: REIMBURSEMENT FOR REGISTERED DIETITIAN SERVICES

Mary Angela Miller, MS, RD, LD, FADA

Medical Nutrition Therapy (MNT)

Medical Nutrition Therapy is the commonly used term to describe the clinical nutrition care that RDs provide to guide patients or clients in the skills needed to prevent or delay the development of a disease or condition.[13] In the process, the RD assesses the patient's nutrition status and develops a care plan that is specific to his or her condition. The plan usually includes diet education, which typically occurs during a series of nutrition counseling sessions. MNT services are provided by RDs (and in some states by licensed nutritionists) in private practice, in hospitals, and in other healthcare facilities and clinics. Many studies show that patients who receive MNT show improvements in their health. Research also shows that MNT saves healthcare costs.[14,15] For example, a person with diabetes who receives MNT may be able to better manage blood glucose levels by following a carbohydrate controlled diet. He or she may not need as many prescriptions or may be able to eliminate diabetes medication altogether. Potentially he or she could avoid a costly hospitalization.

MNT Reimbursement

In the United States, healthcare services are often not paid directly by the consumer to the person or facility that provided the care. Instead, the cost of these services may be reimbursed by a third party such as a health insurance plan provided by an employer or the government. Medicare is a national government program that reimburses health care costs for many citizens. Medicaid is a reimbursement program at the state government level.

continues

Reimbursement for MNT services is important for nutrition professionals working in health care because it is how these services are paid for on an outpatient basis. RDs must be knowledgeable of the MNT reimbursement process in order to be legally compliant with reimbursement regulations, help their clients maximize the benefit of their healthcare plan, and be paid for the services they provide. Dietitians may opt to collect directly from the client. In this scenario the patient pays the cost out of his or her own pocket and then follows up with an insurer to pursue reimbursement. One of the challenges of this approach is that the typical healthcare consumers are not accustomed to paying directly for care. They may decide not to use a service if they have to pay the provider directly.

Third party payers vary widely in the services they cover. Some healthcare benefit plans include coverage for MNT while others do not. For example, Medicare covers MNT services for diabetes and renal disease but not for other conditions.[9] Other healthcare plans may reimburse for more medical conditions but limit the maximum number of MNT counseling sessions they reimburse.[16] In order to appropriately provide and bill for a service, both the client and the dietitian must know the specifics of the client's plan. One way this is accomplished is through precertification. This involves contacting the third party payer and determining, in advance, what services are covered. Often plans require that the patient pay a portion of the cost when he or she has his counseling appointment. Verifying the amount of this co-payment is another element of the precertification process.

One of the critical steps to gaining reimbursement from a third party is to become a provider for that healthcare plan. This is accomplished by contacting the agency, learning its requirements, and then completing and submitting an application for approval.[12] Part of the process includes verifying that the dietitian has the appropriate credentials that comply with competency, quality, and liability standards.[17] RDs may need to provide proof of educational and professional

degrees, licenses, registrations, certifications, and/or mal-
practice insurance. Another part of the application process
may be agreeing to provide the service at a discounted rate.
Becoming a preferred provider may take several months, but
it is worthwhile from a business and marketing perspective.
Not only may it be a requirement for being paid for services,
but also because insurers frequently provide members a list
of their preferred providers and refer patients to them.[18]

Billing for MNT Services

After the MNT service is complete, the dietitian documents
the clinical notes and shares the results with the referring
physician and processes the bill for payment. There are a
variety of codes and forms used in billing. Current Procedural Terminology (CPT) codes describe the type of service
provided. There are unique CPT codes for MNT.[19] International classification of disease (ICD9) codes identify and differentiate among diagnoses.[20] ICD9 codes are determined by
physicians. When a physician refers a patient to a dietitian
for counseling, the ICD9 code should be included in the
referring information. That way the dietitian can record it
when submitting the MNT bill. Accurately completing the
forms is essential for bills to be processed for payment.
Healthcare plans may audit providers to ensure that their
guidelines are being followed.

Typical MNT sessions vary in time. The initial assessment
and teaching session for a new patient may take 90 minutes.
Thirty minutes may be allotted for follow-up sessions with
established patients. MNT bills reflect only the amount of
time spent with a patient. Dietitians cannot bill for the time
they spend in related tasks, such as scheduling appoint-
ments, documenting care plans, or processing payments.

The amount of revenues billed for healthcare services does
not necessarily equal the amount actually reimbursed or collected by the MNT provider. For example, patients may have
already paid a portion of the bill as a co-payment at the time

continues

of service, or the dietitian may have agreed to provide services at a discounted rate as part of the preferred provider agreement. Reimbursement rates can and do vary from 0% to 100%. Collecting 30% to 70% of the billed amount is typical.

Consider the following when setting fees:

- Average percent of revenues anticipated to be collected from client mix.
- Local market rates: what consumers consider reasonable and are willing to pay.
- Geographic differences: third party payment amounts may vary by location.
- Overhead: software, mailing, office supplies, educational materials, rent.
- Facility financial guidelines: guidelines may determine hospitalwide fee schedules.
- Indirect time: scheduling, billing, marketing, documenting; self-employed dietitians estimate they spend about 25% to 50% of their time on these tasks.[21]

Payers may reimburse the dietitian directly at the agreed-upon rate. This is called accepting assignment.[22] If the dietitian is employed and paid by a healthcare facility, he or she then reassigns the reimbursed amount to his or her employer.

Summary

Despite the emphasis on writing a business plan in the chapter title, the reader should know by now that it's not the business plan that makes the business successful. *Planning* is what makes the business successful. Writing a business plan is the final assembly and mechanics of much research and analysis to determine the feasibility of the endeavor. If the business plan is done properly and accurately, it should tell what the expected outcomes will be. Hopefully, the authors have presented an overview of the breadth and depth of work, detail, and accuracy necessary to plan a business and then compile it into a business plan. The time commitment is considerable, the level of knowledge, detail, and work is great, but the rewards are many.

MNT reimbursement is an evolving process influenced by advocacy, legislation and public policy, healthcare users, providers, and third party payers. The healthcare reimbursement process is a complex one that involves learning which services are covered, becoming a preferred provider, and following the guidelines to correctly submit claims and receive payment. Healthcare consumers are more likely to take advantage of services covered by their benefit plans. Because MNT benefits the individual patient and collectively saves healthcare industry dollars, navigating the reimbursement process is a necessary and worthwhile skill.

Student Activities

1. Select a market and do some general market research to determine if the market is underserved, or adequately served, or overserved in your area. Use the Internet, newspaper, Web sites with business and demographic information, and any other resources to prove your case.
2. Assume you are starting a private practice or opening a restaurant. Research your state and local authorities to see what permits, licenses, and regulations the area has that will affect your business. This could include zoning issues, building codes, health codes, business forms, etc.
3. You are considering starting a private practice. Who is the competition? Who can you partner with? How will you increase your visibility to recruit clients?
4. You are considering opening a restaurant. How much and from whom will you get food, beverages (nonalcoholic and alcoholic), supplies, plates, silverware, linens, and equipment? What is the availability of skilled and unskilled labor, and what will you have to pay for this labor?

Web Resources

How to open a successful restaurant
http://sdsd.essortment.com/howtoopenrest_rrsk.htm

Checklist for going into business
http://www.nyssbdc.org/StartBiz/Checklist/Check-List_for_Going_
Into_Business_MP-12.pdf

Virtual restaurant
http://www.virtualrestaurant.com/sample.htm

American Dietetic Association Nutrition Entrepreneurs Practice
Group
State and District Dietetic Association: Reimbursement Teams

Note: Mary Angela Miller would like to acknowledge registered
dietitians Maureen Latanick, Julie Meddles, and Julie Jones for sharing their personal and professional experience regarding reimbursement.

References

1. United States Small Business Administration. (2006). Startup basics. Retrieved April 12, 2006, from http://www.sba.gov.
2. National Restaurant Association. (2006). Retrieved April 12, 2006, fromhttp://www.restaurant.org.
3. Academy of Dispensing Audiologists. (2006). Retrieved April 26, 2006, from http://www.audiologist.org.
4. Miller, Russel. (2006). My 6 best tips for starting a business from the New York state small business development center. (2006, March 15). *The Post-Standard*, Article ID#0603110392.
5. United States Department of Agriculture (USDA). (2006). Steps to a healthier you. Retrived April 20, 2006, from http://www.mypyramid.gov.
6. National Diabetes Information Clearinghouse (NDIC). (2006). National diabetes statistics. Retrieved April 20, 2006, fromhttp://diabetes.niddk.nih.gov/dm/pubs/statistics/index.htm.
7. American Dietetic Association. (2006). About ADA: Who we are, what we do. Retrieved April 15, 2006, from http://www.eatright.org.
8. Conner, Julie C. (1997). Insurance reimbursement savvy: Do you have what it takes to get paid?
9. Infante, M. (2003). Correct billing for Medicare part B MNT. Excerpt from *Medicare MNT Provider*. Retrieved July 12, 2006, from http://www.eatright.org/cps/rde/xchg/ada/hs.xsl/nutrition_3389_ENU_HTML.htm.
10. Mississippi Lawyers Domain (MLD). (2006). Forms of business ownership. Retrieved April 18, 2006, from http://www.mslawyer.com/businesr.htm.

11. Nutrition Entrepreneurs. (2006). Experts in the business of nutrition. Retrieved April 29, 2006, from http://www.nedpg.org.

12. Albarado, M. (1997). Dietitians are working smarter. *Health Care Food & Nutrition Focus, 13*, 3-4.

13. American Dietetic Association and Morrison Health Care, Inc. (1996*). Medical nutrition therapy across the continuum of care.* Chicago, IL: The American Dietetic Association.

14. American Dietetic Association. (1997). *Medical nutrition therapy: A solution that saves!* Chicago, IL: The American Dietetic Association.

15. Carey, M. & Gillespie, S. (1995). Position of the ADA: Cost-effectiveness of medical nutrition therapy. *Journal of American Dietetic Association, 95*, 88-91. Retrieved July 12, 2006, From http://www.eatright.org/cps/rde/xchg/ada/hs/xsl/nutrition_3822_ENU_HTML.htm.

16. Weese, N., Jones, J. & Miller, M. (1993). Successful strategies for reimbursement of outpatient nutrition services. *Journal of the American Dietetic Association, 93*, 458-459.

17. Allen, K. (n.d.). Insurance credentialing for new healthcare practices. Retrieved July 19, 2006, from http://ezinearticles.com/?expert=K Allen.

18. Conner, J. (1997). Insurance reimbursement savvy: Do you have what it takes to get paid? *Ventures, XIII(2),* 14-15.

19. American Medical Association (AMA). (2005*).* Current procedural terminology CPT 2006. Thomson Delmar Learning. Retrieved November 17, 2006, from http://www.amazon.com/CPT-standard-current-procedural-terminology/dp/157947697X.

20. National Center for Health Statistics (NCHS) and the Centers for Medicare and Medicaid Services (CMS). (2006). International classification of diseases (9th ed.). Retrieved November 17, 2006, from http://icd9cm.chrisendres.com/2007/.

21. Duester, K. (1997). Building your business: Setting your fees: A Cost-based approach. *Ventures, XIII(2),* 2-4.

22. American Dietetic Association. (2006). Medicare assignment and payment. Retrieved July 12, 2006, from http://www.eatright.org/cps/rde/xchg/ada/hs.xsl/nutrition_assignpay_ENU_HTML.htm.

APPENDICES

UNITS OF MEASURE

Units of Length

10 millimeters (mm)	= 1 centimeter (cm)
10 centimeters	= 1 decimeter (dm) = 100 millimeters
10 decimeters	= 1 meter (m) = 1000 millimeters
10 meters	= 1 dekameter (dam)

Units of Liquid Volume

10 milliliters (mL)	= 1 centiliter (cL)
10 centiliters	= 1 deciliter (dL) = 100 milliliters
10 deciliters	= 1 liter = 1000 milliliters
10 liters	= 1 dekaliter (daL)
10 dekaliters	= 1 hectoliter (hL) = 100 liters
10 hectoliters	= 1 kiloliter (kL) = 1000 liters

Units of Mass

10 milligrams (mg)	= 1 centigram (cg)
10 centigrams	= 1 decigram (dg) = 100 milligrams
10 decigrams	= 1 gram (g) = 1000 milligrams
10 grams	= 1 dekagram (dag)
10 dekagrams	= 1 hectogram (hg) = 100 grams

Units of Length

12 inches (in)	= 1 foot (ft)
3 feet	= 1 yard (yd)
1 inch	= 2.54 centimeters (cm)

Units of Liquid Volume

2 pints	= 1 quart (qt) or 32 fluid ounces
4 quarts	= 1 gallon (gal) or 128 fluid ounces
	= 8 pints
16 fluid ounces (2 cups)	= 1 pint (pt)

Measurement Units of Volume (Capacity)

Metric capacity

10 milliliters = 1 centilitre	2 teaspoons = 1 dessertspoon
10 centiliters = 1 decilitre	3 teaspoons = 1 tablespoon
10 deciliters = 1 litre	2 tablespoons = 1 fluid ounce
100 centimeters = 1 meter	16 tablespoons = 1 cup

Measurement Units of Mass (Weight)

Metric mass

Imperial weight

1000 grams = 1 kilogram	16 ounces = 1 pound = 454 grams
	1 ounce = 28 grams

Teaspoon (US)	5 milliliters
Tablespoon (US)	15 milliliters
Fluid ounce (US)	30 milliliters
Pint (US)	0.47 liter
Quart (US)	0.95 liter
Gallon (US)	3.79 liters
Ounce (weight)	28.35 grams
Pound	0.45 kilogram
Kilogram	2.21 pounds

Temperature Conversion Between Celsius and Fahrenheit

$°C = (°F - 32) ÷ 1.8$

$°F = (°C × 1.8) + 32$

Condition	Fahrenheit	Celsius
Boiling point of water	212°	100°
A very hot day	104°	40°
Normal body temperature	98.6°	37°
Freezing point of water	32°	0°

SCOOP AND CAN SIZES

Scoop Sizes

Size/No.[1]	Level Measure
6	2/3 cup
8	1/2 cup
10	3/8 cup
12	1/3 cup
16	1/4 cup
20	3-1/3 Tbsp
24	2-2/3 Tbsp
30	2 Tbsp
40	1-2/3 Tbsp
50	3-3/4 tsp
60	3-1/4 tsp
70	2-3/4 tsp
100	2 tsp

[1]Number on the scoop indicates how many level scoopfuls make one quart. For example, eight No. 8 scoops = 1 quart.

Can Equivalents

Use this can size equivalent chart to find out how much of an ingredient you need when your recipe suggests a specific can size rather than a volume quantity.

Numbered Can Sizes/Miscellaneous Can Sizes

Numbered Can Size	Volume	Equivalents
#1	11 oz.	1 1/3 cups
#1 Juice	13 oz.	1 5/8 cups
#1 Tall	16 oz.	2 cups
#1 Square	16 oz.	2 cups
#2	1 lb. 4 oz.	2 1/2 cups
#2 1/2	1 lb. 13 oz.	3 1/2 cups
#2 1/2 Square	31 oz.	scant 4 cups
#3 Squat	23 oz.	2 3/4 cups
#3	33 1/2 oz.	4 1/4 cups
#3 Cylinder	46 oz.	5 3/4 cups
#5	56 oz.	7 1/3 cups
#10	6 1/2 lbs. (104 oz.) to 7 lbs. 5 oz. (117 oz.)	13 cups
#211	12 oz.	1 1/2 cups
#300	14 to 16 oz.	1 3/4 cups
#303	16 to 17 oz.	2 cups

Miscellaneous Can Size	Volume	Equivalents
4 oz.	4 oz.	1/2 cup
6 oz.	6 oz.	3/4 cup
8 oz.	8 oz.	1 cup
Picnic	10 1/2 to 12 oz.	1 1/4 cups
12 oz. vacuum	12 oz.	1 1/2 cups
Baby Food Jar	3 1/2 to 8 oz.	7/16 cup (5.8 tbsp.) to 1 cup, depending on size of jar
Condensed Milk	15 oz.	1 1/3 cups
Evaporated Milk	6 oz.	2/3 cup
Evaporated Milk	14 1/2 oz.	1 2/3 cups
Frozen Juice Concentrate	6 oz.	3/4 cup

APPENDIX C

FOODSERVICE EQUIPMENT

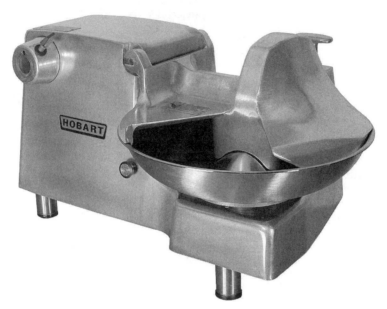

FIGURE C.1 Food Cutter [Hobart Food Cutter 84186]
Photo courtesy of Hobart Food Equipment Group

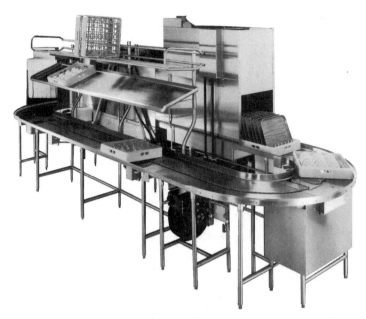

FIGURE C.2   Fast Rack Ware Washing [Hobart Fast Rack Ware Washer]
Photo courtesy of Hobart Food Equipment Group

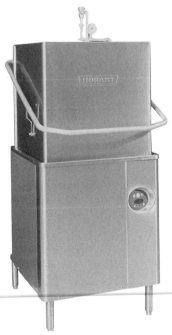

FIGURE C.3   Single Tank Dishwasher
[Hobart Dishmachine AM15]
Photo courtesy of Hobart Food Equipment Group

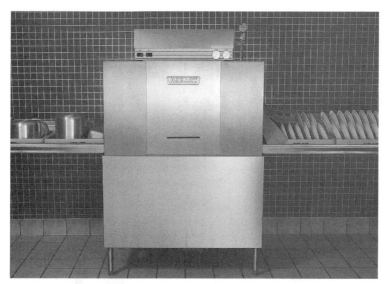

FIGURE C.4   Pass Through Dishwasher [Hobart C-Line Pass Thru Dishwasher]
Photo courtesy of Hobart Food Equipment Group

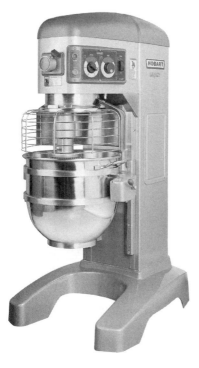

FIGURE C.5   Food Mixer [Hobart Mixer HL600]
Photo courtesy of Hobart Food Equipment Group

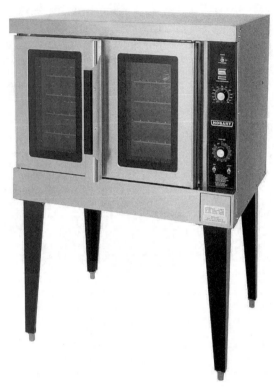

FIGURE C.6   Convection Oven [Hobart Oven HEC501]
Photo courtesy of Hobart Food Equipment Group

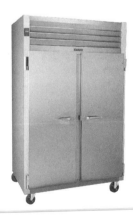

FIGURE C.7   Reach-In Refrigerator [Hobart
Refrigerator G20010]
Photo courtesy of Hobart Food Equipment Group

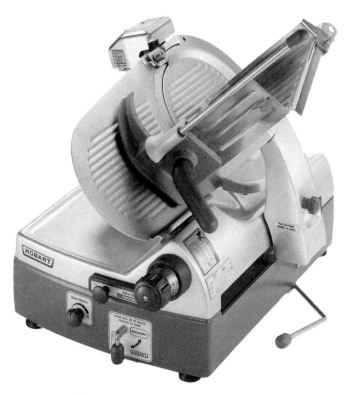

FIGURE C.8   Food Slicer [Hobart Slicer 2912]
Photo courtesy of Hobart Food Equipment Group

APPENDIX D

FOODSERVICE MANAGEMENT REVIEW FOR REGISTERED DIETITIAN'S EXAM

Karlyn Grimes, MS, RD

Types of Foodservice Systems

1. **Describe the advantages and disadvantages of the following types of foodservice systems:**

Conventional

The conventional foodservice system traditionally has been used in most operations. Foods are purchased in various stages of processing, and production, distribution, and service are completed on the same premises. This system is most effective in situations and locales where the labor supply is adequate and inexpensive; where sources of food supplies, especially raw foods, are readily available; and when adequate space is allocated for foodservice equipment and activities.

Advantageously, this system is not dependent on the availability and variety of frozen entrees and other menu items commercially prepared. It is more adaptable to the regional, ethnic, and individual preferences of its customers than is possible with other systems. Also, there is greater flexibility in making menu changes.

On the negative side, the conventional system produces an uneven, somewhat stressful workday caused by meal period demands. Because the menu differs each day, the workloads vary, making it difficult for workers to achieve high productivity.

Commissary

In commissary foodservice systems, foods are purchased with little or no processing but are processed completely in the central facility. Prepared food generally is packaged in bulk and transported to satellite service centers in the local area. Airline foodservice is an example of a commissary foodservice system in which individual meals are packaged to be heated as needed.

This system can realize cost savings due to large volume purchasing and reduced duplication of the labor and equipment that would be required if each serving unit prepared its own food. Quality control may be more effective and consistent with only one unit to supervise.

Food safety and distribution of prepared foods may be concerns. There are also high purchase, maintenance, and repair costs due to the sophisticated and specialized equipment needed for this type of production and distribution.

Ready-Prepared (Cook-Chill)

The ready prepared foodservice system is similar to the commissary system and was originally designed for a singe operation. In this system, foods with varying degrees of processing are purchased, and the amount of production depends upon the state of the purchased food. The food items are either stored chilled or frozen and are readily available at any time for final assembly and heating for service.

The advantages of the ready prepared system are related to reducing the "peaks and valleys" of workloads that may be found in the conventional system. Employee turnover is decreased and recruitment of new employees is enhanced by offering staff a more normal workweek and reasonable hours. There are reductions, production labor costs, improved quality control by decreasing job stress related to production deadlines, and improved nutrient retention by decreasing time food is held within the serving temperature range. Management has close control over menu selections, the quality of ingredients, and portion size and quantity.

One disadvantage is the need for large cold storage and freezer units, which take up a lot of space and add to energy costs. Additionally, appropriate and adequate equipment for rethermalization of foods prior to service is essential and can be costly. Other challenges in this system are retention of nutrient content, microbial safety, and sensory quality of food. Chilling and freezing of food items must be rigidly controlled and length of holding time monitored.

Assembly Serve

Completely processed food items are purchased in the assembly/serve systems, and the only storage, assembly, heating, and service functions are performed in the operation. A huge advantage to this system is the labor savings. Fewer personnel are required, and they do not have to be highly skilled or experienced. Procurement costs are lower due to better portion control, less waste, reductions in purchasing time, and less pilferage. Equipment and space requirements are minimal as are operating costs for gas, electricity, and water.

The availability of a good selection of desired menu items may be limited. Also, the quality of available prepared products and customer acceptability may be a disadvantage. The proportion of protein foods to sauce or gravy in some menu items may not be adequate to meet the nutritional requirements of the clientele.

The Menu

1. Why is the menu considered the primary control of the food-service operation?

The primary goal of a foodservice operation is to serve food that is pleasing to its clientele. The planned menu should be appropriate for the foodservice and consistent with its organizational missions and goals. An important step in preliminary planning is identifying the type of menu to be served and the various food preparation methods required for that menu type. This is the key to equipment needs, which in turn determines the space requirement for the equipment. The menu affects design and layout, as well as personnel skills and staffing levels required. Menu items determine the storage needed, portion sizes, total number of portions, batch size, processing required, utensils needed, necessary work surfaces, and type of equipment required. Before any menu is planned, the amount of money that can be spent for food must be known. Availability of food, style of service, and types of menus should be known as well.

2. **Describe the following types of menus:**

Static

Static or set menu means that the same menus are used each day. This type of menu is found in restaurants and other food-services where the clientele changes daily or where there are enough items listed on the menu to offer sufficient variety.

Cycle

This is a planned set of menus that rotate at definite intervals of a few days to several weeks. The length of the cycle depends on the type of foodservice operation. Cycle menus typically are used in healthcare institutions and schools, offering variety with some degree of control over purchasing, production, and cost. In many noncommercial operations, seasonal cycle menus are common; for example, a 3-week menu for winter, spring, summer, and fall may be repeated during each season.

Single-use

This menu is planned for a certain day or event and is not repeated again in exactly the same form. This type of menu is often used for special functions, holidays, or catering events.

Degree of Choice

Selective menu includes two or more food choices in each menu category such as appetizers, entrees, vegetables, salads, and desserts. A semi-selective menu includes one or more food choices in at least one menu category. A nonselective menu offers no choice of food items.

3. **Describe how the following factors influence menu planning: clientele, nutritional influence, physical facility, personnel, budget, aesthetics, external factors (climate, seasons, etc.).**

Clientele Satisfaction

Sociocultural factors must be considered in planning menus to satisfy and give value to the clientele. Nutritional needs provide a framework for the menu and add to consumer satisfaction. Probably the most important aspect for satisfying clientele are the aesthetic factors of taste and appearance for the menu items. Will the customer be satisfied with the meal and want to return for another one?

Nutritional Influence

Nutritional needs of the consumer should be a primary concern for planning menus for all foodservice operations but are a special concern when living conditions constrain persons to eat most of their meals in one place. For example, in healthcare facilities, colleges and universities, and other types of institutions, most of the nutritional needs of the clientele are provided by the foodservice. Increasing public awareness of the importance of nutrition to health and wellness also has motivated commercial foodservice operators to consider the nutritional quality of menu selections.

Personnel

To produce a given menu, several resources must be considered, a primary one being labor. The number of labor hours, as well as the number and skill of personnel at a given time, determine the type of menu that could be planned. Some menu items may be produced or their preparation completed during slack periods to ease the production load during peak service times; however, the effect on food quality may limit the amount of production in advance of service that could be completed. Employees' days off may need to be considered in menu planning because relief personnel may not have equal skill or efficiency.

Physical Facility

Production capability also is affected by the layout of the food production facility and the availability of large and small equipment. The menu should be planned to balance the use and capacity of ovens, steamers, fryers, grills, and other equipment. Refrigeration and freezer capacity must also be considered.

Budget

The amount of financial resources a facility has available is a very important consideration in menu planning. Obviously, the more money a facility has and/or the wealthier the clientele, the more flexibility there is with menu planning.

Aesthetics

Flavor, texture, color, shape, and method of preparation are other factors to consider in planning menus. A balance should be maintained among flavors. Foods of the same or similar flavor should generally not be repeated in a meal. A variety of flavors in a meal are more enjoyable than duplications.

External Factors

Availability of foods exerts great influence on the selection of menu items. Although most foods are now available in fresh and frozen forms because of the sophistication of the marketing-distribution system, fresh foods produced locally are often of better quality and less expensive during the growing season than those shipped from distant markets. Taking advantage of foods abundantly available during various seasons of the year not only reduces costs but also enhances the acceptability of menu items.

4. Describe the following three methods for pricing menus:

Factor Method

The factor method is often used by foodservice managers because only very simple mathematics is involved. The principal disadvantage is that costs other than food are not known until the end of the month. A considerable amount of anticipated profit might not be realized when using this method. In factor pricing, raw food cost from the standardized recipe is multiplied by an established pricing factor. First, the desired percentage of food cost must be selected and divided into 100 to give a pricing factor. By multiplying the raw food cost by this factor, a menu sales price will result.

Raw Food Cost × Pricing Factor = Menu Sales Price

Prime Cost Method

Prime cost consists of raw food cost and direct labor cost including only those employees involved in preparation of a food item but not service, sanitation, or administrative costs. To make the cost method practical, some assumptions must be made on the percentage of prime cost attributable to raw food, direct labor, and operating margin. Each restaurateur would need to decide what percentage of the selling price would be assigned to the raw food and direct labor costs to give a prime total cost.

Actual Cost Method

This method is used in operations that keep accurate cost records. The initial step as usual, is to establish the food cost from standardized recipes and labor costs, which are the principal variable costs and are actual. Other variable costs, fixed costs, and profit can be obtained as a percentage of sales from the profit-and-loss statement.

Purchasing

1. Describe the following types of middlemen involved in the purchasing process:

Wholesalers

Wholesalers in secondary markets purchase products in large quantities from primary markets and redistribute in smaller quantities to local buyers.

Brokers

Brokers are in business for themselves, but do not take title to the goods being sold. A broker's responsibility is to bring buyers and sellers together.

Commissioners

Similar to a broker except they take title to the merchandise, usually highly perishable produce. Like brokers, they are experienced in the business, know the market and quality necessary to satisfy customers' needs, and are able to rush deliveries.

Manufacturer's Representatives

Manufacturer's representatives do not take title, bill, or set prices. They represent fewer and more specialized lines and a minimum number of manufacturers; they have greater product expertise than brokers. This representative is a salesperson for the manufacturer and is on the company payroll.

Retailers

Retailers are the final middleman in the marketing channel and are the ones who sell the products to the ultimate buyer, the consumer. In both commercial and noncommercial foodservice, the foodservice manager would be considered a retailer.

2. **Define forecasting and its importance in the purchasing process.**

   The goal of forecasting is to estimate future demand using past data. It is a prediction of food needs for a day or other specified periods of time. Forecasting is vital to financial management and facilitates efficient scheduling of labor, use of equipment, and space.

3. **Describe how the following factors can affect the accuracy of forecasts: availability of resources (money, personnel, and raw materials); technological, societal, and governmental changes; economic outlook; and population trends.**

   The forecast is the basis for estimating in advance the quantities of menu items to be prepared and foods to be purchased or requisitioned from the storerooms. Forecasts are often adjusted at the time of actual production due to unseen influences at the time (economic outlook, governmental changes, etc). During these periods of change, the food manager can use his/her intuition to make last minute adjustments to the forecasts. The actual amount of food prepared is based on the number of persons served, portion sizes, and the amount of waste and shrinkage loss in the preparation of foods. Trends in these various factors can affect the accuracy of forecasts.

4. **Describe value analysis and make-or-buy decisions. How are these techniques used by a purchaser to procure required products for minimum cost?**

   Value Analysis: the methodical investigation of all components of an existing product or service with the goal of discovering and eliminating unnecessary costs without interfering with the effectiveness of the product or service.

   Make-or-Buy Decisions: the procedure of deciding whether to purchase from oneself (make) or purchase from vendors (buy) is a continuing process.

   There are several factors that affect the make-or-buy decisions:

   - *Quality*: Evaluate whether quality standard, as defined by the organization, can be achieved.
   - *Equipment*: Assess availability, capacity, and batch turnover time to ensure that product demand can be met.

- *Labor*: Evaluate availability, current skills, and training needs.
- *Time*: Evaluate product set-up, production, and service time based on forecasted demand for the product.
- *Inventory*: Gauge needed storage and holding space.
- *Total Cost*: Conduct complete cost analysis of all resources expended to make or buy product.

5. **What's the difference between informal and formal purchasing?**

   Informal: A commonly used method of buying, especially in smaller foodservice operations. Involves ordering food and supplies from a selected list of vendors based on daily, weekly, or monthly price quotations. This method is often used when time is an important factor.

   Formal: Competitive bidding generally is required when buying for an institution under federal, state, or local jurisdiction. Written specifications and estimated quantities are needed to submit to vendors with an invitation for them to quote prices within a stated time for the items listed. With high-use items, competitive bidding usually culminates in a formal contract between purchaser and vendor.

6. **What is bid buying?**

   Bid buying is characterized by an availability of a sufficient number of vendors willing to compete over price quotes on the purchaser's item specifications. Purchasers using bid buying generally take one of two approaches, either the fixed bid or the daily bid, before initiating a bidding procedure.

7. **What's the difference between a purchase requisition, purchase order, and invoice?**

   Purchase requisition: A list of desired products. Generally originates in a department and is submitted to the purchasing department.

   Purchase order: written requests to a vendor to sell goods or services to a facility.

   Invoice: A list of goods shipped or delivered. Includes prices and service charges.

Receiving, Storage, and Inventory Control

1. **Describe the significance of the following steps in the receiving process:**

   Inspection against the purchase order

   Inspection against the invoice

   Acceptance or rejection of orders

   Completion of receiving orders

   Removal to storage

   The purpose is to ensure that the foods and supplies delivered match established quality and quantity specifications. It also is a time to verify prices. These steps are important to cost and quality control, and warrant careful planning and implementation. The proper storage of food immediately after it has been received and checked is an important factor in the prevention and control of loss or waste.

2. **What's the difference between invoice receiving, blind check receiving, and partial blind receiving?**

   Invoice receiving: A traditional method that involves the receiving clerk who checks the items against the original purchase order and notes any deviations. This method is efficient but requires a careful evaluation by the clerk to ensure that the delivery is accurate and quality standards are met.

   Blind check receiving: Provides an invoice or purchase order, one in which the quantities have been erased or blacked out to the receiving clerk. The clerk must then quantify each item by weighing, measuring, or counting and recording it on the blind purchase order. The blind document is then compared with the original order. This method offers unbiased approach by the receiving clerk but is more time-intensive.

   Partial blind receiving: A less time-intensive version of blind check receiving. In this type of receiving the invoice or purchase order form contains more information about the product in terms of what is to be expected from the order than the forms used in blind check receiving.

3. Describe the following types of storage facilities and equipment:

Table D.1 Types of Storage Facilities and Equipment

Storage Facility/ Equipment	Description/ Ideal Features	Foods Commonly Here	Proper Temperatures
Dry Storage Facility	Located convenient to the receiving and preparation areas. Located at or above ground level. Ventilation is vital.	Non-perishable foods that do not require refrigeration. Paper supplies also.	50–70°F
Coolers	Used for thawing frozen foods, storing meat, dairy, fruits, and vegetables. Separate refrigerators for fruits and vegetables, and dairy, eggs, and meats due to varying ideal temperatures. Cleanliness vital. Remote thermometers.	Fresh foods. Fresh fruits and vegetables.	Fresh produce: 41°F to 45°F; Meat: 32°F to 40°F
Thawers or Tempering Boxes	Units for thawing foods, specifically designed to maintain a steady temp-erature of 40°F regardless of room temperature or product load.	Meats	40°F (steady)
Storage Freezers	Cleanliness. Remote thermometers.	Frozen foods	–10°F to 0°F
Processing Freezers	Units designed to perform the actual freezing of food. Generally not used for storage.	All perishable foods	–20°F or below

4. **Define inventory. Why is the development and maintenance of an inventory system important? What's the difference between physical inventory and perpetual inventory?**

   Inventory is a detailed and complete list of goods in stock. It is a system of communicating needs from the production areas and the storeroom to the buyer. Establishment of a minimum and maximum stock level provides a means of alerting buyers to needs. The minimum is the point at which the inventory should not fall below. Management of inventory is practiced both to determine quantities to keep on hand and to determine the security methods used to control how the stock influences overall foodservice costs.

   Physical inventory: An actual account of the items in all storage areas.

   Perpetual inventory: A running record of the balance on hand for each item in the storeroom.

5. **Define issuing. What's the difference between direct issues and storeroom issues?**

   Issuing is the process used to supply food to the production units after it has been received. Products may be issued directly from the receiving area (direct issues), especially if planned for that day's menus, but, more often, food supplies are issued from dry or low temperature storage (storeroom issues).

6. **Describe the following tools available to assist managers in determining quantities for purchase, inventory levels, and cost of maintaining inventories:**

   ABC Method

   This principle states that effort, time, and money for inventory control should be allocated among products according to their value. Products should be divided into three groups: A = high value, B = med value, C = low value. A-class items should be reviewed continually to estimate requirements, check stock balances, and determine material on order. The inventory level of these important dollar components should be maintained at an absolute minimum. As you go down the classes to B and C, less concern should be directed toward these inventories.

Mini-Maximum Method

In this method, a safety stock is maintained at a constant level both on the inventory record and in the storerooms. The max level consist of the safety stock plus the correct ordering quantity, which is the difference between the safety stock and the max inventory level. The safety stock is essentially the back-up supply to ensure against contingencies, such as a sudden increase in usage rate, failure to receive ordered materials on schedule, receipt of items that do not meet specifications, and clerical errors in inventory records.

Economic Order Quantity Method

Is derived from a sensible balance of ordering cost and inventory holding cost. Ordering cost diminishes rapidly as the size of the orders is increased, and holding cost of the inventory increases directly with the size of the order.

7. **Describe the significance of the following methods for inventory valuation:**

Purchase Price

Involves pricing the inventory at the exact price of each individual product. Used only in small foodservice operations.

Weighted Average Purchase Price

A weighted unit cost is used that is based on both the unit purchase price and the number of units in each purchase.

FIFO

First in, first out. This means of inventory pricing closely approximates the physical flow of goods through an organization. The ending inventory reflects the current cost of goods, because inventory is valued at the dollar amounts for the most recent purchases.

8. **Describe the significance of the following methods for inventory valuation:**

LIFO

Last in, first out. LIFO is based on the assumption that current purchases are largely, if not completely, made for the purpose of meeting current demands of production. The purchase cost of the oldest stock, therefore, should be charged out first.

Generally, the value of the inventory will be the lowest using LIFO and highest using FIFO based on the assumption that current prices will be higher than older ones.

Production Planning and Control

1. **Define production.**
    In the generic sense, it is the process by which products and services are created. In the context of foodservice, production is the managerial function of converting food purchased in various stages of preparation into menu items that are served to customers.

2. **Define production demand forecasting. How does this help with cost control in a foodservice organization?**
    Forecasting is a function of production, but also is needed for procurement. Food products must be available for producing menu items for customers. The primary result for forecasting should be customer satisfaction. Production demand forecasting may be based on historical records or a forecasting model. Production demand forecasting helps to minimize the chance of over or underproduction. Overproduction generates extra costs because production of extra food items is not feasible; underproduction also can increase cost because of additional labor for preparation and often the substitution of a higher priced item.

3. **What are production meetings? What topics are discussed at these meetings?**
    Foodservice managers in small operations, or unit supervisors in large ones, should hold a meeting daily with employees in the production unit. Production meetings facilitate communication between all employees of the foodservice organization. Employees can be encouraged to discuss the effectiveness of the schedules, new recipes, and employee assignments. The meeting should conclude with a discussion of the production schedule for the following three meals.

4. Describe why employee scheduling, standardized recipes, and quality and quantity control are so important to production control?

These are critical dimensions of cost control throughout the foodservice system. In essence, then, quality control means ensuring day-in, day-out consistency in each product offered for service. Quantity control, simply stated, means producing the exact amount needed—no more, no less. Each is directly related to control of costs and thus to profit in a commercial operation or to meeting budgetary constraints in a nonprofit establishment. Over- and underproduction create managerial problems and impact cost. Time and temperature, product yield, portion control, and product evaluation all relate directly to quality, quantity, and indirectly to control of costs. Additionally, employee scheduling and standardized recipes are key to ensuring product consistency.

5. What are the cup and ounce measurements for the following scoop sizes?

Table D.2 Scoop-Size Measurements

Scoop Size	Measure (cup, tsp, tbsp)	Ounces
# 6	⅔ c; 10 T	6
# 8	½ c; 8 T	4–5
# 10	⅜ c; 6 T	3–4
# 12	⅓ c; 5 T	2½–3
# 16	¼ c; 4 T	2–2¼
# 20	3⅕ T	1¾–2
# 24	2⅔ T	1½–1¾
# 30	2⅕ T	1–1⅓
# 40	1⅓T	¾
# 60	1 T	½

Methods of Production

1. **Describe the following pieces of equipment common to foodservice establishments. Put a check in the last column if your food service facility possesses the particular piece of equipment.**

Table D.3 Equipment Descriptions

Equipment	Function/Description	✔
Bain-marie	A large pan containing hot water in which smaller pans may be set to cook food slowly or to keep food warm.	
Blender	Timed mixing control with automatic shut-off; action designed for thorough mixing and aerating of ingredients in a bowl.	
Broiler, Char or Open Hearth	Either gas or electric equipment with a bed of ceramic briquettes above the heat source and below the grid or a heavy cast iron grate positioned horizontally above the heat source. Charcoal or chunks of irregular size ceramic above gas or electric burners.	
Convection Oven	Has a fan on the back wall that creates currents of air within the cooking chamber. It has more space and holds two to three times as much food, reduces cooking time by 30%, and cooks at lower temperatures.	
Deck Oven	Pans of food are usually placed directly on the stacked metal decks.	
Dolly	Attachment included with mixers.	
Dough Mixer	Timed mixing control with automatic shut-off; action designed for thorough mixing and aerating of ingredients in a bowl. Attachments such as dough hook.	

Griddle	Separate griddle units to supplement or substitute for range sections.	
Hot Plate	An electrically heated plate for cooking or warming food or a tabletop cooking device with one or two burners.	
Kettle, Steam Jacketed	Two bowl-like sections of drawn, shaped, welded aluminum or stainless steel with air space between for circulation of steam to heat inner shell. Food does not come in contact with steam.	
Kettle, Tabletop	Set on a table; air space between for circulation of steam to heat inner shell.	
Microwave Oven	An oven in which food is cooked, warmed, or thawed by the heat produced as microwaves cause water molecules in the foodstuff to vibrate.	
Oven-top Fryer	A tank of oil heated by gas or electricity into which foods are immersed.	
Pre-rinse or Pre-wash Sink	One, two, or three compartments. One compartment reserved for pre-rinsing.	
Pressure Cooker	An airtight metal pot that uses steam under pressure at high temperature to cook food quickly.	
Range Oven	A part of a stove, generally called a range, and is located under the cooking surface. Primarily used in smaller operations.	
Roll-in Rack Oven	A type of convection oven that accommodates 16 or 20 full-size baking pans and can be rolled into the oven on casters.	

2. Describe the following cooking methods.

Table D.4 Cooking Methods

Cooking Method	Description	Appropriate Foods for This Method
Moist Heat Methods		
Blanching	Cooking an item partially and briefly, usually in water or fat. Often the foods are then plunged into cold water.	Used in vegetables and fruits to set the color and destroy enzymes or to loosen skins for easier peeling. In certain meats and bones, to dissolve out blood, salt, or impurities.
Boiling	Cook in a liquid that is rapidly boiling.	Certain vegetables and starches.
Braising	Cooking food in a small amount of liquid usually after browning it. Also, refers to cooking at low temperature in a small amount of liquid, without first browning in fat.	Meats and poultry.
Poaching	Cooking food in a small amount of liquid that is hot but not actually bubbling.	Used to cook delicate foods such as fish, eggs, and fruit.
Simmering	Cooking in liquid that is boiling gently.	Soups, sauces, meat, and poultry.
Steaming	Cook foods by exposing them to steam.	Vegetables, fruits, poultry, dumplings, pasta, rice, and cereals.
Stewing	Cooking in liquid that is boiling gently.	Meat, poultry, and fruits.
Dry Heat Methods		
Baking	Cooking food by surrounding it with hot, dry air, usually in an oven.	Generally applied to desserts and bread.

Barbecuing	Cooking on a grill or spit over hot coals or in an oven.	Meat, poultry, and vegetables.
Broiling	Cooking by radiant heat.	Tender cuts of meat (steaks, chops), fish, and poultry.
Charbroiling	Cooking on a grill or spit over hot coals or in an oven where the heat source is from below. A distinctive feature of charbroiling is the flavor imparted as fat and juice drip into the hot briquettes, vaporize into smoke, and then contact the food.	Meat and poultry
Deep Frying	Foods are immersed in oil.	Fish, shellfish, chicken, meat, and vegetables.

Moist Heat Methods

Grilling	Food cooked on an open grid over a heat source, which may be an electric or gas-heated element, or charcoal.	Meat, poultry, fish, and vegetables.
Oven Frying	A variation of oven broiling and involves placing food on greased pans and usually dribbling fat over it before baking in a hot oven. The resulting product is much like fried or sautéed food.	Chicken pieces and fish fillets
Pan Frying	Cooking in a moderate amount of fat in a pan over moderate heat.	Meat, chicken, eggs, potatoes, and onions.
Roasting	Cooking food by surrounding it with hot, dry air, usually in an oven.	Poultry, tender cuts of beef, pork, lamb, and veal.
Sautéing	Cooking quickly in a small amount of fat.	Poultry, fish, and tender cuts of meat.

Foodborne Pathogens

1. **Describe the difference between the four major types of food spoilage:**

   Microbiological

   Food spoilage caused by microorganisms such as bacteria, molds, and yeast is considered microbiological. Microbiological spoiling is found everywhere that temperature, moisture, and substrate favor life and growth.

   Biochemical

   Biochemical spoilage is caused by natural food enzymes, which are complex catalysts that initiate reactions in foods. Off flavors, odors, or colors may develop in foods if enzymatic reactions are uncontrolled.

   Physical

   Temperature changes, moisture, and dryness can cause physical spoilage in foods.

   Chemical

   Chemical spoilage may result from interaction of certain ingredients in a food or beverage with oxygen or light. The reaction of incompatible substances can lead to chemical spoilage, such as the effect of certain metals on foods.

2. **What's the difference between foodborne poisoning/intoxication and foodborne infections?**
   Foodborne intoxications or poisoning are caused by toxins formed in foods prior to their consumption. Foodborne infections are caused by the activity of large number of bacterial cells carried by the food into the gastrointestinal system of the victim.

3. **Fill in the following chart identifying major foodborne illnesses.**

Table D.5 Major Foodborne Illnesses

Foodborne Pathogen	Foods Usually Involved and Time Frame for Onset of Symptoms	How Introduced Into Food	Preventive or Corrective Procedures
Food Poisoning/Intoxication			
Staphylococcus Aureus	Food that requires considerable handling. Ham and other cooked meats, dairy products, custards, potato salads, cream-filled pastries, and other protein foods. Onset of symptoms: 24 to 48 hours.	Humans (skin, nose, throat, infected sores) and animals.	Avoid contamination from bare hands, exclude sick food handlers from food preparation and serving areas, good personal hygiene, sanitary habits, proper heating and refrigeration.
Clostridium Botulinum	Improperly processed canned low acid foods. Onset of symptoms: Several days to a year.	Soil and dirt, water, and spores not killed in inadequately heated foods.	Pressure cook canned foods with pH over 4.0; home-canned foods boil 20 minutes after removal from the can or jars; cook foods thoroughly after removing before serving; discard all food in swollen, unopened cans.
Clostridium Perfringens	Meat that has been boiled, steamed, braised, or partially roasted, allowed to cool several hours, and subsequently served either cooled or reheated. Onset of symptoms: 24 hours.	Natural contamination of meat.	Rapidly refrigerate meat between cooking and use.

continues

Table D.5 continued

Foodborne Pathogen	Foods Usually Involved and Time Frame for Onset of Symptoms	How Introduced Into Food	Preventive or Corrective Procedures
Food Poisoning/Intoxication			
Salmonella	Poultry, poultry salads, meat and meat products, milk, shellfish, eggs, egg custards and sauces, other protein foods. Onset of symptoms: 1 to 2 days.	Fecal contamination by food handlers; raw contaminated meat and poultry, liquid eggs, and unpasteurized milk.	Avoid cross-contamination, refrigerate food, cool cooked meats and meat products properly, and avoid fecal contamination from food handlers by practicing good hygiene.
Listeria Monocytogenes	Unpasteurized milk and cheese, vegetables, poultry and meats, seafood and prepared ready-to-eat foods, including cold cuts and fermented raw meats and sausages. Depends on treatment-high mortality in susceptible populations.	Human, domestic and wild animals, fowl, soil, water, mud. Contaminated cole slaw, milk, and cheese.	Use only pasteurized milk and dairy products, cook foods to proper temperatures, avoid cross-contamination. Wash leafy vegetables and fruit adequately
Campylobacter Jejuni	Raw poultry, raw vegetables, unpasteurized milk, untreated water. Onset of symptoms: 4 to 7 days.	A pathogen of cattle, sheep, pigs, and poultry. Found in the flesh of these animals and thus may be introduced into the kitchen with the food supply.	Avoid cross contamination, cook foods thoroughly.

Food Service and Management Rotation

1. Describe the following laws and regulations involved in the employment process.

Unemployment Compensation

Employees who have been working in employment covered by Social Security Act and who are laid off may be eligible for compensation during their unemployment period up to 26 weeks. When workers become unemployed through no fault of their own, states provide them with certain weekly benefits. Each state has its own unemployment insurance law that defines the terms and benefits of the program.

Workman's Compensation

In general, these laws provide for income and medical benefits to victims of work-related accidents, reduce court delays arising out of personal injury litigation, encourage interest in safety and rehabilitation, eliminate payment fees to lawyers and witnesses, and promote study of accident causes.

National Labor Relations Act (Wagner Act, 1935)

This act placed the protective power of the federal government behind employee efforts to organize and bargain collectively through representatives of their choice. It established the right of a union to be the exclusive bargaining agent for all workers in a bargaining unit.

Taft Hartley Relations Act (Labor Management Relations Act, 1947)

This law amends the Wagner Act. The major thrust of the legislation was to balance the powers of labor and management. Specific activities were defined as unfair union practices in the Taft Hartley Act.

Labor Management Reporting and Disclosure Act (1959)

This was passed because the Taft Hartley Act did not cover labor racketeering. This act requires that labor organizations hold periodic elections for officers, that members be entitled to due process both within and outside the union, that copies of labor agreements be made available to covered employees, and that financial dealings between union officials and companies be disclosed to the U.S. Department of Labor.

Fair Labor Standards Act (1938)

The Fair Labor Standards Act established minimum wages for hourly employees and overtime wage requirements. Through the years, amendments to the act have enlarged the number of work groups covered by the law and have steadily increased the minimum wage. The act requires employers to pay time-and-a-half the regular rate received by employees for all hours worked in excess of 40 hours a week. The act also defines specific occupations that are exempt from minimum wage and overtime requirements.

Civil Rights Act (1964)

States that "No person in the United States shall, on the ground of race, color, or national origin be excluded from participating in, be denied the benefits of, or be subjected to any program or activity receiving Federal Financial assistance."

Age Discrimination Act (1967)

Promotes the employment of the older worker, based on ability instead of age. It prohibits arbitrary age discrimination in employment and helps employers and employees find ways to meet problems arising from the impact of age on employment.

Equal Employment Opportunity Act (1972)

The umbrella term that encompasses all laws and regulations prohibiting discrimination and/or affirmative action.

2. Define the following concepts involved in job design.

Job Description

An organized list of duties that reflects required skills and responsibilities in a specific position. It may be thought of as an extension of the organization chart in that it shows the activities and job relationships for the positions identified on the chart.

Job Analysis

Often referred to as the base of human relations management because the information collected serves so many functions. It is the process of obtaining information about jobs by determining what the duties and tasks or activities of those jobs are.

Job Specification

A written statement of the minimum standards that must be met by an applicant for a particular job. It covers duties involved in a job, the working conditions, and personal qualifications required of the worker to carry out the assigned responsibilities successfully.

Work Schedule

An outline of work to be performed by an individual with stated procedures and time requirements for his or her duties. Work schedules are especially helpful in training new employees and are given to the employee after the person has been hired and training has begun. This is one means of communication between the employer and employee. Work schedules should be reviewed periodically and adjustments made as needed to adapt to changes in procedures.

3. Describe the following types of personnel actions.

Promotion

Commonly implies an increase in responsibility and salary. Sometimes promotion carries only the opportunity for experience in a desired field. It may mean shorter hours and greater assurance of security. Regardless, it is an expression of appreciation in an individual's worth.

Transfer

Often a worker who is found unfit for one job may do well in another. In some cases, a minor shift may enable the worker to become a contented and valuable employee. Transfer of an employee who is not finding satisfaction in the current job to another job within the organization offering a different challenge or opportunity has salvaged many workers.

Separation

Involves either voluntary or involuntary termination of an employee. In instances of voluntary termination or employee resignations, many organizations attempt to determine why employees are leaving by asking them to complete a questionnaire or by conducting an exit interview.

Compensation (salary vs. wage)

Compensation is the financial reimbursement given by the organization to its employees in exchange for their work. It includes salaries or wages and benefits. *Salary* is the term used to refer to earnings of managerial and professional personnel. *Wage* refers to hourly earnings of employees covered by the Fair Labor Standards Act.

Benefits (statutory vs. compensatory vs. supplementary)

Compensatory benefits include paid time off, such as vacation, sick leave, holidays, military and jury duty, and absences due to death in the family or other personal leave. *Statutory benefits* include Social Security, Unemployment Compensation, and Workers' Compensation for injury on the job, disability, retirement, or death. *Supplementary benefits* include life insurance, medical insurance, etc.

4. **Describe the following motivational theories, strategies, and studies commonly used as leadership tools.**

Maslow's Hierarchy of Needs

This theory suggests that a person is motivated by his or her desire to satisfy specific needs. These needs are arranged in a hierarchical order. Maslow theorized that only an unsatisfied need motivates behavior. When the need is satisfied, the need is no longer a primary motivator. Higher order needs cannot become motivating forces until preceding lower order needs have been satisfied and people want to move up the hierarchy.

Herzberg's Theory

Developed the two-factor theory of motivation, which focuses on rewards and outcomes of performance that satisfy needs. Two sets of rewards or outcomes are identified: those related to job satisfaction and those related to job dissatisfaction. Those related to satisfaction are called motivators, and those related to dissatisfaction are called maintenance or hygiene factors.

Macgregor (Theory X and Y)

This theory suggests that the basic attitude of a manager toward employees has an impact on job performance. Theory X attitude was held by the traditional and "old-line" managers and is pessimistic about employees' abilities and skills. Theory Y was the attitude held by the emerging managers of the 1960s and 1970s and is optimistic in nature.

Hawthorne Studies (Western Electric)

Western Electric Company conducted some experiments at its Hawthorne Plant to determine the relationship between the physical working environment and productivity. Lighting was one variable that was tested. Researchers were surprised to find that no matter how they varied the intensity of the lighting, productivity increased. They concluded that the level of performance had nothing to do with the lighting intensity but rather was a result of the interest shown in the worker as a person rather than as a machine. Thus, the human relations theory era was born.

5. Describe the difference between the following leadership styles.

Autocratic

Employees are motivated by fear, threats, punishments, and seldom by reward. Almost all decisions are made by top management, and only occasionally do communications move up from employees to the manager.

Bureaucratic

Bureaucratic leadership is where the manager manages "by the book". Everything must be done according to procedure or policy. If it isn't covered by the book, the manager refers to the next level above him or her. This manager is really more of a police officer than a leader. He or she enforces the rules.

Diplomatic

A diplomatic leadership style guides and encourages groups to make decisions. In early work on leadership styles, this type was considered the most desirable and productive. Current research does not necessarily support this conclusion. This style works best when people are lacking information. Employees can provide input to help make the best possible decision. It also works well with a large number of experienced, cooperative people.

Participative

A participative leader operates on a basis of trust and responsibility. Employees discuss the job with their superiors, and communication flow up, down, and laterally. Decisionmaking is spread evenly through the organization.

Free Rein

This leader exercises little direct control but is the prime source of information, suggestions, and authority. This works best if the staff are well trained, responsible and professional. This is successful in public works when people working in the field have to make decisions with little direct supervision. Within certain limits, individuals are allowed to set their own goals. This often results in outstanding performance.

6. **Describe the five primary management functions: Planning, Organizing, Staffing, Leading/Directing, and Controlling.**

   - *Planning*: The function of management that involves developing the activities required to accomplish organizational objectives and the most effective ways of doing so. Involves vision, strategic planning, procedures, and rules.
   - *Organizing*: The function of management that involves the development of the formal structure through which work is divided, defined, and coordinated. The chief function of the organizing process is the establishment of relationships among all other functions of management.
   - *Staffing*: The personnel function of employing and training people, and maintaining favorable work conditions.
   - *Directing*: The continuous process of making decisions, conveying them to subordinates and ensuring appropriate actions.
   - *Controlling*: Involves coordinating, reporting, and budgeting. The functional activity of interrelating the various parts of a process to create a smooth work flow. Keeping supervisors, managers, and subordinates informed concerning responsibility through records, research, inspection, and other methods. Budgeting includes the fiscal planning, accounting, and controlling activities.

7. **What's the difference between the following types of work schedules?**

   Master Schedule

   Serves as an overall plan for employee scheduling. It shows days on and off duty and vacation days.

   Shift/Staggered Schedule

   The shift schedule will indicate the position and hours worked and may indicate the number of days worked per week. It also lists relief assignments for positions when regular workers are off. It shows the staffing pattern of the operation. The staggered schedule provides for employees to begin work at varying times, generally resulting in better use of labor force.

   Production Schedule

   Also called the production worksheet, the production schedule is the major control in the production subsystem because it activates the menu and provides a test of forecasting accuracy. It is highly individualized and may vary in form.

8. **What are the two major costs in a foodservice operation? Which is the least controllable? The most manageable?**

   Foodservice operation control usually involves two main costs: food and labor. They are often referred to as prime costs and usually contribute the bulk of the costs in foodservice operations. Food costs vary depending on the season and weather conditions, and due to supply and demand. Labor costs are somewhat consistent for specific job responsibilities, but may vary within and between states. The minimum wage makes labor costs more consistent. Also, overtime compensation is predetermined by various employment laws and regulations making this component of labor costs more consistent. As a result, food costs are generally considered the least controllable and labor costs more manageable.

FOODSERVICE WORKER JOB DESCRIPTIONS

Federal Wage System Job Grading Standard for Food Service Working, 7408

From the U.S. Office of Personnel Management, February 1992

Work Covered

This standard covers nonsupervisory work involved in serving food and beverages and preparing simple food. It includes setting and waiting on tables where food service is informal; attending food counters; portioning and serving food; assembling trays for hospital patients; recording and retrieving patient diet and other food-service information using a computer or manual file system; washing dishes, pots, pans, glasses, and silverware; transporting food, equipment, and supplies by manual or motorized carts; and assisting in food preparation by peeling potatoes, cutting vegetables, assembling and tossing salads, measuring and weighing ingredients, brewing coffee and tea, and mixing bulk fruit juices. In addition, the work typically includes sweeping, washing, mopping and buffing floors, and washing walls and ceilings.

Work Not Covered

This standard does not cover work that primarily involves:

- Performing laboring duties that require mainly physical abilities and effort and involve little or no specialized skill or prior work experience, such as loading and unloading trucks at loading docks, moving kitchen equipment and supplies, and collecting and disposing of trash. This work is excluded from the series when it is performed full time or when it represents the highest skill and qualification requirements of the job. (See Job Grading Standard for Laboring Series, 3502.)

- Performing custodial duties such as sweeping, scrubbing, and waxing floors; washing windows, walls, and ceilings; dusting and polishing furniture and fixtures; and emptying waste cans. This work is excluded from the series when it is performed full time or when it represents the highest skill and qualification requirements of the job. (See Job Grading Standard for Custodial Working Series, 3566.)
- Preparing regular and special diet bakery products such as bread, rolls, cakes, cookies, pies, doughnuts, pastries, puddings, fillings, and icings. (See Job Grading Standard for Baking Series, 7402.)
- Preparing regular or special diet foods and meals such as soups, gravies, sauces, meats, poultry, fish, shellfish, vegetables, desserts, and other foods. (See Job Grading Standard for Cooking Series, 7404.)
- Setting tables in a dining room with tablecloths, silverware, glasses, and napkins; serving the requested items in the prescribed manner; and cleaning the tables upon completion of the meal. (See Job Grading Standard for Waiter Series, 7420.)

Titles

Jobs covered by this standard are to be titled *Foodservice Worker.*

Foodservice Worker, Grade 1

General: Grade 1 foodservice workers perform routine manual tasks with few steps that are easily learned and controlled. They work in one or more functional areas of the kitchen such as food preparation, dish and pot washing, dry and refrigerated storage and receiving, and the serving line.

Foodservice workers at grade 1 set up glasses, silverware, dishes, trays, napkins, condiments, and cold menu items such as salads, desserts, bread, and cold beverages on a serving line. They carry trays for ambulatory and wheelchair patients. They remove dishes and trays from tables after meals. They wash tables and counters and vacuum and shampoo carpets. Foodservice workers sort, wash, peel, and cut fresh fruits and vegetables. They operate, break down, and clean all electrical equipment assigned to the area for food preparation. They clean kitchen equipment such as work tables, sinks, and refrigerators. Foodservice workers at this level separate food waste and trash from dishes, glasses, and silverware in the dishwashing area. They load and operate dishwashers and silverware washing machines. They store sanitized dishes, glasses, and silverware.

Food service workers perform cleaning tasks in the food service area such as sweeping and mopping kitchen floors, cleaning windows and washing walls, and cleaning and sanitizing trash cans.

Skill and Knowledge: Grade 1 foodservice workers have an understanding of basic food handling techniques. They have skill and knowledge to perform routine manual tasks involving few steps. They have an understanding of personal hygiene standards and safe work procedures such as wearing a hairnet and a clean uniform daily, stacking dishes carefully to avoid mishaps, and wiping up spilled food or liquid promptly to prevent falls. They have the knowledge to read and understand written material such as time and duty schedules, safety data sheets for hazardous chemicals, menus, recipes, and basic work instructions. They have knowledge of basic arithmetic such as addition, subtraction, multiplication, division, fractions, and decimals.

Responsibility: Grade 1 foodservice workers receive limited assignments of a repetitive nature from their immediate supervisor or a higher grade employee. Work assignments and instructions at this level are typically oral. They are told when and how the work should be done. The work is performed the same way each time and is easily observed and checked.

Physical Effort: Foodservice workers at this grade level perform work requiring light to moderate physical effort. They are subject to continuous standing and walking, and frequent stooping, reaching, pushing, pulling, and bending. They frequently lift or move objects weighing up to 9 kilograms (20 pounds) unassisted (e.g., pushing small carts of dirty dishes) and occasionally lift or move objects weighing more than 9 kilograms (20 pounds) (e.g., filling beverage dispensers) with the assistance of other workers.

Working Conditions: The work is performed in kitchen areas where the steam and heat from cooking and dishwashing equipment often cause uncomfortably high temperatures and humidity. The work area is well lighted but usually noisy from foodservice activities, and there is danger of slipping on floors where food or beverages have been dropped. Foodservice workers are regularly exposed to hot liquids, sharp cutting blades, hot working surfaces, and extreme temperature changes when entering walk-in refrigeration or freezing units.

Foodservice Worker, Grade 2

General: Grade 2 foodservice workers perform tasks with several steps or a sequence of tasks that require attention to work operations. They follow set procedures in accomplishing repetitive assignments and follow an established sequence of work.

Foodservice workers at grade 2 set up cafeteria lines, steamtables, dining room tables, and side service stands with hot and cold food items including meats, vegetables, salads, desserts, bread, butter, and beverages. They serve food cafeteria style by placing uniform portions of food on customers' plates. They break down and clean their assigned area when the meal is finished and return food to the main kitchen. They set up dining room tables for service, place food and beverages on tables, and replenish items as necessary. They return soiled trays and dishes to the dishroom after meals. They deliver meal trays to the patient's bed. Foodservice workers brew coffee according to the number of servings required. They assemble and toss fresh fruit or green salads in quantity, using prepared dressings and portion into standard serving sizes. They apportion other food items (e.g., gelatins, juices, and desserts) into standard serving sizes using the proper utensils and containers. They make cold sandwiches using prepared ingredients and pack box lunches. Foodservice workers at this level set up and operate a mechanical dishwasher, including the continuous conveyor belt feeding dishwasher. They remove inspection doors, strainer pans, screens, and spray arms for preventive maintenance and cleaning.

Grade 2 foodservice workers scrape, soak, scour, and scrub the heavier cooking utensils such as mixing bowls and pots that, because of their large size and weight, are awkward to handle.

Foodservice workers perform heavy-duty cleaning tasks throughout the foodservice and related areas, such as cleaning ceilings and transoms; cleaning exhaust hoods; cleaning spaces under and behind kitchen equipment, including moving the equipment; washing floors and walls with powered cleaning equipment; cleaning walk-in refrigerators and freezers; and sanitizing garbage rooms. Foodservice workers at this level may unload food from delivery trucks. They move heavy garbage cans when collecting and transferring trash from the work area to the disposal area.

Skill and Knowledge: Grade 2 foodservice workers have skill and knowledge to perform tasks involving several procedures. They have ability to concentrate on work assignments despite interruptions and distractions. They have knowledge of basic arithmetic in order to count the number of tables and meal trays required or determine the number of servings a container will yield. They have a working knowledge of sanitation standards, such as the need to keep wiping cloths in a sanitizing solution. They have a working knowledge of procedures to prevent contamination, such as the need to clean equipment previously used for raw food before further use and the need to use a chemical sanitizer or maintain proper water temperature when cleaning dishes.

Responsibility: Grade 2 foodservice workers receive assignments from their immediate supervisor, who provides specific instructions when changes in the work routine or new assignments are made. They are expected to work as scheduled, knowing what steps or sequence of tasks are needed to complete the work. Some judgment is used by these workers in maintaining established standards of sanitation, safety, and service. They are responsible for the correct operation and care of equipment such as mechanical dishwashers, potwashers, tray conveyors, and coffee urns.

The supervisor is available to resolve problems and answer questions. The work is periodically checked to verify that it is being accomplished on time and according to instructions.

Physical Effort: In addition to the physical effort described at grade 1, some foodservice workers at this level may be required to perform heavy work, such as scouring and scrubbing large-size cooking utensils and pushing heavy carts and trucks in unloading, storing, and delivering supplies. They also may be required to work on ladders and use powered cleaning equipment. They frequently lift or move objects weighing up to 18 kilograms (40 pounds).

Working Conditions: The working conditions are the same as those described at grade 1.

Foodservice Worker, Grade 3

General: Foodservice workers at grade 3 select and place food items on patient trays as they proceed down the tray assembly line according to a regular or modified menu, individual diet cards, or patient selections. They can identify obvious discrepancies between the prescribed diets and the food items designated by the menu. They decide what food items to serve for the most common diets when the diet card identifies only the kind of diet called for, such as a liquid diet or diabetic diet. They set up their assigned station on the tray line with the correct supplies and food items, and break down and clean the station after the serving period. Some workers deliver trays to the patient's bed and report the patient's comments and complaints to the supervisor or dietitian. Foodservice workers at this level provide assistance to cooks in the food preparation area by weighing, measuring, and assembling ingredients according to standardized recipes. In some work situations, they prepare uncooked food items such as sandwich spreads and salad dressings.

Skill and Knowledge: Grade 3 foodservice workers apply knowledge of special procedures in preparing food and serving patients. They have skill to organize their work assignments in a logical sequence, execute tasks quickly and accurately, and meet strict meal schedules. They read and understand diet cards when working on the tray assembly line. They know color codes that signify regular or modified diets and special diet card notations. They memorize the most frequently used modified diets to place food items and beverages on the patient's tray, especially where the diet card indicates only the kind of diet and does not provide a precise listing of foods.

They understand food terminology, measurements, and serving information in standardized recipes and regular and modified menus. They apply knowledge of general sanitation principles to safeguard food against spoilage and waste. For example, they are knowledgeable of the temperature range where the potential of bacterial growth in food is greatest and the requirement to keep hot food in heated holding equipment or immediately refrigerate it.

They have knowledge and skill to apportion food items according to approved portion control practices, i.e., they use the correct measuring utensil or a portion control scale regularly and do not rely on visual estimates of food quantity. They have a thorough understanding of the routine methods and procedures used in all functional areas of the foodservice operation and skill to train lower grade workers in such methods and procedures.

Responsibility: Grade 3 foodservice workers complete assignments individually or as part of a team under the general supervision of the immediate supervisor. Assignments are made either orally or in writing. Detailed instructions are provided only for special projects. The work involving diet tray assembly is usually performed as a team with the worker being expected to know the commonly used diets in order to place items on a tray. Completed diet trays are checked by a higher level foodservice worker. Work involving actual food preparation is accomplished under the guidance of a cook who provides technical instruction and checks work in progress and upon completion for conformance with acceptable foodservice practices. Foodservice workers know daily routines and work from guides such as diet cards, menus, portion control charts, standardized recipes, and employee assignment sheets. Questions on unusual or difficult tasks are referred to a higher grade worker or supervisor for clarification and advice. Work at this level is evaluated in terms of accuracy and timely completion of assignments.

Physical Effort: The physical effort is the same as described at grade 2.

Working Conditions: The working conditions are the same as those described at grade 1.

Foodservice Worker, Grade 4

General: Grade 4 foodservice workers perform duties that require proficiency in special procedures and a broad knowledge of service operations, such as food preparation, dishwashing, dry and refrigerated storage, and food and beverage serving.

Foodservice workers at grade 4 make the final check of diet trays assembled by lower grade workers for completeness, correct food temperature, and to verify that food items on the tray are appropriate for the prescribed diet. They conduct the daily patient census by distributing menus to patients. They provide patients with basic information about modified diets, such as explaining to a patient on a sodium-restricted diet that canned vegetables must be eaten in moderation because they are typically high in salt, or telling a patient on a diabetic diet that, according to the exchange lists, cheese may be substituted for meat. Some grade 4 foodservice workers prepare individual and bulk nourishments and special feedings for patients. They follow directions in assembling, measuring, weighing, or mixing ingredients for basic formulas and other supplemental feedings. They take nourishment inventories, replace expired bulk items, and label and distribute individual nourishments to appropriate patients or nursing stations. They apply special sanitary techniques in preparing formulas and tube feedings such as sterilizing equipment and sanitizing work areas. Food service workers at this level weigh and measure food items and recipe ingredients. They use portion control scales and measuring devices to apportion individual items according to standardized recipes. They determine the quantities of ingredients needed to prepare required yields. They make conversions from the metric system to the U.S. standard system. They assemble, label, and arrange completed recipe items in preparation for use by cooks. Some grade 4 foodservice workers use a computer terminal to record and retrieve recipe, menu, and inventory data and to produce printouts of such information for various work units in the kitchen.

Skill and Knowledge: Grade 4 foodservice workers apply skill and knowledge in planning and organizing their work to complete assignments. They are knowledgeable of special procedures and sanitation principles necessary in the preparation of tube feedings to prevent bacterial contamination. They have skill in making precise measurements and accurately weighing recipe ingredients for special feedings. They have knowledge of proper techniques for measuring the volume of dry, liquid, and fat ingredients and in the use of portion control scales. They have skill in arithmetical computations using decimals, fractions, and percentages to determine the quantities of ingredients needed to prepare the required yields. They have a basic understanding of recipe construction. They have skill in measuring and weighing ingredients to adjust recipe yields according to standard procedures. Foodservice workers at this grade apply a thorough knowledge of basic modified diets when providing the final check on patient trays to verify that the food items are correct for the prescribed diet. They have a working knowledge of some diet principles, such as the diabetic exchange lists for meal planning. In some work situations, workers at this level are able to use a computer to enter and retrieve basic information, such as diet orders or recipe, menu, and inventory data. Foodservice workers at this level may carry out the function of a small work unit (e.g., in the nourishment unit they decide what supplies are needed, obtain supplies from other areas of the kitchen, prepare the number and kind of nourishments ordered from an ingredients list, label and distribute nourishments, and clean and sanitize the work area).

Responsibilities: Grade 4 foodservice workers receive limited supervision from their immediate supervisor. The supervisor provides oral and written instructions on changes in procedures and special requirements. Food service workers perform routine work independently in accordance with written guides and established policy. They use judgment in recognizing work objectives and in planning and organizing duties to accomplish those objectives. They refer questions on new work situations to the supervisor. Workers at this level may assist lower grade employees and provide training on technical work matters. The supervisor spot checks work in progress to be sure that set procedures are being followed and that work will be accomplished according to a specific time schedule.

Physical Effort: The physical effort is the same as described at grade 2.

Working Conditions: The working conditions are the same as those described at grade 1.

INDEX